Free Radicals, Lipid Peroxidation and Cancer

NFCR Cancer Symposia

No. 1 Free Radicals, Lipid Peroxidation and Cancer.
Based on the Proceedings of a Symposium held at Brunel University, 8-10 July, 1981
Edited by D.C.H. McBrien and T.F. Slater

Free Radicals, Lipid Peroxidation and Cancer

Edited by

D.C.H. McBrien
and
T.F. Slater

Department of Biochemistry
Brunel University
Uxbridge, England

1982

ACADEMIC PRESS

A Subsidiary of Harcourt Brace Jovanovich, Publishers
London New York
Paris San Diego San Francisco
São Paulo Sydney Tokyo Toronto

ACADEMIC PRESS INC. (LONDON) LTD.
24/28 Oval Road
London NW1

United States Edition published by
ACADEMIC PRESS INC.
111 Fifth Avenue
New York, New York 10003

British Library Cataloguing in Publication Data
Free Radicals, Lipid Peroxidation and Cancer.—
(N.F.C.R. cancer symposia; no. 1)
1. Cancer—Congresses
I. McBrien, D.C.H.   II. Slater, T.F.
III. Series
616.99'4   RC261.A2

ISBN 0-12-481780-7

LCCCN 81-68970

Printed in Great Britain

PARTICIPANTS

ADAMS, G.E. *Royal Marsden Hospital, Institute for Cancer Research, Clifton Avenue, Belmont, Surrey, England.*

ASMUS, K.-D. *Hahn-Meitner Institut für Kernforschung, GmbH, 1 Berlin 39, West Germany.*

BENEDETTI, A. *Istituto di Patologia Generale, University of Siena, 53100 Siena, Italy.*

BENEDETTO, C. *1st University Clinic of Obstetrics and Gynaecology, Via Ventimiglia 3, Torino, Italy.*

CHEESEMAN, K. *Biochemistry Department, Brunel University, Uxbridge, Middlesex UB8 3PH, England.*

CONNORS, T.A. *MRC Unit for Toxicology, Woodmansterne Road, Carshalton, Surrey SM5 4EF, England.*

DIANZANI, M.U. *Institute of General Pathology, University of Turin, Corso Rafaello 30, Torino 10125, Italy.*

ESTERBAUER, H. *Institut für Biochemie der Universität Graz, A-8010 Graz, Halbärthgasse 5/1, Austria.*

GARNER, A. *Biochemistry Department, Brunel University, Uxbridge, Middlesex UB8 3PH, England.*

LOHMANN, W. *Institut für Biophysik der Justus Liebieg-Universität-Strahlenzentrum, D-6300 Giessen, West Germany.*

LOWN, J.W. *Department of Chemistry, University of Alberta, Edmonton, Alberta TG6 242, Canada.*

MAGEE, P.N. *The Fels Research Institute and Department of Pathology, Temple University School of Medicine, 3420 North Broad Street, Philadelphia, Pennsylvania 19140, USA.*

MARSH, D. *Max-Planck Institute for Biophysical Chemistry, Abt. Spektroskopie, D-3400 Göttingen-Nikolausberg, West Germany.*

MASON, R.P. *Laboratories of Environmental Biophysics, National Institute of Environmental Health Sciences, Research Triangle Park, North Carolina 27709, USA.*

McBRIEN, D.C.H. *Biochemistry Department, Brunel University, Uxbridge, Middlesex UB8 3PH, England.*

NÖHAMMER, G. *Institut für Biochemie der Universität Graz, A-8010 Graz, Halbärthgasse 5/1, Austria.*

PLAYER, T.J. *Department of Biochemistry, University of Birmingham, Birmingham, UK.*

POLI, G. *Institute of General Pathology, University of Turin, Corso Rafaello 30, Torino 10125, Italy.*

RILEY, P.A. *Department of Biochemical Pathology, University College Hospital Medical School, University Street, London, WC1E 6JJ, England.*

SCHAUENSTEIN, E. *Institut für Biochemie der Universität Graz, A-8010 Graz, Halbarthgasse 5/1, Austria.*

SEARLE, A.J., *Biochemistry Department, Brunel University, Uxbridge, Middlesex UB8 3PH, England.*

SLATER, T.F. *Biochemistry Department, Brunel University, Uxbridge, Middlesex UB8 3PH, England.*

STIER, A. *Max-Planck Institut fur Biophysikalische Chemie, Abt. Spektroskopie, D-3400 Gottingen-Nikolausberg, West Germany.*

SWARTZ, H.M. *University of Illinois College of Medicine, Medical Sciences Building, Urbana, Illinois 61801, USA.*

SYMONS, M.C.R. *Department of Chemistry, University of Leicester, Leicester, England.*

TOMASI, A. *Istituto di Patologie Generale, University of Modena, 41100 Modena, Italy.*

TS'O, P.O.P. *Department of Biochemical and Biophysical Sciences, Division of Biophysics, The Johns Hopkins University, Baltimore, Maryland 21205, USA.*

WILLSON, R.L. *Biochemistry Department, Brunel University, Uxbridge, Middlesex UB8 3PH, England.*

NONPARTICIPATING CO-AUTHORS

BENSCH, K.G. (On leave of absence from Stanford University, California.) *Institut für Biophysik, Justus-Liebig-Universität Giessen, D-6300 Giessen, West Germany.*

SAPPER, H., PLEYER, A., SCHREIBER, J. and KANG, S.O. *Institut für Biophysik, Justus-Liebig-Universität Giessen, D-6300 Giessen, West Germany.*

LÖFFLER, H. *Zentrum für Innere Medizin, Justus-Liebig-Universität Giessen, D-6300 Giessen, West Germany.* (Present address: Zentrum für Innere Medizin der Universität, Kiel, West Germany.)

PRALLE, H. *Zentrum für Innere Medizin, Justus-Liebig-Universität Giessen, D-6300 Giessen, West Germany.*

SCHWEMMLE, K. and FILLER, R.D. *Zentrum für Chirurgie, Justus-Liebig-Universität Giessen, D-6300 Giessen, West Germany.*

GRAVELA, E. *Istituto di Patologia Generale, University of Turin, Corso Rafaello 30, Torino 10125, Italy.*

JOSHUA, A.V. and CHEN, H.-H. *Department of Chemistry, University of Alberta, Edmonton T6G 2G2, Alberta, Canada.*

CLAUSS, R., LÜCKE, A. and REITZ, I. *Max-Planck-Institut für Biophysikalische Chemie, Am Fassberg, 3400 Göttingen, West Germany.*

HARRELSON, W., KALYANARAMAN, B. and MOTTLEY, C. *National Institute of Environmental Health Sciences, Laboratory of Environmental Biophysics, P.O. Box 12233, Research Triangle Park, N.C. 27709, USA.*

PETERSON, F. and HOLTZMAN, L. *Veterans Administration Hospital, Minneapolis and Departments of Medicine and Pharmacology, University of Minnesota, Minneapolis, MN 55455, USA.*

LESKO, S.A., YANG, S.-U. and ZHENG, R. *Division of Biophysics, Johns Hopkins University, 615 North Wolfe Street, Baltimore, Maryland 21205, USA.*

MORGAN, B.D.G. *University College Hospital, Gower Street, London, WC1, England.*

O'NEILL, T., DEWEY, D.L. and GALPINE, A.R. *Mount Vernon Hospital, Northwood, Middlesex, England.*

PREFACE

This book is a record of the proceedings of the first of a series of symposia on cancer topics that are organised and supported by the N.F.C.R. Cancer Research Association and the National Foundation for Cancer Research.

The National Foundation for Cancer Research was founded seven years ago by Dr F.C. Salisbury and Mrs Tamara Salisbury to provide research funds for innovative programmes of cancer research. Although based in Bethesda, Maryland, USA, it supports cancer research at the highest level in many different countries including the United Kingdom.

The N.F.C.R. Cancer Research Association is a new United Kingdom-based charity that has close scientific links with the National Foundation for Cancer Research. The N.F.C.R. Cancer Research Association has among its aims and objectives: (a) to supplement the proven and valuable work of other cancer charities by giving pump-priming funds to initiate creative new approaches in specifically selected areas of cancer research; (b) to catalyse new directions of research where some positive initial evidence is required prior to submitting a major grant application; (c) to promote the exchanges of scientists between laboratories in different countries where the scientific programmes are closely related to the areas of interest of the N.F.C.R. Cancer Research Association and would profit from detailed discussions; (d) to encourage the exchange of ideas and information on topical and rapidly developing areas by organising small symposia on relevant subjects.

The last objective mentioned above has led to the decision to hold annual symposia on cancer research topics whereby acknowledged experts in each field can discuss results over a three-day period in the presence of a selected informed audience. In general, the number of speakers will be approximately 15 with a similar number of invited discussants. The proceedings of each symposium, together with edited discussion, will be published as soon as possible after each meeting.

As organisers and editors of the first N.F.C.R. symposium we wish to record our sincere gratitude to our many colleagues at Brunel University who have helped us extensively with administrative, technical and other matters. We are specially grateful in these respects to Mrs W. Ditschler, Mrs A. Aboud, Dr A. Garner, Dr R.L. Willson, Mr K. Cheeseman, Dr A. Tomasi, Ms Sheila Billing, Dr Maria Lai, Mr A. Searle, Mr M. O'Connell, Mr D. Cukier, Mr P. Richardson (Catering Officer), Mr Beattie (Accommodation Secretary) and Mrs V. Britain (Lodgings Office). We thank our colleague Dr Jeffrey Mahood for compiling the index. We also gratefully acknowledge the expert help and assistance of the staff of Academic Press and Mrs Penny Brown who retyped the papers for publication.

We record with pleasure that Dr and Mrs Salisbury were present at this symposium, and cemented firmly the ties between the National Foundation for Cancer Research and the N.F.C.R. Cancer Research Association.

December, 1981 T.F. Slater D.C.H. McBrien

CONTENTS

3. ACTIVATED INTERMEDIATES

Chairman's Introduction

T.F. SLATER

The importance of metabolic activation in the mechanism of action of many carcinogenic substances has been recognised for a considerable time since the pioneering work of the Millers in the United States. More recently it has been realised that metabolic activation of chemical carcinogens may lead to free radical intermediates with high chemical reactivity. There is considerable current interest in evaluating the importance of such radical intermediates in the carcinogenic action or actions of the relevant carcinogens.

Free radicals can best be studied directly by the technique of electron spin resonance. A discussion and evaluation of the application of electron spin resonance to problems of cancer occupied the first section of this symposium. An introductory account of electron spin resonance was provided by Professor Martyn Symons, an acknowledged expert in electron spin resonance procedures. The application of electron spin resonance to the examination and analysis of free radical constituents in tumours has produced a number of confusing and conflicting reports. Professor Swartz has made a careful and critical study of this area of cancer research and his survey presented to the symposium is important and timely. The electron spin resonance section includes also two current studies as well as the two reviews just mentioned. Professor Lohmann described his recent work on human leukaemia and Dr Chiara Benedetto her collaborative study, involving the Universities of Turin, Graz and Brunel, on carcinoma of the cervix. This first section of the symposium highlighted the pitfalls and benefits in applying electron spin resonance to a study of chemical carcinogenesis and to the examination of samples of human tumour tissue.

The activation of toxic agents to give free radical intermediates can lead to a variety of types of cellular damage including membrane disturbance through lipid peroxidation. Lipid peroxidation is now recognised to produce a rich variety of products with interesting biochemical and pharmacological properties. It is also generally the case that lipid peroxidation is much reduced in many types of cancer, whereas prostaglandin synthesis, which also involves a free radical oxidation of a polyunsaturated fatty acid, may be increased in extent. The second section of the symposium concentrated on lipid peroxidation with respect to free radical activation mechanisms. The recent exciting advances made in the analysis and biochemical properties of aldehydic products of lipid peroxidation were described by Professors Esterbauer and Dianzani; some of the aldehydic products are sufficiently effective on rapidly dividing cells to have some promise as anti-tumour agents at least for study in experimental systems. This latter aspect was described in the paper from Professor Schauenstein. The general depression of lipid peroxidation in tumour tissue samples was described in Dr Player's contribution and the discussion brought out the need to study intensively the distribution and extent of antioxidants in tumour cell fractions. The section on lipid peroxidation also included detailed contributions on the stimulatory effect of carbon tetrachloride on lipid peroxidation in microsomal and isolated hepatocyte systems given by Kevin Cheeseman and Giuseppe Poli.

The third and longest section of the symposium was concerned with activated intermediates in relation to tissue damage and chemical carcinogenesis. A description of the current status of studies dealing with the activation of carbon tetrachloride was given by Professor Slater who outlined some recent work done at Brunel University using the fast reactions technique of pulse radiolysis. This approach was developed by Dr Robin Willson who specially emphasised the important role that iron-catalysed reactions may have in such free radical events. Professor Lown's presentation was an exciting account of current work dealing with the participation of certain clinically used anti-tumour agents in generating free radical intermediates. The cytotoxic and carcinogenic action of aromatic amines and nitrosamines were surveyed by Professors Stier and Magee. Other examples of free radical intermediates arising from metabolic processes were described by Dr Mason and Professor Ts'o; these presentations included important accounts of spin trapping and of the formation of free radicals from polycyclic hydrocarbons. Finally, Dr Patrick Riley from University College London gave a convincing presentation of how free radical reactions may be involved in a primary fashion in the considerable clinical responses seen in some malignant melanomata treated with 4-hydroxy-anisole. This third section of the symposium presented overall a striking amount of evidence concerning the active role of free radical intermediates in various types of cell damage and cancer.

There is no doubt that there is much current interest in the role of free radicals in cancer and cell injury in general. This symposium reinforces such interest and will be, I believe, a valuable contribution to the literature on this important topic.

Electron Spin Resonance Studies of Cancer: A Status Report

H.M. SWARTZ

INTRODUCTION

This paper will focus on the overall status of studies of cancer employing Electron Spin Resonance (ESR) and related techniques to investigate the role of paramagnetic molecules, especially free radicals, in cancer and cancer therapy. Considerable progress in several fields makes such a status report feasible and even desirable. Whenever possible, I shall attempt to relate this paper to the subsequent papers presented at this symposium.

The following statements outline my view of the current status of ESR studies of cancer. The body of the paper will consider each in detail.

1. Free radicals are not involved systematically in cancer.
2. Free radical reactions are important in many specific processes, including activation of some chemical carcinogens, radiation effects, and the action of some chemotherapeutic agents.
3. Free radicals involved in significant reactions are likely to have intermediate reactivity.
4. Highly reactive radicals can be important under special circumstances.
5. The ascorbyl radical has a special role and potential importance in studies of complex biological systems.
6. Oxygen-related free radicals may have important roles in a number of processes related to cancer.
7. Free radicals do play a role in experimental studies of some specific types of cancer.

8. Paramagnetic metals have important roles in both experimental studies and in chemical reactions associated with cancer.
9. Technological and methodological advances will increase further the usefulness of ESR studies of cancer.

1. FREE RADICALS ARE NOT INVOLVED SYSTEMATICALLY IN CANCER

The original basis for ESR studies of cancer was a somewhat vaguely defined hypothesis that the reactions of free radicals are intrinsically related to cancer and/or carcinogenesis (Swartz, 1972, 1979). After more than 30 years of study it is clear that while free radicals are involved in many specific instances, they do not have an obligatory or general role. Many of the papers of this symposium directly or indirectly touch upon this conclusion.

The papers of Stier *et al.* (1982), Magee (1982), and most explicitly, Mason *et al.* (1982) provide substantive data that although many active carcinogens are free radicals, many are not, and some related non-carcinogenic compounds do form free radicals in tissues. As one understands this principle, it assists in the design of experiments in which the actual active forms of a particular carcinogen and its mechanism of carcinogenesis can be better studied, without the distraction of trying to fit the data into a grand scheme involving free radicals (see following section).

Similarly, studies of free radical levels in tissues indicate that there is no consistent relationship of these levels to cancer. The very exciting studies of Emanuel and Saprin (see Swartz, 1972; Emanuel, 1976, for an introduction to this literature) which indicated a possible systematic role of free radicals, now seem best understood in terms of experimental changes that reflect the ability of ascorbic acid to form stable free radicals via both radical and nonradical pathways (Swartz and Dodd, 1981; Dodd and Swartz, 1980) (see Section 5). In fact, if one looks at different systems under the proper conditions one can find evidence for an increase, decrease, or no change in the level of free radicals in virtually any stage of tumour development.

Finally, as one examines the theoretical bases for anticipating an obligatory role of free radicals in cancer, it becomes apparent that while it was appropriate to make such proposals 30-40 years ago, they fail to hold up in the light of our current understanding of cancer.

The multiple types of cancer and the known properties of both normal and malignant cells leave no room for a general mechanism of control of cells based on free radicals *per se*. It is possible, of course, that some malignancies are associated with metabolic alterations such as a change in the level or type of reducing substances such as SH groups and that these redox changes may be reflected indirectly by experimental studies that use the level or type of free radical as an assay system.

2. FREE RADICAL REACTIONS ARE INVOLVED IN A NUMBER OF SPECIFIC TYPES OF CANCER, CARCINOGENESIS, AND CANCER THERAPY

With the understanding that alterations in free radicals are not a general phenomenon, the study of free radicals in specific cancers may be of considerable value for both fundamental understanding and for treatment. Pigmented melanomas provide an excellent example. Melanin is a stable free radical and its presence can be used to help diagnose this type of tumour (Sarna and Swartz, 1979). The pathway to produce the melanin can also be utilised to produce toxic intermediates that may aid in therapy as discussed in the symposium by Riley. Section 7 provides details of other cancers in which free radicals have a role.

The role of free radicals in some types of carcinogenesis is now established. This often involves one electron oxidations, especially by cytochrome P_{450}. The papers in this symposium by Magee, Mason *et al.*, Stier *et al.*, and Lesko *et al.* provide excellent examples of involvement of free radicals in the metabolic activation of some carcinogens.

Recently it has become apparent that free radicals play a role in some types of therapy. The general cytotoxic role of large numbers of reactive free radicals, especially hydroxyl radicals, is the basis of radiation therapy. More specific roles of free radicals in therapy are now also being recognised. The studies with melanoma have already been mentioned (Riley *et al.*, 1982). A theory of action of bleomycin, involving free radical production at DNA is discussed in the paper of Lown (1982). Other anticancer drugs may also involve free radicals in either their tumouricidal actions or their side reactions (e.g. adriamycin).

3. FREE RADICALS INVOLVED IN SIGNIFICANT REACTIONS ARE LIKELY TO HAVE INTERMEDIATE REACTIVITY

This is an important principle that is only recently generally becoming understood. Relatively stable free radicals have received considerable attention because they can be detected readily but they are unlikely to be important because, as their long lifetimes indicate, they react slowly. Such radicals may dominate the ESR spectra and thereby cause considerable experimental confusion. Some of the less reactive semiquinones are examples of such radicals. Very reactive free radicals, such as the hydroxyl radical, are also unlikely to be important because, unless they are generated in large numbers or at the site of action (see Section 4), they will be used up in harmless reactions with cell constituents whose loss in small numbers will not affect cell function.

Radicals of intermediate reactivity may live long enough to get to critical sites, while having sufficient reactivity to cause damage when they get there - perhaps by rather specific reactions. Semiquinone radicals are receiving increasing attention in this regard. Intermediates in melanin synthesis, some antitumour agents (e.g. adriamycin and bleomycin) and even some normal metabolites (e.g. ubiquinone and even ascorbic acid) may exist in semiquinone forms. It may be especially important that the fully oxidised (quinone) and fully reduced (hydroquinone) forms can, in themselves, undergo a redox reaction, producing semiquinones. This type of equilibrium produces an additional mechanism to transport reactive molecules to sensitive sites. If the semiquinone is the reactive molecule, this can occur by having the semiquinone formed at the site. If the oxidised or reduced form is very reactive (e.g. ascorbic acid is a very strong reducing agent) the semiquinone (e.g. the ascorbyl radical) may generate the reactive molecule at the site where it undergoes a dismutation reaction (e.g. 2 ascorbyl radicals → ascorbate plus dehydroascorbate).

4. HIGHLY REACTIVE RADICALS CAN BE IMPORTANT UNDER SPECIAL CIRCUMSTANCES

Although in general highly reactive radicals such as the hydroxyl radical may be of lesser importance in reactions in complex biological systems because they react before they can diffuse very far from their site of production, in at least four general cases they can cause significant damage.

(a) If Produced at Specific Critical Sites.

If a hydroxyl radical or other very reactive species is produced at a critical site, the probability of the occurrence of significant damage is very high. Such a circumstance is illustrated in the paper by Lown *et al.* (1982) on DNA damage by bleomycin. Bleomycin binds to DNA and it also binds metals, especially iron and copper. It appears that these metals complexed to bleomycin can catalyse the production of a strong oxidising species similar to the hydroxyl radical via a Fenton-like reaction. Because of the site of binding of bleomycin, the reactive molecule has a significant probability of damaging DNA. Analogous reactions may occur with other systems in which drugs bind to important sites (e.g. nucleic acids, membranes, or key enzymes) and then either themselves become converted to active radicals or their metal complexes generate such radicals.

The possibility of such reactions makes it essential to understand thoroughly the mechanisms of production of reactive species in biological systems. Thus it is not sufficient to know that the production of superoxide anions can lead to the production of strongly oxidising species similar to hydroxyl radicals. In order to evaluate the biological importance of such reactions and to modify them, we need to know the details of the reaction including the chemical composition of the reactive molecules. Only with such detailed knowledge can one reasonably evaluate the probability of a deleterious reaction occurring at a critical site.

(b) If Produced Randomly and in Large Quantities

Most reactive radicals produced in metabolic or pathological processes are generated at or near specific sites (e.g. a particular enzyme) rather than at random. As discussed above, unless this site also has a critical target very near to it, the reactive radical will not be able to diffuse to critical targets. If, however, the reactive radicals are produced at random then there is a finite probability of their occurrence at critical sites and, indeed one can use this principle to calculate the size and number of the critical targets (e.g. "target theory" in radiation biology). Such random production of hydroxyl radicals is the mechanism of much of the therapeutic effects of radiation which is used for cancer therapy, as well as the basis for the side effects of medical and environmental ionising radiation. It is unlikely that other sources of reactive radicals in biological systems will produce them so randomly and in such large numbers.

(c) Produced as Products from Less Reactive Precursors

A significant amount of the radical related damage from carbon tetrachloride seems to occur via such a mechanism in which the less reactive $CCl_3^{\cdot}$ radical is converted to the more reactive $CCl_3O_2^{\cdot}$ by the direct addition of molecular oxygen (Slater, 1982). In such a case the site of the addition reaction will determine the area where damaging reactions can occur and this may result in production near a critical target. The $CCl_3^{\cdot}$ plus oxygen reaction probably is the prototype of other potentially damaging reactions in which molecular oxygen converts less reactive precursors to more reactive products. This emphasises the need for more knowledge of the detailed distribution of both molecular oxygen and various radicals, especially in regard to their partition between aqueous and lipid environments. Reaction rates in the latter may differ significantly (e.g. Symons, 1982).

(d) Production of Longer-Lived But Still Reactive Products

If very reactive radicals generate moderately reactive products these can diffuse and cause damage at sites distant from their production. For example, hydroxyl radicals can generate longer-lived radicals in tris buffer and these latter radicals have been detected by spin traps indicating both their capacity for diffusion and their reactivity (McCay *et al.*, 1980). It is quite possible that a chain of radicals could result from an initial attack by a strong oxidising radical, resulting in effects at some distance. Membranes which have a combination of some order and a nonaqueous environment might provide an especially favourable environment for such propagation.

5. THE ASCORBYL RADICAL HAS A SPECIAL ROLE AND POTENTIAL IMPORTANCE IN STUDIES OF COMPLEX BIOLOGICAL SYSTEMS

Its natural occurrence and chemical properties result in the ascorbyl radical having an especially prominant role in ESR studies of cancer (Swartz, 1979; Swartz and Dodd, 1981). It is the product of one electron oxidation of ascorbic acid and because of its relative stability, can be detected readily. In fact, it appears to be the usual final radical product in a number of experimental circumstances, so it is frequently observed in ESR studies. It is the signal observed in the lyophilised blood system studied by Lohmann *et al.* (1982). Because it is an intermediate in a naturally occurring redox system:

$$\text{ascorbic acid} \underset{\text{red}}{\overset{\text{oxid}}{\rightleftharpoons}} \text{ascorbyl radical} \underset{\text{red}}{\overset{\text{oxid}}{\rightleftharpoons}} \text{dehydroascorbic acid}$$

its magnitude may reflect the redox equilibrium of the biological system. This must be a very complex reflection, however, because of the multiple redox factors in biological systems and the subcellular distribution of the various members of the equilibrium. Its ability to participate in cyclic redox reactions, often in association with metals (e.g. Lown *et al.*, 1982), adds to the importance and complexity of its role. Lohmann presents data suggesting that its magnitude may provide very useful empirical data on the clinical state of leukaemia and may eventually provide insights into biochemical changes that occur in certain types of this disease.

The reactivity of ascorbate and its metabolic products and their metal complexes plays a role in many of the results reported in several papers in this symposium. They can accelerate or retard many of the reactions involved in lipid peroxidation: e.g. Magee (1982) presents data on the inhibition by ascorbate of methylation of DNA. Because the most reduced form (ascorbate) and the most oxidised form (dehydroascorbate) are so reactive, it is even possible that the ascorbyl radical can serve as a relatively inert form of these to allow diffusion to more distant sites where, upon combination with another ascorbyl radical, one molecule of each of the oxidised and reduced forms is produced.

Finally, there is some preliminary evidence that the ascorbyl radical itself can covalently link to DNA (Harms-Ringdahl, 1981). If these reports are substantiated, it may turn out that there are circumstances where the generally low reactivity of the ascorbyl radical enables it to diffuse long distances and then cause very specific damage at a critical site. In view of the usual location of DNA far from potential sources of ascorbyl radicals, even with such specificity of reaction this still might be unimportant under most circumstances.

6. OXYGEN-RELATED FREE RADICALS MAY HAVE IMPORTANT ROLES IN A NUMBER OF PROCESSES RELATED TO CANCER

In the last few years a dramatic increase in interest and knowledge of oxygen-related radicals has occurred. This area has become too broad and dynamic a field to permit its summation here, but I shall touch on several aspects that seem to be of particular pertinence to the discussions of this paper. The term oxygen-related radicals is chosen because the precise nature of the reactive radicals and their precursors is not known yet and may include metal complexes that have not yet been defined. In order to fully understand these reactions and their importance we need to develop detailed knowledge both of the chemical species involved and their concentrations at various locations within the cell.

Many of the previous sections of this paper apply to the oxygen-related radicals, such as their production at specific sites, the high reactivity of some of these species (especially the hydroxyl radical), and the potential of the production of products of intermediate reactivity. A common theme of several of the papers in this symposium is the role of oxygen addition to form radical chains or cycles (e.g. Slater; Lesko *et al.*; Lown *et al.*; Mason *et al.*; and Benedetto). Some of the reactions discussed in these papers indicate the possibility of forming large quantities of superoxide anions. The direct reactivity of superoxide is relatively low but there is abundant evidence that it can lead to reactive products in complex biological systems via a complex and poorly understood chain of events. As indicated above, until we understand these chains, it will be very difficult to develop rational means to control the damage that can occur.

A number of papers in the "Lipid Peroxidation" part of the symposium emphasise a concept that is essential for an understanding of the role of oxygen-related free radicals: the important reactive molecules may be nonradical products such as aldehydes and their derivatives. In a further complication, the nonradical product may later generate addition free radical products and metal ions also may be involved.

7. FREE RADICALS DO PLAY A ROLE IN EXPERIMENTAL STUDIES OF SOME SPECIFIC TYPES OF CANCER

This section attempts to delineate some specific instances in which free radicals may play a role in the experimental study of cancer although the reactions of the free radicals may or may not be important. Three specific cases and one general case are discussed.

(a) Leukaemia and the Ascorbyl Radical

The data presented by Lohman *et al.* (1982) indicate possible useful clinical applications of the level of ascorbyl radicals in lyophilised blood. These may prove useful even though the ascorbyl radical appears to be generated by the process of sample preparation and probably only indirectly reflects a complex redox process. His studies provide much more thorough data that support an earlier preliminary report of a similar nature (Kruglyakova *et al.*, 1972). Recent studies (Gutierrez and Swartz, 1979; Gutierrez *et al.*, 1979; Swartz and Gutierrez, 1977) indicate that changes in the amount of ascorbyl free radical in lyophilised samples do not occur in all types of cancer so the finding of changes in leukaemia may provide insights specific to that type of malignancy.

(b) Cervical Cancer

The paper by Benedetto (1982) confirms and extends an earlier report by Slater and Cook (1970) that the cervix has relatively characteristic ESR spectra and that these change with the development of malignancy. They speculate that one of the observed ESR signals may reflect prostaglandin metabolism and lipid peroxidation and they provide data consistent with this hypothesis. This ESR signal appears to have sufficient structure that its nature may be determined spectroscopically.

It is interesting to note that this signal usually is observed only after manipulation of the sample (by grinding). This is somewhat analogous to the situation for the ascorbyl radical in leukaemia where a very useful correlation may occur even though the observed radical is generated by lyophilisation and probably is only an indirect indicator of the biochemical and pathological processes involved in the tissue. It is not yet clear whether the free radical signal observed in cervix is produced *de novo* by grinding or whether it is formed by transfer of an unpaired electron from a paramagnetic metal ion.

(c) Melanoma

The involvement of free radicals in melanomas is quite complex. Melanin is a stable free radical that reflects very complex chemical equilibria (Sealy *et al.*, 1980). The quinone-semiquinone-hydroquinone equilibrium has been discussed in detail in an earlier section and the following section discusses its perturbation by metal ions. Riley, in this symposium, describes a possible exploitation of the enzymic mechanism (tyrosinase) for producing melanin: an artificial substrate (4-hydroxyanisole) may be converted by tyrosinase to a reactive free radical which directly or indirectly selectively damages cells that contain this enzyme. Oxygen radicals may also be involved in melanins and hence in melanomas, inasmuch as melanin consumes oxygen and produces both superoxide anions and hydrogen peroxide (Sealy *et al.*, 1980; Sarna *et al.*, 1980).

(d) Alterations in Protective Mechanisms Affecting Levels and Reactions of Free Radicals

Several of the papers in the symposium deal directly or indirectly with a concept that is needed to understand the role of free radicals in complex biological systems: the effect of alteration of protective mechanisms on the types and amounts of observable free radicals. Changes in the amount and *distribution* of reducing and oxidising substances including transition metals and some enzymes will significantly alter the level and nature of free radical reactions (e.g. in this symposium, Poli and Gravela, Willson, Player, and Lesko *et al.*). I emphasise the word distribution because I believe that the critical changes may turn out to be alteration in intracellular distributions rather than the overall content of key constituents. Currently, we often lack the means to determine quantitatively intracellular distributions but the means to do so are developing (e.g. Nöhammer, in the discussion of this symposium, in regard to aldehydes) and may help resolve some of the apparent contradictions in experimental results in this field.

8. PARAMAGNETIC METALS HAVE IMPORTANT ROLES IN CANCER IN BOTH EXPERIMENTAL STUDIES AND CHEMICAL REACTIONS

Previous sections have touched on this topic and therefore this section will be brief. Key concepts include:

(a) Paramagnetic Metals May Cause Experimental Confusion in ESR Studies of Complex Biological Samples

Some valence states of iron, copper, manganase, and other transition elements are paramagnetic and therefore may have detectable ESR spectra and these can be confused with free radicals. This is especially a problem when their spectra include a component at or near the g = 2.00 region where spectra of free radicals usually occur. These may usually be distinguished by their shape and power saturation but some confusion is possible, especially if there are complexes involving both free radicals and metal ions.

(b) Interactions with Free Radicals

There are at least two important types of interactions of trace metals with free radicals that are important to our discussion. They can generate free radicals by participation in redox reactions (e.g. $H_2O_2 + Fe^{2+} + H^+ \rightarrow Fe^{3+} + OH^{\bullet} + H_2O$) and they can interact with free radicals forming new species. Examples of the former are discussed by Lown for iron-bleomycin and by Lesko *et al.* Important examples of the latter include the possible generation in the cell of reduced iron by superoxide ($O_2^{\bullet -} + Fe^{3+} \rightarrow O_2 + Fe^{2+}$) and the shift of equilibria in quinone-semiquinone-hydroquinone equilibria:

Quinone (Oxidised) $\rightleftharpoons$ Semi-Quinone (Free Radical) $\rightleftharpoons$ Hydroquinone (Reduced)

Semi-Quinone (Free Radical) + Trace Metal $\rightleftharpoons$ Semi-Quinone-Metal Complex (Free Radical)

The latter reaction has been demonstrated in orthoquinones involved in melanin (Sealy *et al.*, 1980).

(c) Direct Role on Reactions

Many of the trace elements detectable by ESR can undergo a variety of redox and electrostatic reactions with components of cells. These reactions can range from changing conformation of proteins to irreversible oxidations of reactive groups. This area of chemistry is too large and complex to be discussed here other than to note it must be considered in the evaluation of experimental results in which transition metal ions are present in the system - especially if there are data (such as ESR spectra) that indicate that the metal ions are changing valence state or ligands.

(d) As Indicators of Other Processes

Changes in the amount and/or type of paramagnetic trace elements may provide indirect evidence of changes in the biological system. The valence state of transition elements may be affected by changes in the redox balance of the cell - such an effect has been suggested as an empirical parameter indicating the viability of tissues (Swartz *et al.*, 1971). Changes of paramagnetic trace elements in blood or tissues may occur with cancer and other diseases, and might be useful for following the course of disease as indirect indicators of its state. Some of the causes of such changes in blood are known (Mailer *et al.*, 1974) so that their indirect nature is clear, while in many cases they are not known (Dodd, 1980). It is tempting to speculate that eventually we might be able to use changes in the valence states of paramagnetic elements, perhaps in conjunction with levels of ascorbyl radicals, to measure a parameter related to the overall redox state of a complex biological system.

9. TECHNOLOGICAL AND METHODOLOGICAL ADVANCES WILL INCREASE THE USEFULNESS OF ESR STUDIES OF CANCER

Recent technological developments already have added significantly to our ability to get useful information from ESR studies of complex biological systems and it is likely that we are only on the threshold of the full extent and exploitation of such developments. These are grouped below in rather arbitrary categories. Taken as a whole, the list of potential techniques is impressive and, I believe, an accurate indication of the real possibilities. Some of the techniques have been used already and are described in papers presented in the symposium.

(a) Resolution of Spectra by Complex Techniques

An unfortunate characteristic of many ESR studies of complex biological systems is the paucity of the detailed spectroscopic features needed for straightforward definitive interpretation of the spectra. The use of multiple resonance techniques such as ENDOR and ELDOR has provided information not attainable by conventional ESR techniques - such as the presence of a freely rotating methyl group or the exchangeability of the water near a free radical. The use of multiple frequencies is another spectroscopic technique that has been productive in studies of complex biological materials including the use of high frequencies to resolve anisotropic features of free radicals (Gutierrez and Swartz, 1979) and low frequencies to suppress such features (Froncisz *et al.*, 1979) and thereby permit the resolution of hyperfine features.

(b) Resolution of Time-Dependent Processes

Several different methodological developments now enable one to use ESR to study fast processes in complex systems. Special pulsed spectrometers are now available in a few laboratories with the capabilities of measuring events and motions with times as short as 10 μsec. Active intermediates can be studied directly in conventional spectrometers as well as by converting the reactive species to more stable (and hence, observable) intermediates by the technique of spin trapping. (The latter technique was used and is described in several of the papers in this symposium.) Techniques such as saturation transfer spectroscopy (STS) and spin labelling enable one to follow motions in complex structures such as membranes over time scales ranging from 10^{-4} sec to 10^{-10} sec.

(c) Enhanced Sensitivity

Another characteristic problem of ESR studies of complex biological systems is the low concentration of free radicals and other paramagnetic species in these systems, combined with our inability to concentrate them without destroying the nature of the system. Recent developments in computer processing are beginning to overcome this problem using a variety of data manipulation techniques including sophisticated averaging, resolution enhancement, and spectral subtraction.

Another set of developments in cavity design have already greatly increased the scope and sensitivity of possible experiments and some developments in progress include concepts that may add significantly to the capabilities of the technique. The use of TM and large access cavities have significantly increased the amount of biological sample that can be used. Cavities under development include some with the potential of studying intact tissues *in vivo* by surface probes or by cavities designed to permit the introduction of parts of animals into the cavity while retaining high sensitivity. If these developments are successful, then it should be possible to study free radical and other paramagnetic changes at the critical times when the biochemical lesions that lead to cancer may occur.

(d) Measurements of Oxygen

Quite recently ESR techniques have been developed that give the promise of providing better data on intracellular and extracellular oxygen concentrations - data that are essential for the study of many aspects of carcinogenesis and lipid peroxidation. These techniques are based on the effect of oxygen on the relaxation time of paramagnetic species. Certain spin labels have hyperfine structure that is affected by oxygen and this can be used to measure extracellular oxygen in suspensions of viable cells. One may also use an analogous approach to measure intracellular oxygen if the cells contain a paramagnetic substance with the proper relaxation time. Melanin is such a substance and we have used it to measure intracellular oxygen, both in melanoma cells and in CHO cells, that have phagocytised melanin.

REFERENCES

Benedetto, C. (1982). In this Symposium.
Dodd, N.J.F. (1980). *In* "Metal Ions in Biological Systems" (Ed. A. Sigel), Vol. 10, pp.95-131, Marcel Dekker, New York.
Dodd, N.J.F. and Swartz, H.M. (1980). *Br. J. Cancer* 42, 349-351.
Emanuel, N.M. (1976). *Q. Rev. Biophys.* 9, 283-307.
Froncisz, W., Scholes, C.P., Hyde, J.S., Wei, Y., King, W.E., Shaw, R.W. and Beinert, H. (1979). *J. Biol. Chem.* 254, 7482-7484.
Gutierrez, P.L. and Swartz, H.M. (1979). *Br. J. Cancer* 39, 24-34.
Gutierrez, P.L., Swartz, H.M. and Wilkinson, E.J. (1979). *Br. J. Cancer* 39, 330-336.
Harms-Ringdahl, M. (1981). Presented at 1981 Radiation Research Society Meeting in Minneapolis, Minnesota.
Kruglyakova, K.E., Klochko, E.V., Kassirskii, I.A. and Emanuel, N.M. (1972). Proceedings of the IV International Biophysics Congress, Vol.4, p.196.
Lesko, S.A., Ts'o, P.O.P., Yang, S.-U. and Zheng, R. (1982). In this Symposium.
Lohmann, W., Bensch, K.G., Sapper, H., Pleyer, A., Schreiber, J., Kang, S.O., Loffler, H., Pralle, H., Schwemmle, K. and Filler, R.D. (1982). In this Symposium.
Lown, J.W., Joshua, A.V. and Chen, H.-H. (1982). In this Symposium.
Magee, P.N. (1982). In this Symposium.
Mailer, C., Swartz, H.M., Konieczny, M., Ambegaonkar, S. and Moore, V. (1974). *Cancer Res.* 34, 637-642.
Mason, R.P., Harrelson, W.G., Kalyanaroman, B., Mottley, C., Peterson, F.J. and Holtzman, G.C. (1982). In this Symposium.
McCay, P.B., Noguchi, T., Fong, K.-L., Lai, E.K. and Poyer, J.L. (1980). *In* "Free Radicals in Biology" (Ed. W.A. Pryor), Vol.4, pp.155-186, Academic Press, New York.
Player, T.J. (1982). In this Symposium.
Poli, G. and Gravela, E. (1982). In this Symposium.
Riley, P.A., Morgan, B.D.G., O'Neill, T., Dewey, D. and Galpine, A.R. (1982). In this Symposium.
Sarna, T., Duleba, A., Korytowski, W. and Swartz, H.M. (1980). *Arch. Biochem. Biophys.* 200, 140-148.
Sarna, T. and Swartz, H.M. (1979). *Folia Histochem. Cytochem.* 16, 275-286.
Sealy, R., Felix, C., Hyde, J.S. and Swartz, H.M. (1980). *In* "Free Radicals in Biology" (Ed. W.A. Pryor), Vol.4, pp.209-259, Academic Press, New York.
Slater, T.F. and Cook, J.W.E. (1970). *In* "Cytology Automation", (Ed. D.M.D. Evans), Livingston, Edinburgh.
Slater, T.F. (1982). In this Symposium.
Stier, A., Clauss, R., Lücke, A. and Reitz, I. (1982). In this Symposium.
Swartz, H.M. (1972). *Adv. Cancer Res.* 15, 227-252.
Swartz, H.M. (1979). *In* "Submolecular Biology and Cancer", Ciba Foundation Symposium 67, pp.107-124, Excerpta-Medica, Amsterdam.
Swartz, H.M., Darin, J.C. and Lewis, J.D. (1971). *Proc. Eur. Biophys. Congr.* 2, 557-561.
Swartz, H.M. and Dodd, N.J.F. (1981). *In* "Oxygen and Oxy-Radicals in Chemistry and Biology" (Eds. M.A.J. Rodgers and E.L. Powers), Academic Press, New York.

Swartz, H.M. and Gutierrez, P.L. (1977). *Science* 198, 936-938.
Symons, M.C. (1982). In this Symposium.
Willson, R.L. (1982). In this Symposium.

DISCUSSION

Slater: You started by showing an interesting slide linking reactive radicals to vitamin E to vitamin C to NADH; I believe the reasons that NADH was put on at the end of the sequence were two-fold. Firstly that Staudinger had shown many years ago (Schneider and Staudinger, 1965) that there is an active dependent NADH system that regenerates vitamin C from the vitamin C radical and secondly, of course, there is a fairly low daily requirement for vitamin C, and if the vitamin C radical was not repaired in some way we might rapidly become vitamin C deficient or scorbutic. What do you have to say about this?

Swartz: I plead ignorance. I think you know more than I on it and I don't have anything useful to add.

Ts'o: Would you say a few more things about the new technological advances enabling the measurement of oxygen radicals in living cells?

Swartz: What a nice question! There are certain spin labels in which there is a hyperfine pattern which can be resolved in its entirety only under oxygen free conditions, and the amount of resolution is directly proportional to oxygen. In fact one can get a calibration curve relating the amount of oxygen to some experimental parameter. Here in our laboratory we used the K parameter, which is the ratio of some of these peak heights, and the nice thing is it is valid at oxygen concentrations that occur under physiologically important conditions. I know of some work of Leukewich who is measuring the oxygen depletion in two melanoma cell lines, a melanotic cell line and an amelanotic cell line. This is in a respiring cell culture and one is looking then at the depletion of oxygen in a very non-perturbing yet accurate way by looking at the change in the hyperfine pattern. These are extracellular cell probes. In melanin containing cells you can get an intracellular probe by looking at the power saturation of the melanin, which is also affected by oxygen. So you can simultaneously measure both extracellular and intracellular oxygen, and certainly from the point of view of a radiation biologist to be able to do this inside cells under physiological conditions has great excitement.

Generally the measurement of oxygen in tumours and the measurement of oxygen in cell cultures is indirect and the usual methods, even using micro-electrodes, are very perturbing.

Ts'o: So you are measuring the oxygen tension, using the resolution of the hyperfine?

Swartz: That is correct.

Ts'o: But it is not a measure of the oxygen radical?

Swartz: It's not oxygen radicals, it's just a technique for measuring oxygen.

Ts'o: Do you see any new method for measuring the concentration of oxygen radicals inside the living cell?

Swartz: I think that spin trap techniques and perhaps, also, some of the pulse spectrometers will be able to resolve some of the oxygen radicals. A number of years ago Fessenden and Smaller demonstrated that pulse spectrometers could look at transients as short-lived as hydroxyl radicals. There's a new generation of ESR spectrometers that Jim Hyde is developing that will have the time resolution and facility of operation to enable us to start looking at some of the oxygen radicals on a more systematic basis.

Slater: The use of ESR hyperfine measurements in relation to O_2 concentration is a very interesting development. This comes from the technique first proposed by a group in Poland, I believe?

Swartz: That's right. Originally it was some Russian work but then that was picked up by the Polish workers. I think it was Restanoff, but I'm not completely sure who originally proposed the method, and then Leukewich and Sarna applied it to biological problems. I have done some work with this method in collaboration with Sarna in Kracow.

Stier: Could you give us more details about more recent technological advances with regard to the surface probes? How large are they?

Swartz: I have the frustrations of not being regularly in the National Biomedical ESR laboratory any more and therefore cannot push things in the directions that I want. What they have found is that a type of cavity called the lumped circuit is such that it puts out a microwave field in the form of a cylinder and this field extends from the end of the cavity and is such that there is not as severe a problem of the usual absorption of the electrical component and so one can use this in the presence of a large amount of water. Theoretically, although we have not done the experiment yet, one can place this probe on the surface and it concentrates the microwaves such that one obtains a spectrum from the surface outside the cavity. Placing the sample inside, we are able to get, at low frequency (around 2 GHz), a sensitivity on a Varian weak pitch sample, which is the same as one gets at 9 GHz. So it's a concentrated component of the electro-magnetic wave extending outside the cavity which would be a cylinder if the theoretical considerations were correct, but more probably a cone potentially in size up to 3 or 4 Mm. One could think about exciting experiments in which one looked at surface tumours which are easy to generate and one might be able to look at more dynamic aspects of changes without having to remove the sample, without having to compromise the circulation.

Esterbauer: You said that the hydroxyl radical is not important because it reacts in a complex system too fast. If it experiences a protein, isn't there a new radical generated? And don't you then get a chain that can spread out over a long distance? That is my first question. And now my second question is: in the redox system of a cell there are thiols, for example glutathione is very important, and isn't there some evidence that there are thiol radicals corresponding to alkoxy radicals? Is there anything like a thiol radical?

Swartz: You are of course correct in both statements. Indeed, when the hydroxyl radical reacts something is left and if what is left is a radical of some intermediate activity, indeed the damage can spread. I would say though that to the extent that radiation biology provides a useful analogue, one can discount in terms of cell killing in radiation biology almost all of the hydroxyl radicals except those that directly affect DNA. So that the amount of damage that is done is unlikely to be important unless it is at a critical site. Now if the hydroxyl radical is at a site that is particularly good for amplification (I think the membrane is certainly an exciting area from the point of view of inducing lipid peroxidation, getting out the kinds of products that your laboratory has worked on), that is a way of amplifying and spreading them. So that over-dramatically perhaps I said they are not important but my next principle was that they are important under certain conditions. But what I was really trying to do was to over-react to what I think has been an over-reaction which is "My God, it's a hydroxyl radical - it must be important". I feel that if it's a hydroxyl radical it's unimportant unless proven otherwise, because you've got to prove that it's occurring somewhere where something significant can happen. Regarding the thiol radicals, your second question, they certainly do occur, they seem to be particularly stable and I am not aware of much evidence in terms of biologically important reactions that go on from the thiol radical. It seems to be a very useful end point, certainly in radiation protection. Once one gets the energy transferred to the sulphydryl group and creates a thiol radical this seems to disappear probably by generating disulphides and Jed Adams may be able to give much more detail than this but as far as I know there is not much damage that occurs, once you get that unpaired electron on to the sulphydryl group, except of course for the using up of the sulphydryl, and that may be very significant.

Adams: The general statement that the most reactive radicals are not going to be the most important is a rather sweeping statement. Take the OH radical which actually may not be all that important. However, any free radical that reacts with a solute must leave another radical behind and it would follow that that radical would be less reactive. A second point is that one does not always have to invoke diffusion as a means of initiating a chemical reaction particularly in the highly ordered heterogeneous systems in cells. There is evidence that electron transfer reactions involving electrophiles can occur by long-range energy or electron migration. One cannot assume that reactions of very reactive radicals are limited to a very small volume.

Swartz: I would certainly agree.

Slater: When you say "long-range" do you mean intermolecular or do you mean intracellular?

Adams: Intracellular. I am very impressed by some of the Swedish work of Graslund involving orientated DNA molecules. This work provided good support for the proposal that thermal electron migration in DNA can occur over large distances.

Slater: This is consistent with the theoretical studies on electron conduction in DNA, by, for example, Ladik's group in Erlagen (Ladik, 1979).

Swartz: In support of what you are saying there's some very old experimental data that Mike Omerod did with very long-range transfer to the sulphydryl group and eventually the unpaired electron ended up and there seemed to be a very long-range intramolecular transfer and that unpaired electron does find the sulphydryl group eventually.

Adams: It is certainly true that the yield of disulphide anions in some irradiated proteins in solution is larger than you would calculate simply on a stoichiometric approach by taking the reactivities of the various parts of the protein chain.

Swartz: You can even dissect those reactions out by temperature and you can watch the transfer occur and you can do your irradiation in liquid nitrogen temperatures and see a slightly larger amount than you would anticipate and as you slowly warm up you can see the so-called thiyl radical increase until it becomes manifold what one would anticipate and I would really support all of what you've said and it's clear that I did make an overly sweeping statement.

Asmus: I was interested in the comments you made on the $OH^{\bullet}$ radical and I would certainly agree that the free $OH^{\bullet}$ radical is not the species that causes most of the damage at a site which is different from the site where the $OH^{\bullet}$ radical is initially formed. We know that since the $OH^{\bullet}$ radical is an electrophilic agent, it likes to add to any centre of high electron density, which could be an heteroatom like nitrogen or sulphur or, for example, any atom which provides a free electron pair. When it is attached, this addition product could be considerably long-lived and thus have a chance to migrate and to enter a reaction at a completely different site. This is particularly true also for metal ions which brings up the old question of what really is produced if we form $OH^{\bullet}$ radicals in a Fenton-type reaction. Is it a free $OH^{\bullet}$ radical? I would rather think it is an $OH^{\bullet}$ radical attached to the metal ion. And now you can start discussing how free it is or whether, in fact, you are already dealing with the oxidised metal ion? We have to keep in mind the fact that these species have considerable life times and when I say considerable life times I mean the microsecond to millisecond time range. This would also be long enough for migration from one place to the other. I would like to make another comment on the thiyl radical which has been mentioned. I agree its reactivity is relatively low compared to other radicals. But we recently conducted a study from the purely chemical point of view on the formation of thiol radicals in the presence of phosphite and we could establish an equilibrium between a phosphite radical and a thiyl radical (Schafer and Asmus, 1981). Phosphite radicals, once they are formed through this equilibrium, can undergo both oxidising and reducing reactions, substitution and addition reactions. So thiyl radicals indirectly could be the source of new chemical reactions, and all these processes are relatively slow which means that these radicals are long lived and in consequence could be transported to some other site of reaction which may be fairly far away. I don't know whether you have phosphite or phosphite radicals in your system. But you might consider the formation of phosphite radicals in the presence of phosphate since their oxidation state lies between that of phosphate and phosphite.

Magee: I was interested in your remarks about most of the hydroxy radicals not having much significance. I think there is a parallel with carcinogenesis by some of the directly acting carcinogens because we found that if you inject methylnitrosourea into rats intravenously you can demonstrate that every cell in the animal's body is probably methylated (Swann *et al.*, 1968; Kleihues *et al.*, 1971), and yet the animal will usually finish with only three macroscopically detectable tumours at the most, and usually only one tumour, assuming the dose to be adequate. This suggests that you can have a very large amount of reactive intermediate generated in the body but the end result may be extremely specific and it may be that there is only one particular spot in the DNA that must be hit to do the trick. I think there is quite a parallel between that and what you were saying.

Willson: I was very interested in your mention of an ascorbate DNA interaction. I was wondering what sort of mechanism you envisage? We have done many pulse radiolysis experiments showing that many organic radicals will react with ascorbic acid. We assume that the organic radicals are being repaired. We have shown that the product from the reaction of OH$^{\cdot}$ with dGMP does interact with ascorbate. You can see the change in the spectrum from that of the dGMP radical cation (possibly the protonated OH$^{\cdot}$ adduct) to that of the ascorbyl radical. Thus there is the possibility of a radical already on the DNA interacting with ascorbate to give you the ascorbyl radical. Do you know of any evidence for the reaction of a radical plus an ascorbyl radical forming a covalent adduct?

Swartz: I'm not aware of any.

REFERENCES to Discussion

Kleihues, P. and Patzschke, K. (1971). *Z. Krebsforsch.* 75, 193-200.

Ladick, J.D. (1979). *In* "Submolecular Biology and Cancer", Ciba Foundation Symposium No. 67 New Series, pp.58-78. Excerpta Medica, Amsterdam.

Schafer, K. and Asmus, K.-D. (1981). *J. Phys. Chem.* 85, 852-855.

Schneider, W. and Staudinger, H. (1965). *Biochim. Biophys. Acta* 96, 157-159.

Swann, P.F. and Magee, P.N. (1968). *Biochem. J.* 110, 39-47.

Biochemical Studies on Human Uterine Cancer

C. BENEDETTO

INTRODUCTORY REMARKS

Carcinoma of the uterine cervix and of the endometrium are major contributors to female deaths by cancer in the U.K. and many other countries. Table 1 gives data from Annual Reports of the Department of Health and Social Security, London, in relation to mortality rates for gynaecological and other types of cancer in women. It can be seen that cancers of the cervix and endometrium (grouped together as uterine cancers in the official statistics) account for more than 3,000 deaths per year in England and Wales. Moreover, it can be seen from these data that there has been a decline in the mortality rate due to uterine cancers over the last 10 years. Similar findings have been reported from the United States and Canada: in British Vancouver, for example, a substantial decrease in the *incidence* of invasive cancer of the cervix has been linked to the success of long-term screening with the Papanicolaou procedure (Boyes and Worth, 1976). Early diagnosis of the lesion, with improvements in the clinical treatment over the last 50 years or so (Stallworthy and Wiernik, 1976) are associated with a net decrease in mortality rate. Figure 1 shows data from an American study (Kessler, 1979) illustrating the fall observed over the last 20 years in the *mortality* rate of patients with carcinoma of the cervix. Despite such encouraging changes in the incidence of invasive cancer (associated with a relative increase in the incidence of carcinoma *in situ* resulting from efficient screening procedures) and in the associated mortality rate, it is evident that cancers of the cervix and endometrium are still major and distressing problems. The incidence of invasive cancer, and deaths due to gynaecological cancer are even higher in some countries than those figures summarised above

TABLE 1 Cancer deaths in England over the period 1970–1979.

Cancer site	1952		1970		1972		1976		1979	
	M	F	M	F	M	F	M	F	M	F
Total cancer	45,429	42,213	59,158	50,184	60,783	51,554	63,367	54,792	64,349	56,112
Oesophagus	1,475	850	1,586	1,206	1,659	1,231	1,821	1,400	1,920	1,465
Stomach	8,066	6,343	6,706	5,079	6,670	4,845	6,419	4,595	6,072	4,392
Pancreas	-	-	2,527	2,242	2,592	2,330	2,681	2,615	2,869	2,677
Trachea, bronchus and lung	11,981	2,237	23,729	5,165	24,466	5,694	25,140	6,634	25,251	7,539
Breast	59	8,285	68	10,089	80	10,564	64	11,091	77	11,367
Cervix uteri	-	2,547	-	2,171	-	2,083	-	2,065	-	1,944
Uterus	-	1,477	-	1,398	-	1,362	-	1,418	-	1,102
Prostate	3,007	-	-	-	3,965	-	4,348	-	4,568	-

Values for 1952 refer to deaths in England and Wales (total cancer deaths in Wales were approx. 6% of total cancer deaths in England in 1969). The values are from the Department of Health and Social Security Annual Reports "on the State of the Public Health", London, Her Majesty's Stationery Office. Abbreviations: M, male; F, female.

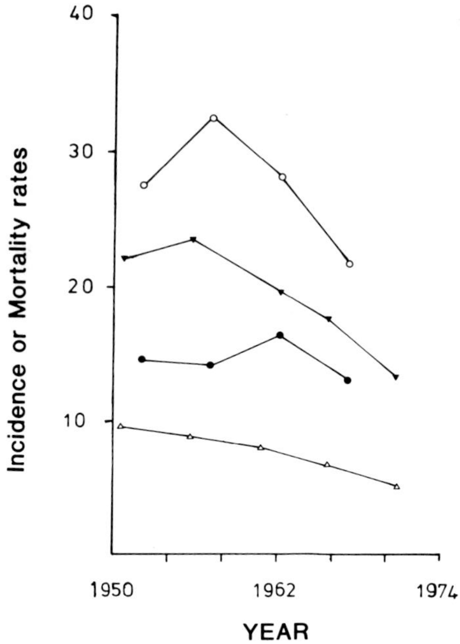

FIG. 1 Mortality from and incidence rates of cervical cancer in white and non-white women in U.S.A. (data from Kessler, 1979). The mortality rates and incidence are for 100,000 females adjusted for the total U.S.A. population, 1950. O — O, invasive cancer (non-whites); ▼ — ▼, mortality (non-whites), ● — ●, invasive cancer (whites); Δ — Δ, mortality (whites).

for the United States and the United Kingdom: in Bulawayo, for example, the incidence is reported to be 80 times higher (Muir, 1975) than in Israeli women, who have a relatively very low incidence rate (2.7 per 100,000) for this type of cancer (see Table 2).

Many forms of cancer commonly show an increasing incidence with age into the sixth and seventh decades (Cairns, 1978); cancer of the cervix, however, not infrequently affects young women in the third and fourth decades of life (see Adelstein and White, 1977) often when they are mothers of young families. In consequence, there are severe sociological and familial consequences of this form of cancer.

An additional worrying aspect of the overall problem of cancer of the cervix is the rapid increase in sexually transmitted diseases in young persons (Catterall, 1981) and the possible effect this will have on its incidence. There is now considerable evidence, admittedly

TABLE 2 Incidence of various types of cancer with range of variation from country to country.

Type of Cancer	Area of high incidence	Area of low incidence	Cumulative risk[3] %	Range of variation in incidence
FEMALE				
Cervix uteri.	Bulawayo	Israel	10	30[1]
Corpus uteri.	U.S.A.Conn.	Japan	2	10[2]
Ovary	Denmark	Japan	2	8[2]
Breast	U.S.A.Conn.	Uganda	7	5[2]
MALE				
Penis	Uganda	Israel	1	300[2]
Oesophagus	Bulawayo	Vas	20	176[1]
Liver	Bulawayo	Bombay	8	95[1]
Bronchus, lung	Liverpool, UK	Ibadan	11	72[1]
Prostate	Alameda (negro)	Israel (non-jews)	7	21[1]

[1]Muir (1975); [2]Doll (1977); [3]Cumulative risk (Doll, 1977) refers to the situation at age 75 y in the absence of other causes of death.

indirect, that points to a role (either primary or secondary) for infective agents in the pathogenesis of cancer of the cervix. Most of these studies relate to the damaging influence of *Herpes hominis* type 2 (Poste and Waterson, 1975). Direct virus transmission experiments in the rat have demonstrated effects on the cervix ranging from basal cell hyperplasia, to dysplasia (Tobin *et al.*, 1979), but see the recent study by Cassai *et al.* (1981) that has produced negative evidence for herpes involvement.

A relatively recent phenomenon is the apparent shift in the relative incidences of gynaecological cancers in favour of an increased emphasis on endometrial cancer compared to cancer of the cervix (Gusberg, 1980; Jick *et al.*, 1980): this has led to the use of phrases such as "the epidemic of endometrial cancer" (Jick *et al.*, 1980). Epidemiological analysis points towards the use of estrogen-replacement therapy as an important factor in this shift of emphasis. Gusberg (1980) has reviewed reports showing that the relative risk of endometrial cancer was between 3.8 and 38.0 in patients who had used estrogens for a long term compared to an age-matched control group. Jick *et al.* (1980) have estimated that more than 15,000 cases of endometrial cancer in the United States were caused by replacement estrogens during the period 1971-1975.

In contrast to the increased incidence of endometrial cancer that has been related to estrogen therapy, there are indications that estrogen-users who develop endometrial cancer have a more favourable prognosis for the course of the disease (Jick *et al.*, 1980; Collins *et al.*, 1980).

The above discussion has referred to two important possibilities in the pathogenesis of uterine cancer: estrogen-use in relation to endometrial cancer, and herpes infection in relation to cancer of the cervix. A number of other factors have been isolated as contributory to the incidence of these diseases. With cancer of the cervix, for example, the age at first coitus, age at first marriage, age at first pregnancy, pregnancy outside marriage, number of children and of sexual partners, cigarette smoking, social class, oral contraceptives, personal hygiene and circumcision of the male partner are all features that have been reported to affect the incidence of cervical abnormalities and cancer of the cervix. Two recent studies that can be consulted for background references are by Harris *et al.* (1980) and Terris *et al.* (1980).

The former study points to common aetiological factors for invasive cancer, carcinoma *in situ* and the different degrees of dysplasia. These results support the findings of Meisels *et al.* (1977), and Wright *et al.* (1978), but contrast with those of Terris *et al.* (1980). The latter authors reported that the epidemiology of carcinoma *in situ* was related to that of invasive cancer, whereas all dysplasias, considered together without reference to their degree, did not behave in an epidemiological sense like invasive cancer. These differences in the results of different groups of investigators may reflect the histopathological problems underlying a uniform diagnosis of dysplastic lesions (Editorial, 1975). For some additional discussion of the possible relationship of cervical dysplasias to carcinoma *in situ* see Briggs (1979).

With endometrial cancer the incidence rate increases sharply at about the age of 40 and reaches a maximum in the middle or late 50s (Elwood *et al.*, 1977). Factors reported to be important in affecting the incidence of endometrial cancer are somewhat similar to those reported for breast cancer and include: an early menarche, and a late menopause; a high estrone:estriol ratio; dysfunctional bleeding; failure of ovulation; increased relative body weight (i.e. obesity); diabetes; hypertension, and nulliparity (see Elwood *et al.*, 1977; Wynder *et al.*, 1966; Gusberg, 1980).

The above remarks have briefly summarised much evidence in the literature concerning the importance of, and pathogenetic factors in gynaecological cancers of the cervix and endometrium. The requirement for a reliable, relatively inexpensive mass screening method that can recognise such cancers at an early stage, and thereby permit effective treatment before metastatic dissemination occurs, is evident. The Papanicolaou smear test fulfils most requirements in these respects but the published data show a somewhat disturbing variation in the proportion of false negatives in groups of patients from different clinics (see Rees *et al.*, 1970).

A number of other approaches to routine screening have been tried over the last 20 years or so, ranging from automated cell imaging procedures to attempts to find specific biochemical disturbances in gynaecological cancer cells that could be used in automatic screening methods (for general references see Evans, 1970; Riggott, 1971; Ploem, 1980). 6-Phosphogluconate dehydrogenase activity in samples of vaginal fluid, for example, is much elevated in invasive cancer (Rees *et al.*, 1970) and the percentages of false negative and false positive results were low and acceptable for screening purposes. However, the method gave a 25% false negative finding in carcinoma *in situ*, possibly due to the low and variable desquamation of the *in situ* cancer cells into vaginal fluid (Rees *et al.*, 1970). Possibly this percentage could be improved by the use of a cytochemical procedure for the enzyme activity, linked to rapid automated cell scanning with data sorting of the cytoplasmic intensities.

The 6-phosphogluconate dehydrogenase test mentioned above depends on a much greater activity being present in tumour cells compared to normal cells: in other words, the result depends on a *quantitative* difference. In consequence, there is always the likelihood that there will be overlap between the control and tumour population values, and this creates a problem of where to place a value-line that separates the two groups of data. Clearly, the bigger the average difference in enzyme activities between the control and tumour values the better is the accuracy of discrimination. An even more useful opportunity would occur if the difference between the groups were *qualitative* in nature.

One such qualitative possibility was considered for diagnosis of cancer of the cervix following a report on mouse tumours by Brennan *et al.* (1966). They reported that the electron spin resonance (ESR) spectrum obtained from a mouse tumour was a triplet, whereas the corresponding response in the normal case was a single line. Thus, there was a qualitative and easily recognisable difference. It is now known, however, that such a qualitative difference in ESR response was largely artefactual, and came from degradation reactions during tissue preparation (Muruyama *et al.*, 1971). However, before the artefactuality of the triplet response was known, Slater and Cook (1970) had applied ESR techniques to samples of normal and malignant cervix and endometrium and had found a striking *quantitative* difference: normal tissue gave an unexpectedly strong ESR signal, indicating a high content of paramagnetic species, whereas the cancer samples gave a much diminished or undetectable response.

The report of Slater and Cook (1970) was the incentive for this present study for it was realised that larger numbers of human uterine samples required testing for their ESR response, and a detailed study on the behaviour of the paramagnetic or free radical species was considered to be necessary to gain insight into the chemical nature of the radical species involved.

EXPERIMENTAL PROCEDURES

Tissue Samples

Samples of uterus and cervix were obtained from normal patients, and from cancer patients who had not received previous radiotherapy or cytotoxic drug therapy, at operations for hysterectomy or cone biopsies.

All tissue specimens were approx. 2 cm long and 0.3 cm thick, weight approx. 150 mg; the samples were immediately frozen in liquid nitrogen within a few minutes after obtaining them. Some samples were inserted directly into quartz ESR tubes (internal diameter approx. 3 mm) prior to freezing (these were later examined by ESR) and are termed "intact samples"; other samples were first frozen in plastic tubes and were later powdered under liquid nitrogen and then transferred to quartz ESR tubes for ESR analysis; these are termed "powder" samples. Histological examination of the tissue was made using small pieces taken from an immediately adjacent and macroscopically similar site to that used for ESR analysis. The samples of cervix were always taken so as to most probably include the squamocolumnar junction which is known to change in position with age and childbirth (Briggs, 1979). In Table 3 are shown the number of cases studied in each clinical condition by ESR analysis. The mean age (and range in years) for the normal patients and those with cancer were respectively 44 (38-66) and 53 (29-80) years.

Samples of cervix and uterine horn, liver, lung and seminal vesicle were taken from adult albino rats, and were immediately frozen after being placed in quartz ESR tubes.

ESR Analysis

Samples were examined usually at $-130^{\circ}C$, using a Varian E-104 spectrometer with a variable temperature cavity, the microwave power was 10-50 mW, the gain approx. 10^3, scan range 2000 G, modulation 16 G. Variations of procedure from the above descriptions will be described below at the appropriate position under Results. Diphenyl-picryl-hydrazyl was used as an internal and external reference standard (g = 2.0036).

Microspectrophotometry

Serial frozen section of human cervix were prepared using a cryostat at $-20^{\circ}C$ and were stained serially with 2,2'-dihydroxy-6,6'-dinaphthyl-disulphide (DDD) for reactive thiol groups, by the procedure of Barrnett and Seligman (1952) modified by Esterbauer (1972, 1973), Esterbauer *et al.* (1973) and Nohammer (1977), and with haematoxylin-eosin. Microspectrophotometric measurements were performed using a

TABLE 3 Histological classification of the cases studied by ESR analysis

Number of cases	Histological diagnosis
CERVIX	
22	normal
5	metaplasia
7	cystic glandular transformation of the exocervix
13	parakeratosis
4	erosion
3	carcinoma *in situ*
5	invasive carcinoma
ENDOMETRIUM	
33	normal
5	endometrial atrophy
6	endometrial hyperplasia
15	fibroleiomyoma
13	adenocarcinoma
3	mesonephric carcinoma

computer programme APAMOS 3T at a wavelength of 560 nm with a scanning microspectrophotometer (C. Zeiss, Oberknochen, FRG).

RESULTS

Our results have confirmed the preliminary data of Slater and Cook (1970) in demonstrating (i) that frozen powdered samples of normal human cervix and endometrium yield very strong ESR signals; (ii) that the corresponding signals in samples of malignant tissues are much reduced or undetectable. We have found (Benedetto *et al.*, 1981) that the normal tissue samples from human patients almost always give powerful ESR signals; the occasional weak signal is possibly the result of accidental warm-up of the sample during handling procedures (Benedetto *et al.*, 1981; for the temperature response of the ESR signal see below). In arbitrary units of signal intensity (signal height in cm at constant gain) the mean value (± SEM) obtained from

TABLE 4 Human tissues examined by ESR spectroscopy, and ESR major signal heights (in arbitrary units) at 10 mW power.

Tissue	Intact samples			Powdered samples		
	No.	% negative	signal height	No.	% negative	signal height
Normal cervix	26	11	3.3 ± 0.6	24	8	3.3 ± 0.5
Normal endometrium	15	7	3.1 ± 0.7	18	6	2.3 ± 0.4
Normal cervix and endometrium	41	9	3.2 ± 0.5	42	7	2.8 ± 0.3
Carcinoma *in situ* and invasive cancers	15	73	0.4 ± 0.4	16	56	1.6 ± 0.6

The number of samples that gave no significant signals in the regions g = 2.11-2.15 (intact samples) and g = 2.002-2.003 (powdered samples) are shown as percentages of negative signals. Mean values ± SEM.

41 *powdered* samples of normal cervix and endometrium was 3.2 ± 0.5, whereas the mean value obtained from 15 samples of invasive cancer and carcinoma *in situ* was 0.4 ± 0.4; with *intact* samples the corresponding values were 2.8 ± 0.3 and 1.6 ± 0.6 (Table 4). There are clearly marked reductions in signal intensities in the cancer samples even though some such samples gave signals in the normal range. The reason for the latter is probably related to the virtual impossibility of excluding significant amounts of "normal tissue" from the cancer samples that were macroscopic in nature (for further discussion see Benedetto *et al.*, 1981): despite such difficulty in the sampling process, two of the three samples of carcinoma *in situ* examined did not give any signal. Intact samples of normal endometrium and cervix give strong ESR signals centred around g = 2.11-2.15 (Fig. 2a,b) whereas quite different signals (g = 2.002-2.035) appear in the powdered samples (Fig. 2d,e). Tumour samples generally gave much reduced signals, as already mentioned, and two illustrations are given in Fig. 2c and 2f.

The major change in signal shape and g-value when the intact samples are ground to powder under liquid nitrogen could be construed to indicate that the grinding process destroyed one species (g = 2.11-2.15) and, artefactually produced another (g = 2.002-2.035). However,

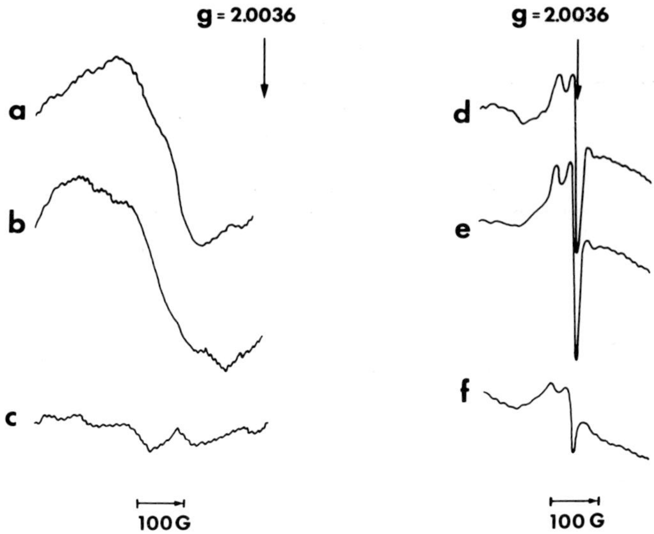

FIG. 2 ESR spectra of samples of normal human cervix and endometrium and of carcinoma of the cervix. Spectra a, b and c show results for frozen intact samples of normal endometrium, normal cervix and carcinoma of the cervix respectively. Spectra d, e and f show results for frozen powders of normal endometrium, normal cervix and carcinoma of the cervix respectively. The conditions used were: scan range, 2000 G; power, 50 mW; gain, 6.3×10^2; cavity temperature, -130°C; field setting for a, b and c, 3230 G and for d, e and f, 3350 G.

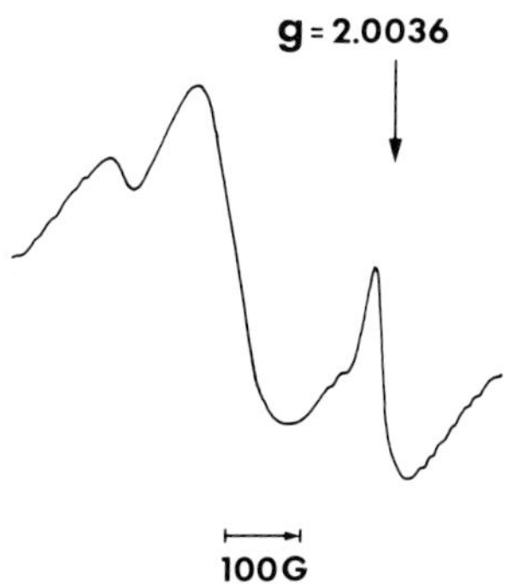

FIG. 3 ESR spectrum of frozen intact normal endometrium that shows both types of major signal in the regions near to g = 2.14 and g = 2.002. Conditions used: power, 50 mW; gain, 2×10^2; scan range, 2000 G; cavity temperature, -130°C; field setting, 3100 G.

it is germane to this point to note that we generally observed a good correlation between the signal intensities in the intact and the powdered samples (Benedetto *et al.*, 1981), and that in some intact tissue samples both types of signal were observed (Fig. 3). In consequence, we prefer the view (as a working hypothesis) that the act of grinding under liquid nitrogen *interconverts* the g = 2.11-2.15 species to the other (g = 2.002-2.035).

Both types of signal, in the intact and in the powdered samples, from normal and malignant tissue, were sensitive to changes in cavity temperature; the signals rapidly decreased in intensity when the temperature increased above -80°C, and disappeared at 0°C. Some recovery on re-cooling was seen with intact samples only. An indication that the major signals in intact samples at g = 2.11-2.15 was a composite envelope of several contributory signals can be seen from Fig. 4a where a change in temperature resulted in some fine structure appearing in this range of g-values.

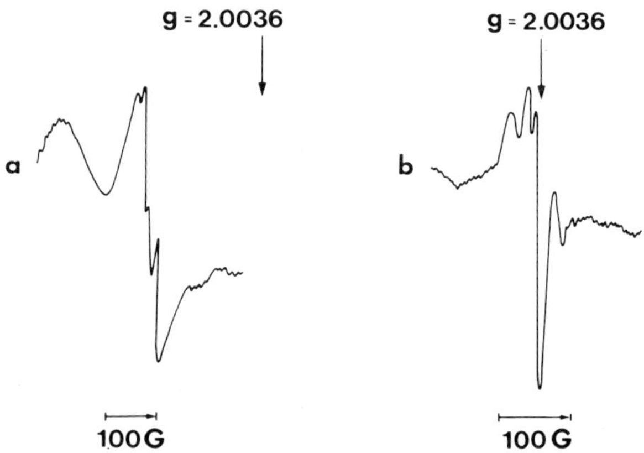

FIG. 4 Fine structures appearing with changes in cavity temperature and at low microwave power. Spectrum a shows the ESR signal in a frozen intact sample of normal cervix at a cavity temperature of -80°C. The increase in temperature from -130°C to -80°C results in the appearance of additional structure to the broad signal centred near to g = 2.14. Conditions used: scan range, 2000 G; power, 50 mW; gain, 10^3; modulation, 16 G; field setting, 3230 G. Spectrum b shows the ESR signal in a frozen powdered sample of normal endometrium at 1 mW power; other conditions: scan range, 2000 G; gain, 4 x 10^2; temperature, -130°C; modulation, 16 G; field setting, 3350 G. The fine structure disappeared with microwave power above 5-10 mW leaving the basic peroxy-type spectrum shown in Fig. 2 for frozen powders.

All samples examined showed relatively little saturation of signal response with increasing microwave power: the intact samples gave no indication of saturation up to 150 mW, whilst the powdered samples showed some extent of saturation above 10 mW (see Benedetto *et al.*, 1981). Again, it was observed that some fine structure was contained within relatively broad peaks, and Fig. 4b shows this for a powdered sample of normal endometrium at 1 mW power: a complex signal is observed that is saturated by increasing the microwave power.

Very similar spectra to those reported above for powdered human samples of normal cervix and endometrium were obtained with frozen powders of rat cervix and seminal vesicles; these studies were done in collaboration with Dr. Aldo Tomasi. No similar signals were observed in samples of rat liver or kidney, but a small and similar signal was seen in samples of rat lung. The strong signals in seminal vesicles were considerably reduced in intensity by an intraperitoneal injection of 100 mg/kg body weight of indomethacin; this latter result suggests that the species responsible for the ESR signal is arising via a cyclo-oxygenase catalysed step.

Plate I gives some recent data obtained in collaboration with Dr. G. Nöhammer concerning the content of reactive -SH in epithelium and stroma of sections of normal and malignant cervix. It can be seen that I(a) in normal cervix sections there is a significant difference in reactive -SH between epithelium and stroma after a 7 h staining with DDD reagent; I(b) in the tumour sections the ratio of staining in the epithelium to that in the stroma is considerably decreased not only in the cancer area, but also in the epithelium adjacent to the malignant lesion.

DISCUSSION

The results that I have described confirm those of Slater and Cook (1970) in demonstrating unequivocally that samples of normal human cervix and endometrium give very strong ESR signals both with intact and powdered materials. Moreover, these present studies have established that there is indeed a significant *quantitative* difference between the normal and malignant samples in relation to their ESR features.

The latter demonstration is consistent with a number of other reports already in the literature, and which show clearly that tumour samples in general have a smaller content of free radicals (as detected by ESR) than their control normal tissues: this point has been discussed comprehensively and cogently by Swartz (1972, 1979).

The strong ESR signal in normal intact cervix or endometrium, *g*-value between 2.11 and 2.15, appears to us to result from a metal-associated paramagnetic species. Our reasons for this belief are based on the *g*-value and the power-saturation characteristics of the signal. For reasons discussed below, we consider the metal ion to be most probably Fe^{2+}.

In *powdered* samples of cervix and endometrium the *g*-values, the anisotropy of the signal, and the power-saturation behaviour are consistent with the major species being an organic peroxy-radical $RO_2^{\bullet}$. For background references on the ESR behaviour of organic peroxy-radicals see Chien and Boss (1967), Kuznetsov and Radtsig (1972); and Ysebaert-Vanneste *et al.* (1972). The peroxy-radical in powdered samples of cervix and endometrium could be formed artefactually during grinding under nitrogen, since mechanical grinding is known to be capable of generating new radical species (Urbanski, 1967). However, we favour a different explanation based on the conversion by grinding of an iron-based paramagnetic species present in intact samples to an organic peroxy-radical in the frozen powder. Firstly, we noted a correlation between the intensity of the g = 2.11-2.15 signal in intact samples with the g = 2.002 signal in subsequently ground-up powders; this is consistent with an interconversion process. Secondly, we observed *both* signals in some intact samples indicating that the generation of the presumed peroxy-radical can occur physiologically, and without grinding.

Uterine tissues are known to be active in prostaglandin dependent reactions, and in prostanoid synthesis (Samuelsson *et al.*, 1978; Ellwood *et al.*, 1980; Massobrio *et al.*, 1981); lipid peroxidation also occurs readily in such tissues during incubations *in vitro* (Falkay *et al.*, 1977). Both enzyme processes (prostaglandin biosynthesis and lipoxygenase activity) involve, or are stimulated by, iron complexes (De Groot *et al.*, 1975; Pistorius *et al.*, 1976; Hemler *et al.*, 1976; Rao *et al.*, 1978; Van der Ouderaa *et al.*, 1979) so that the ESR signal observed in the intact sample *may* represent a ferrous-oxygen complex in close association with a polyunsaturated fatty acid (PUFA) required as substrate for the enzymic cyclo-oxygenase or lipoxygenase reactions. Mechanical grinding under nitrogen *may* alter the molecular associations such that the product is essentially a fatty acid peroxy species. A diagrammatic view of this suggestion is shown in Fig. 5.

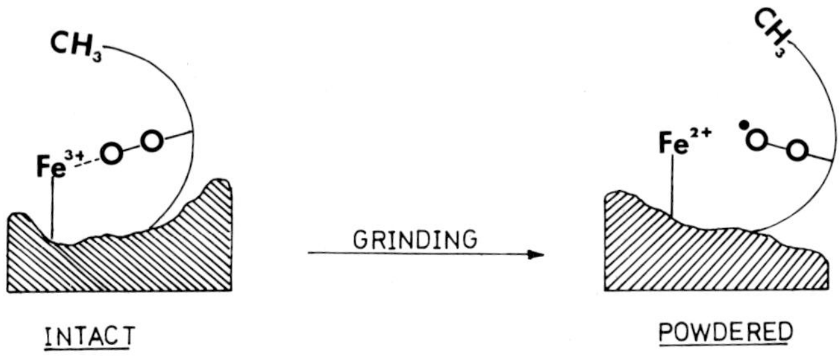

FIG. 5 Diagrammatic view of the effect of mechanical grinding on the molecular association between a ferrous-oxygen complex and a polyunsaturated fatty acid required as substrate for the enzymic cyclo-oxygenase or lipoxygenase reactions.

Some evidence in favour of the above scheme involving cyclo-oxygenase is our finding that corresponding signals (g = 2.002) in *powders* of rat tissues were observed only in those tissues examined that are known to be active in the synthesis of prostaglandins: cervix, seminal vesicles. The same type of ESR signal was observed also, but to a lesser extent, in lung. Moreover, we have recently observed (A. Tomasi, C. Benedetto and T.F. Slater, unpublished experiments) that treatment of male rats with the cyclo-oxygenase inhibitor indomethacin reduces the signal seen subsequently in powdered samples of seminal vesicles.

Some arguments *against* the powdered sample species arising from prostaglandin-type reactions, however, can be based on the general finding that prostaglandin synthesis is increased in cancer samples (see Karmali, 1980) whereas our observation of ESR signal intensities show decreases. This seeming incompatibility would be explained if it could be shown that the "transit-time" of PUFA through the intermediate peroxy-radical to the cyclic endoperoxide PGG_2 is decreased in tumours, thereby *decreasing* the steady-state peroxy-radical concentration as measured by ESR (Fig. 6) and increasing the concentration of end-products.

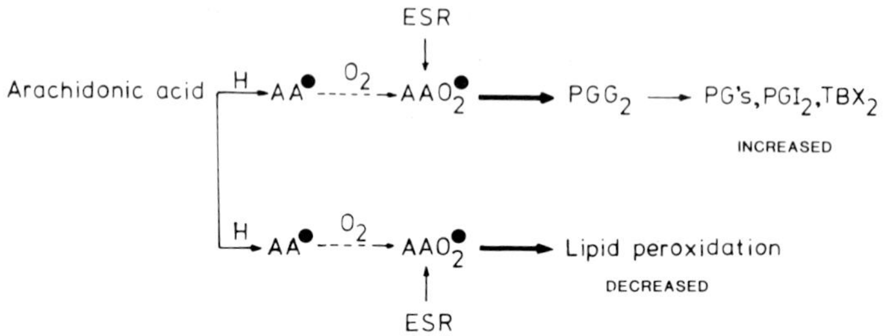

FIG. 6 Prostaglandin and lipid peroxidation pathways in tumours.

Returning now to the human samples as examined by ESR, we did not observe any significant influence of the phase of the menstrual cycle of the patients on the ESR signals seen in normal tissues. In contrast to this, however, studies on the rat (A. Tomasi, unpublished experiments) show marked ESR changes in cervix samples over the oestrus cycle. Non-malignant conditions examined such as cervicitis, parakeratosis, etc. did not show any recognisable differences in ESR behaviour to normal.

Our studies, so far, with samples of carcinoma *in situ* have been restricted to only three samples. Nonetheless, the results are intrinsically interesting and potentially important. No significant ESR signals were observed in two of the three samples of carcinoma *in situ* examined. Since most of the tissue content of such samples is probably "apparently normal" tissue (the *in situ* lesion is generally microsopic) then it would be expected that the ESR response should be strong, and reflect the major contribution of normal tissue to the sample. The absence of signal in two of the three samples studied suggests that a small tumour cell population may have biologically and chemically detectable effects on the surrounding normal tissue, even over a considerable distance in cellular terms. In this context, we can note that liver tumours can cause considerable effects on neighbouring liver tissue, for example in cytochrome P_{450} content (Sultatos and Vessell, 1980). More importantly, in relation to our own studies on carcinoma of the cervix, our recent work with Professor Schauenstein and Dr. Nöhammer has demonstrated a decrease in the reactive -SH content of "normal" epithelium adjacent to malignant lesions. Such effects as demonstrated by ESR and microspectrophotometry, if confirmed by studies with many more *in situ* samples, are of intrinsic biological and pathological importance, in our opinion.

ACKNOWLEDGEMENTS

This work was supported by the National Foundation for Cancer Research. I am very grateful to Professor T.F. Slater and to Professor M.U. Dianzani for their encouragement and scientific support and Professor Slater for providing Fig. 6. Also, I thank Dr. A. Tomasi and Dr. G. Nöhammer for their collaboration.

REFERENCES

Adelstein, A.M. and White, G.C. (1977). *In* "Understanding Cancer: A Guide for the Caring Professions" (Eds. I. Burn and R.Ll. Mayrick), pp.24-30, Her Majesty's Stationery Office, London.

Barnett, J.R. and Seligman, A.M. (1952). *Science* 116, 323-327.

Benedetto, C., Bocci, A., Dianzani, M.U., Ghiringhello, B., Slater, T. F., Tomasi, A. and Vannini, V. (1981). *Cancer Res.* 41, 2936-2942.

Boyes, D.A. and Worth, A.J. (1976). *In* "The Cervix" (Eds. J.A. Jordan and A. Singer), pp.404-411, W.B. Saunders Co. Ltd., London.

Brennan, M.J., Cole, T. and Singley, J.A. (1966). *Proc. Soc. Exp. Biol. Med.* 123, 715-718.

Briggs, R.M. (1979). *Obstet. Gynaecol. Surv.* 34, 70-99.

Cairns, J. (1978). *In* "Cancer: Science and Society", pp.6-14, W.H. Freeman and Co., San Francisco.

Cassai, E., Rotola, A., Meneguzzi, G., Milanesi, G., Garsia, S., Remotti, G. and Rizzi, G. (1981). *Eur. J. Cancer* 17, 685-693.

Catterall, R.D. (1981). *Lancet* (i), 315-319.

Chien, J.C.W. and Boss, C.R. (1967). *J. Am. Cancer Soc.* 89, 571-575.

Collins, J., Allen, L.H., Donner, A. and Adams, D. (1980). *Lancet* (ii), 961-964.

De Groot, J.J.M.C., Veldink, G.A., Vliegenthart, J.F.G., Boldingh, J., Wever, R. and Van Gelder, B.F. (1975). *Biochim. Biophys. Acta* 377, 71-79.

Doll, R. (1977). *In* "Origins of Human Cancer" Book A, pp.1-12 (Eds. H.H. Hiatt, J.D. Watson and J.A. Winsten), Cold Spring Harbor Laboratory Conference on Cell Proliferation, Vol. 4, Cold Spring Harbor Laboratory, U.S.A.

Editorial (1975). *Br. Med. J.* (i), 294.

Ellwood, D.A., Mitchell, M.D., Anderson, A.M.B. and Turnbull, A.C. (1980). *Br. J. Obstet. Gynaecol.* 87, 210-214.

Elwood, J.M., Cole, P., Rothman, K.J. and Kaplan, S.D. (1977). *J. Natl. Cancer Inst.* 59, 1055-1060.

Esterbauer, H. (1972). *Acta Histochem.* 42, 351-355.

Esterbauer, H. (1973). *Acta Histochem.* 47, 94-105.

Esterbauer, H., Nöhammer, G., Schauenstein, E. and Weber, P. (1973). *Acta Histochem.* 47, 106-114.
Evans, D.M.D. (Ed.) (1970). *In* "Cytology Automation", Second Tenovus Symposium, E. and S. Livingstone Ltd., Edinburgh.
Falkay, H., Herczeg, J. and Sas, M. (1977). *Biochem. Biophys. Res. Commun.* 79, 843-851.
Gusberg, S.B. (1980). *N. Engl. J. Med.* 302, 729-731.
Harris, R.W.C., Brinton, L.A., Cowdell, R.H., Skegg, D.C.G., Smith, P.G., Vessey, M.P. and Doll, R. (1980). *Br. J. Cancer* 42, 359-369.
Hemler, M., Lands, W.E.M. and Smith, W.L. (1976). *J. Biol. Chem.* 251, 5575-5579.
Jick, H., Walker, A.M. and Rothman, K.J. (1980). *Am. J. Public Health* 70, 264-267.
Karmali, R.A. (1980). *Prostaglandins Med.* 5, 11-28.
Kessler, I.I. (1979). *Obstet. Gynaecol. Surv.* 34, 790-794.
Kuznetsov, A.N. and Radtsig, V.A. (1972). *Chem. Phys. Lett.* 17, 377-380.
Massobrio, M., Benedetto, C. and De Andrea, G. (1981). *Minerva Endocrinol.* 6, 1-30.
Meisels, A., Begin, R. and Schneider, V. (1977). *Cancer* 40, 3076-3081.
Muir, C.S. (1975). *In* "Persons at High Risk of Cancer" (Ed. J.F. Fraumeni, Jnr.) pp.293-304, Academic Press, New York.
Muruyama, T., Kataoka, N., Negase, S., Nakada, N., Sato, H. and Sasaki, J. (1971). *Cancer Res.* 31, 179-184.
Nöhammer, G. (1977). *Acta Histochem.* 59, 317-328.
Pistorius, E.K., Axelrod, B. and Palmer, G. (1976). *J. Biol. Chem.* 251, 7144-7148.
Ploem, J.S. (1980). *In* "Trends in Enzyme Histochemistry and Cytochemistry" Ciba Foundation Symposium 73, new series (Eds. D. Evered and M. O'Connor), pp.275-299, Excerpta Medica, Amsterdam.
Poste, G. and Waterson, A.P. (1975). *In* "Gynaecological Malignancy: Clinical and Experimental Studies (Eds. M.G. Bush and R.W. Taylor), pp.87-108, Bailliere Tindall, London.
Rao, G.H.R., Gerrard, J.M., Eaton, J.W. and White, J.G. (1978). *Prostaglandins Med.* 1, 55-70.
Rees, K.R., Slater, T.F., Gibbs, D.F. and Stagg, B.H. (1970). *Am. J. Obstet. Gynaecol.* 107, 857-864.
Riggott, J.M. (Ed.) (1971). *In* "The Early Diagnosis of Cancer of the Cervix", University of Hull, U.K.
Samuelsson, B., Goldyne, M., Grandstrom, E., Hamburg, M., Hammerstrom, S. and Malmsten, C. (1968). *Ann. Rev. Biochem.* 47, 997-1029.
Slater, T.F. and Cook, J.W.R. (1970). *In* "Cytology Automation" (Ed. D.M.D. Evans), pp.108-120, E. and S. Livingstone, Edinburgh.
Stallworthy, J. and Wiernik, G. (1976). *In* "The Cervix" (Eds. J.A. Jordan and A. Singer), pp.474-493, W.B. Saunders Co. Ltd., London.
Sultatos, L.E. and Vesell, E.S. (1980). *Proc. Natl. Acad. Sci. U.S.A.* 77, 600-603.
Swartz, H. (1972). *Adv. Cancer Res.* 15, 227-252.
Swartz, H. (1979). *In* "Submolecular Biology and Cancer" Ciba Foundation Symposium 67, new series. (Eds. G.E.W. Wolstenholme, D.W. Fitzsimons and J. Whelan), pp.107-124, Excerpta Medica, Amsterdam.
Terris, M., Wilson, F. and Nelson, J.H. (1980). *Am. J. Epidemiol.* 112, 253-257.

Van der Ouderaa, F.J., Buytentiek, M., Sukkerveer, F.J. and Van Dorp, D.A. (1979). *Biochim. Biophys. Acta* 572, 29-42.
Wright, N.H., Vessey, M.P., Kenward, B., McPherson, K. and Doll, R. (1978). *Br. J. Cancer* 38, 273-279.
Wynder, E.L., Escher, G.C. and Mantel, N. (1966). *Cancer* 19, 489-520.
Ysebaert-Vanneste, M., Vanneste, W.H. and Mason, H.S. (1972). *Biochim. Biophys. Acta* 267, 268-274.

DISCUSSION

Slater: Before opening this very interesting paper for general discussion I should like to invite Dr Nöhammer to show just a couple of slides which follow on the last aspect that Dr Benedetto described relating to reactive SH.

Nöhammer: I propose to make some comments which will describe the "additional microspectrometrical measurements" which Dr Benedetto mentioned at the end of her paper. The measurements were intended to assist in interpreting the ESR measurements. Our group in Graz, led by Professor Schauenstein, started these particular microspectrometrical investigations about two years ago. Most of the samples which we investigated came from the Institute of Professor Dianzani in Turin, the rest were prepared by Professor Bajardi in Graz. The sections of the samples of uterus were stained using histochemical methods that have been developed, optimised and quantified by our group (Esterbauer, 1972, 1973; Esterbauer *et al.*, 1973; Nöhammer *et al.*, 1973; Nöhammer, 1977; Nöhammer *et al.*, 1981; Schauenstein *et al.*, 1980). The staining methods used for these investigations were originally developed for our own investigations concerned with quantitative cytospectrometry of the cells from cervical smears (Nöhammer *et al.*, 1977; Schauenstein *et al.*, 1977; Bajardi *et al.*, 1977, 1978). We started those investigations about eight years ago in collaboration with Professor Bajardi.

One of the staining methods we used is DDD-7h-staining for so-called reactive protein-SH-groups (SH_r). I shall present some preliminary results with microspectrometrical measurements of sections from the cervix uteri, stained with DDD for reactive SH.

In portio sections taken from normal cases, the stratified squamous epithelium is well stained and well preserved. An abrupt decrease of the optical density from the epithelium to the stroma is particularly noticeable (see Plate 1 in this paper). The basal line clearly separates two areas of quite different optical densities. Our microspectrometrical measurements comprise more or less equal parts of the epithelium and the proximate adjoining stroma. The total measured area was about 1 mm^2 per single case and single type of epithelium.

TABLE 1 Sulphydryl staining in cervix from normal cases

	n	Epithelium*	Stroma*	ES-ratio
Normal epithelium	21	0.362 ± 0.148	0.133 ± 0.061	2.829 ± 0.778
Metaplastic epithelium	7	0.529 ± 0.196	0.160 ± 0.045	3.341 ± 0.894

n = number of separate sections examined. *Values are the means ± Std. Dev. of the extinctions (μm^2).

Table 1 shows preliminary results from "normal" cases (with mild and severe chronic cervicitis, parakeratosis and metaplasia). We measured the mean optical density, as the sum of all single extinctions per area unit, divided by the number of all single measurements. The absolute value of the mean optical density depends on the thickness of the single sections. Because of the variable thickness of the sections, for comparison of the different types of epithelium we used the mean epithelium-stroma-ratio. (Together with each single part of an epithelium we measured a more or less equal part of the immediately adjoining stroma so that we could calculate the ratio between the mean optical densities of the epithelium and the stroma (ES-ratio)). The mean ES-ratios of the distinct groups and types of epithelium are listed in Tables 1 and 2. We have made a distinction between normal epithelium and the so-called benign metaplastic squamous epithelium. The metaplastic epithelium is characterised by lack of glycogen accumulation within the intermediate cell layer. Also in this group are cases with basal cell hyperplasia. From 23 normal cases investigated, the ES-ratios of both the normal and the metaplastic epithelium are about 3.

TABLE 2 Sulphydryl staining in cervix from cases with cervical neoplasia

	n	Epithelium*	Stroma*	ES-ratio
Normal epithelium	11	0.283 ± 0.186	0.130 ± 0.088	2.253 ± 0.363
Metaplastic epithelium	8	0.368 ± 0.361	0.141 ± 0.095	2.249 ± 0.945
Dysplastic++ epithelium	17	0.320 ± 0.222	0.182 ± 0.106	1.648 ± 0.456
Carcinoma *in situ*	8	0.276 ± 0.180	0.208 ± 0.125	1.312 ± 0.169
Invasive carcinoma	3	0.250 ± 0.044	0.153 ± 0.040	1.673 ± 0.291

n= number of sections examined. *Values are the means ± Std. Dev. of the extinctions (μm^2).

With sections from cases with carcinoma *in situ* (CIS), stained with DDD for SH_r if you locate the area of the carcinoma and try to find the basal line, you can see a striking difference in comparison with the normal cases (see Plate 1 in this paper). The ES-ratio has now changed strongly.

Table 2 shows these changes in the ES-ratios of cases with cervical neoplasia. You can see the decrease of the ES-ratios of all types of epithelium of the neoplasia cases compared with the normals. Two facts should be emphasised: (1) The mean ES-ratio in the case of CIS is lower than for normals. (2) The mean ES-ratios of the dysplastic epithelia and especially of the metaplastic epithelia are decreased significantly compared with those of the normal cases.

Finally, I should mention that these preliminary results (from 23 normal and 19 neoplasia cases) confirm the supposition that in the case of a malignant transformation of the cervical epithelium quasi-normal parts of the surrounding tissue have also changed biochemically. We are able to demonstrate these changes for the first time as a decrease of the ES-ratio. The decrease of the ES-ratio of the metaplastic epithelium of neoplasia cases compared with the corresponding ES-ratio of the normals points to the possibility of early cancer diagnosis. But this is a project for the future and its realisation requires first of all a careful statistical comparison of these preliminary results that come from a collaboration with Professor Bajardi, Dr C. Benedetto, Professor M.U. Dianzani, Professor E. Schauenstein, Professor T.F. Slater and myself.

Slater: The reason I asked Dr Nöhammer to speak immediately after Dr Benedetto's presentation is that the ESR work described by Dr Benedetto is now moving very rapidly towards the micro-spectrophotometric project of Dr Nöhammer. We will now proceed with the discussion on Dr Benedetto's work.

Lohmann: You ascribe one of your signals to Fe^{2+} that means to the high spin state of iron Fe^{2+}. How can you exclude Fe^{3+} either in the low spin or high spin state?

Slater: Perhaps I could ask Professor Symons, who is collaborating with us on this problem, if he has any comments on this point of Professor Lohmann's concerning iron 2^+ or iron 3^+ as being responsible for this strong signal.

Symons: I'm not sure really about the question, but I think you are detecting iron 3^+ rather than iron 2^+. It's very rare that iron 2^+ would give a signal about 4 K if at all. Relaxation processes are very efficient and very often the signal has moved right out of range of the spectrometer. So I would suspect a form of iron 3^+, possibly low spin. I should need to see the spectrum.

Benedetto: The *g* values in question lie in the range 2.11 to 2.15.

Symons: Then it sounds like low spin iron 3^+.

Mason: I have a two-part question, the first part of which is how do you prepare your powder samples? and when you have answered that I can ask the second part.

Benedetto: As I said very briefly what we call powdered samples are samples taken immediately after operation, put into plastic tubes in liquid nitrogen, powdered under liquid nitrogen always before ESR analysis, and transferred the powder into ESR turbes prior to ESR analysis. The actual powdering was done by hand using a pestle and mortar.

Mason: The species that you describe as peroxy radicals could conceivably arise from the physical stress placed on the sample leading to bond cleavage, and then reaction of carbon centred radicals with liquid oxygen, which is always a contaminant of liquid nitrogen. You can check for such possibilities by dissolving $^{17}O_2$ in liquid nitrogen. Liquid O_2 has the higher boiling point and will stay there for a while, and in this case the peroxy radicals formed during the grinding, as a result of the grinding, will have a different ESR spectrum in the presence of liquid nitrogen containing $^{17}O_2$ (see Dimmey and Gordy, 1980).

Benedetto: We thought, at a certain point, that the signal we were seeing in powdered samples could be due to an artefact, in a way, on grinding. But the reason why we now think it's probably not an artefact is the fact that we saw a similar signal to that in powdered samples in some intact samples, so we think that this is something which could be present physiologically, and not only produced as a result of the actual mechanical process. But, of course, your suggestion is very valuable.

Slater: If I could add one other thing, we only see this type of "powdered signal" in very few tissues: we see it in normal cervix and endometrium, in normal seminal vesicle and, to a very small extent, in lung. We don't see it in liver, or spleen, or brain, or in muscle, and we don't see it very much in tumour tissue. In all of those cases, of course, there is the same amount of liquid oxygen dissolved in the liquid nitrogen, and the grinding process is the same. Moreover, as Dr Benedetto said the fact that we see both signals in some intact samples, where no grinding has occurred, leads us to presume that what we are looking at basically is a conversion of some paramagnetic species mainly contributing to the intact signal into another species giving a g-value as observed mainly in powdered samples. Although we think this conversion can occur to a limited extent physiologically, we feel the process is much accentuated by the mechanical grinding process. In this sense, the peroxy-type signal seen in powders is artefactual, but we feel it is telling us something interesting and important about the paramagnetic behaviour of normal and abnormal cervix.

Mason: Peroxy radicals are always presumed to exist naturally as well.

Slater: But the signals we see in powdered samples of normal cervix suggest a very high concentration.

Mason: We have a collaboration with Dr Thomas Eling concerning the free radicals of prostaglandin synthetase, and there are a couple of results which might be of interest to you. One is that we were able to spin trap the arachidonic acid carbon-centred radical, the first intermediate in the scheme you showed (Mason *et al.*, 1980). Secondly, we became interested in oxygen-centred free radical described by Egan, Kuehl and co-workers at Merck. This is the species that arises from reactions of prostaglandin G2. In fact, it arises from the reaction of either prostaglandin G2, any organic hydroperoxide, or even hydrogen peroxide, with haemoproteins. It forms an oxidised free radical containing haemoprotein; the ESR signal has a *g*-value of 2.005 (Kalyanaraman, B., Mason, R., Tainer, B.E. and Eling, T.E., unpublished work). It's quite easily observable at liquid nitrogen temperature, its line width is about 25 gauss peak-to-peak, and, upon warming to room temperature, the signal disappears. Its saturation properties are something like the free radicals that you have been observing, and since we were interested in relating the results to prostaglandins, this might be of some interest to you.

Benedetto: Thank you very much.

Adams: Could I make a general point that concerns problems that arise when one is dealing with excised tissue. We are also involved with drug metabolism studies where we analyse excised tumour tissue. We have run into problems due to the rapid speed at which excised tissue becomes hypoxic, and this can obviously generally affect the metabolic state of the tissue. We have to place the tissue in liquid nitrogen immediately after excision. If one is concerned with some consequence of the redox state of the cell as you are, and particularly concerned with SH levels, the problem of induced hypoxia has to be controlled. Do you have any thoughts on this?

Benedetto: We thought of that and the only thing we have looked at up until now is just to see if there was an influence of the time between the actual hysterectomy or cone biopsy and the moment that we put the sample into liquid nitrogen.

Adams: Do you do it, or do the surgeons do it?

Benedetto: No, I do it. I am quite certain of the time, and of course, we have observed this in a relative sense, we did not leave the samples for more than two or three hours, of course, compared to our normal procedure where we work as fast as possible. We couldn't really see any significant effect.

Adams: Tissue can become hypoxic in a matter of minutes, post surgery.

Benedetto: This was a very gross or coarse check.

Slater: Perhaps I could add, we see identical behaviour in the rat where we can get the tissue frozen within a few seconds after exposing the tissues under anaesthetic. So, we take your point. In fact, it's very difficult to control this factor better than simply working as fast as possible, and that is what we try to do, with Dr Benedetto taking the samples immediately in the theatre and then rapidly freezing with all the subsequent operations under liquid nitrogen.

Of course, hypoxia is relative in the sense that if one uses freeze clamping which we have done now for nearly 20 years in relation to nucleotide redox levels, one can essentially preserve the redox state of certain tissue components such as the nicotinamide adenine dinucleotises for example. In other cases, as you have said, like with Professor Beinert's studies on non-haem iron, one has to try to work even faster if that is possible. On the other hand, it is probable that with less sensitive indicators of the tissue redox-state, like the ESR signals that we have seen here, we can probably get away with seconds or even minutes, because we don't see any change, as Dr Benedetto said. If we store normal tissue at room temperature for minutes where surely it becomes virtually completely anoxic, then we don't see the change from the normal to the malignant condition that we see in the human samples. So that leads us to conclude, basically, that hypoxia is not the cause of the effects that Dr Benedetto has reported. But, nonetheless, we take the point that all tissue taken at human operations is sure to be oxygen-deficient. But the effects on redox couples are going to be relative depending on which parameter you measure.

Swartz: I would interpret it slightly differently. I think it does support the results, but the point is that it can't be a differential hypoxia of the tumour because probably normal and tumour are both fully hypoxic. No matter how quickly you work and, therefore, the difference is a real one and, therefore, certainly not related to the different vascular supply or different rates of hypoxia of the two tissues.

Slater: Can I suggest one extra piece of evidence that what we are looking at has some physiological significance - it is the change in the ESR signals that Dr Benedetto has reported over the oestrus cycle. Whereas if it was completely artefactual and dependent entirely on the development of anoxia we would not expect to see that. Perhaps I could invite Dr Tomasi to show two slides where in the experimental condition the signals show clear oestrus cycle-dependence.

Tomasi: A strong free radical signal arising from normal human cervix, which is modified in neoplastic cervix samples, has been reported using both intact tissues or tissues which have been ground under liquid nitrogen (Slater and Cook, 1970; Benedetto *et al.*, 1981).

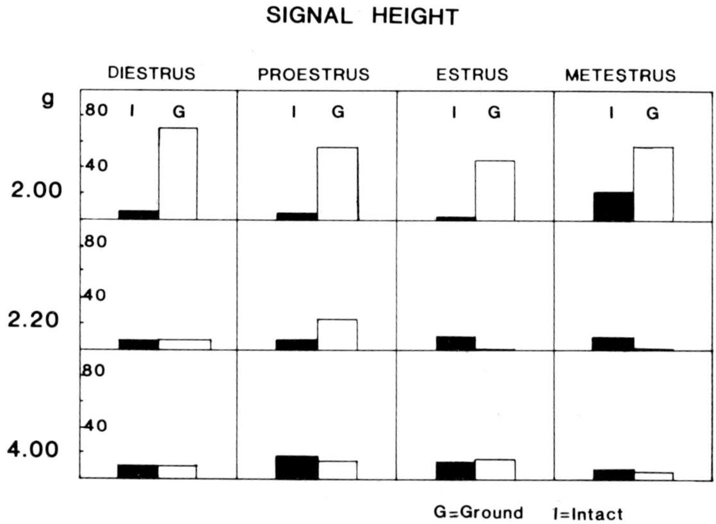

FIG. 1 Variations in the intensity of the three main signals at different stages of oestrus (mean of 5-12 experiments). The stages of oestrus were classified according to Hamilton (1947). Intact samples of cervix frozen in liquid nitrogen are shown in the solid columns, the open columns represent samples of uterine cervix frozen and ground in liquid nitrogen. The usual instrument conditions were: microwave power = 25 mW, modulation amplitude = 10 G, cavity temperature = 123 K.

I want briefly to report on an electron spin resonance (ESR) study performed on rat uterus and cervix, the results of which are comparable to those from tissues of human origin. Moreover, we checked the possible influence exerted on the signal by the oestrus cycle and by an inhibitor of prostaglandin synthetase. The oestrus stage was determined using the Papanicolaou method for smear staining. Figure 1 shows the behaviour of the three main ESR signals at different stages of oestrus. Intact rat cervix does not show significant variations in the absorptions at g = 2.20 and g = 4. The free radical signal at g = 2.00 is almost absent during oestrus, increases during the metoestrus, and decreases slowly during the two remaining stages. The signal arising from ground tissue shows an important difference at g = 2.00; the anisotopic signal is identical to that obtained from

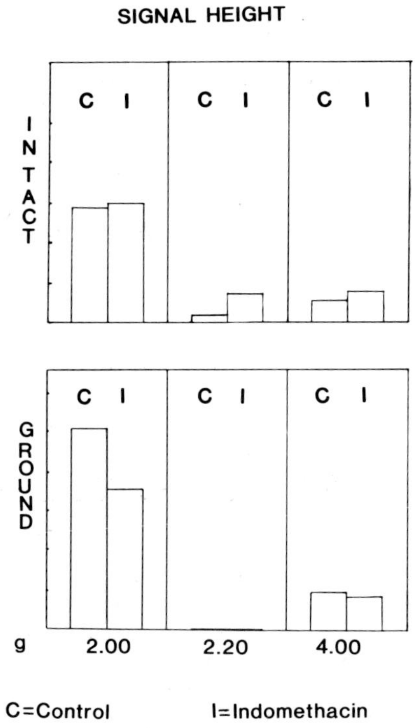

FIG. 2 The effect of indomethacin-incubation on cervix is shown (mean of three experiments). Cervix cut into small pieces was incubated in Ham's medium F-12 with or without indomethacin (100 μM) at 37°C for 10 min, then frozen in liquid nitrogen and recorded as r ground at the same conditions as in Fig. 1.

human samples (Benedetto, 1981). The absorptions at $g = 2.20$ are labile and disappear during oestrus and metoestrus. After incubating small pieces of rat uterus and cervix in the presence of indomethacin (100 μM) an increase of the signal at $g = 2.20$ is evident (Fig. 2). I believe this is further evidence for the contribution of prostaglandin synthetase to the observed signal.

REFERENCES to Discussion

Bajardi, F., Schauenstein, E., Nöhammer, G. and Unger-Ullmann, C. (1977). *Acta Cytol.* 21, 573-577.
Bajardi, F., Schauenstein, E., Nöhammer, G. and Unger-Ullmann, C. (1978). *Z. Krebsforsch.* 91, 291-299.
Barrnett, J.R. and Seligman, A.M. (1952). *Science* 116, 323-327.
Benedetto, C., Bocci, A., Dianzani, M.U., Ghiringhello, B., Slater, T.F., Tomasi, A. and Vannini, V. (1981). *Cancer Res.* 41, 2936-2942.
Dimmey, L.J. and Gordy, W. (1980). *Proc. Natl. Acad. Sci. USA* 77, 343-346.
Esterbauer, H. (1972). *Acta Histochem.* 42, 351-355.
Esterbauer, H. (1973). *Acta Histochem.* 47, 94-105.
Esterbauer, H., Nöhammer, G., Schauenstein, E. and Weber, P. (1973). *Acta Histochem.* 47, 106-114.
Hamilton, C.E. (1947). *Anat. Rec.* 97, 47-60.
Mason, R.P., Kaylanaraman, B., Tainer, B.E. and Eling, T.E. (1980). *J. Biol. Chem.* 255, 5019-5022.
Nöhammer, G. (1977). *Acta Histochem.* 59, 317-328.
Nöhammer, G., Schauenstein, E. and Weber, P. (1973). *J. Histochem. Cytochem.* 21, 1082-1089.
Nöhammer, G., Schauenstein, E., Bajardi, F. and Unger-Ullmann, C. (1977). *Acta Cytol.* 21, 341-344.
Nöhammer, G., Desoye, G. and Khoschsorur, G. (1981). *Histochemistry* 71, 291-300.
Schauenstein, E., Nöhammer, G., Bajardi, F. and Unger-Ullmann, C. (1977). *Acta Cytol.* 21, 345-349.
Schauenstein, E., Desoye, G. and Nöhammer, G. (1980). *Histochemistry* 68, 75-90.
Slater, T.F. and Cook, S.R.W. (1970). *In* "Cytology Automation" (Ed. D.M.D. Evans), pp.108-120. Livingstone, Edinburgh.

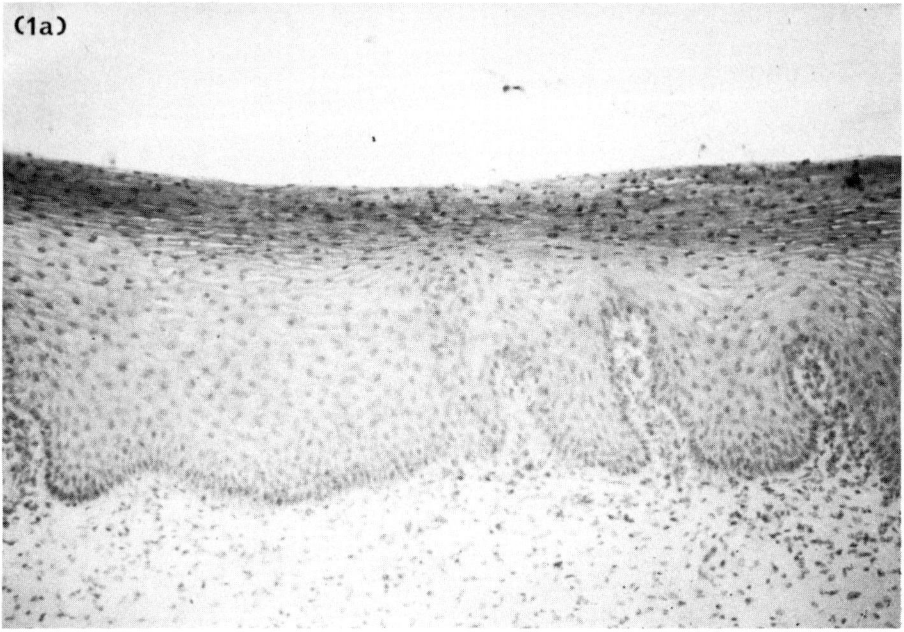

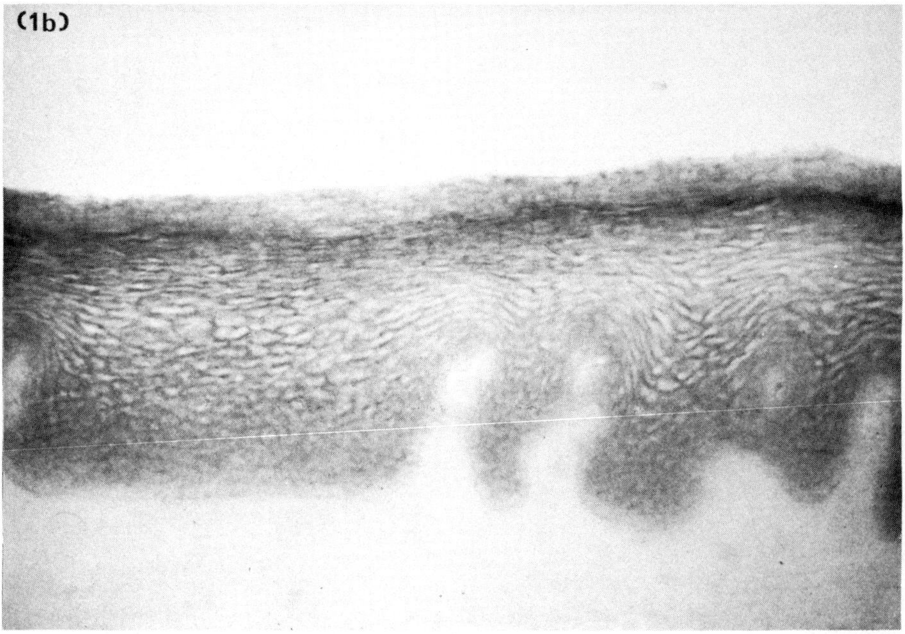

PLATE I Content of reactive -SH groups in epithelium and stroma of serial sections of normal and malignant cervix. (1) Sections of normal cervix stained with haematoxylin-eosin and 2,2'-dihydroxy-6,6'-dinaphthyldisulphide (DDD) in 1a and 1b respectively.

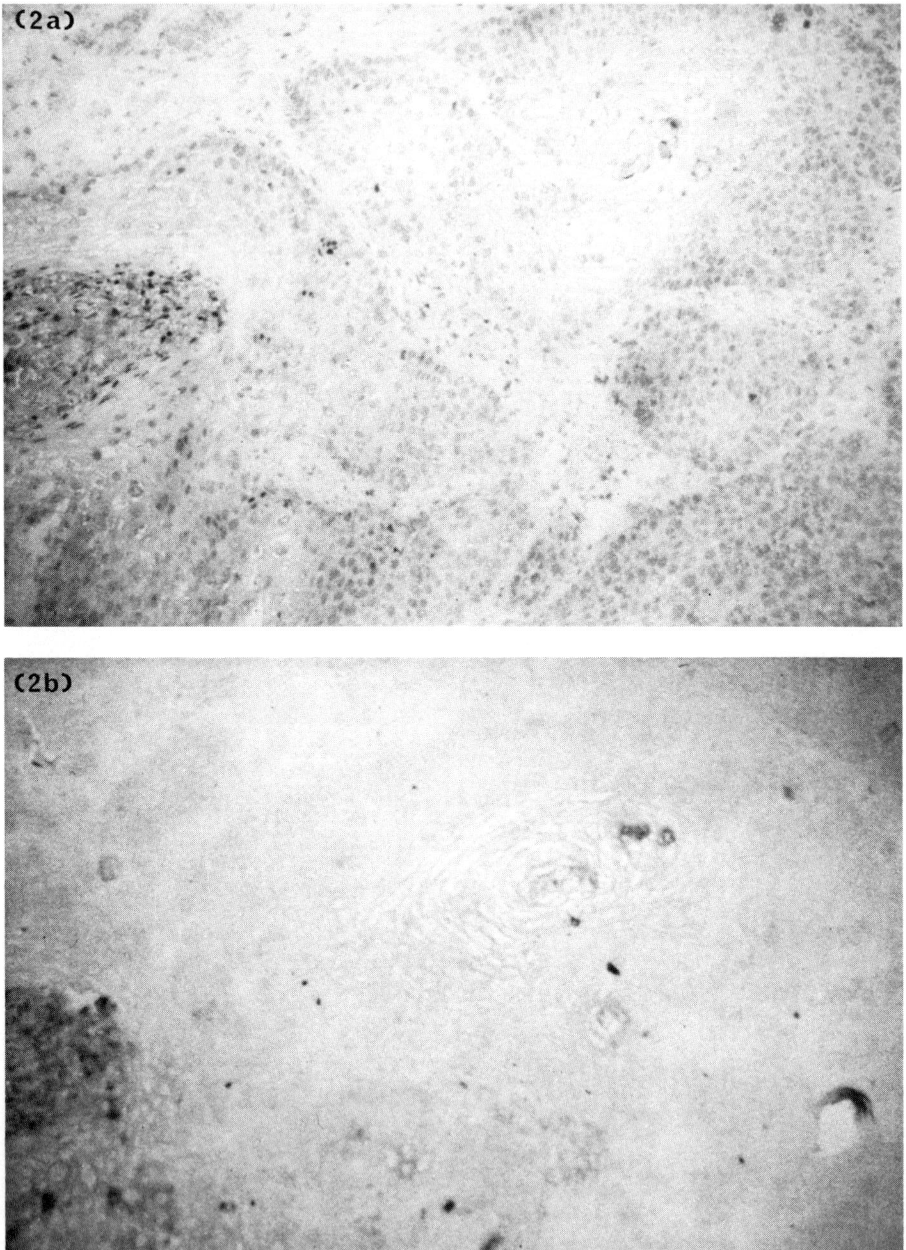

PLATE I (Continued) (2) Sections of invasive carcinoma of the cervix stained with haematoxylin-eosin and DDD in 2a and 2b respectively.

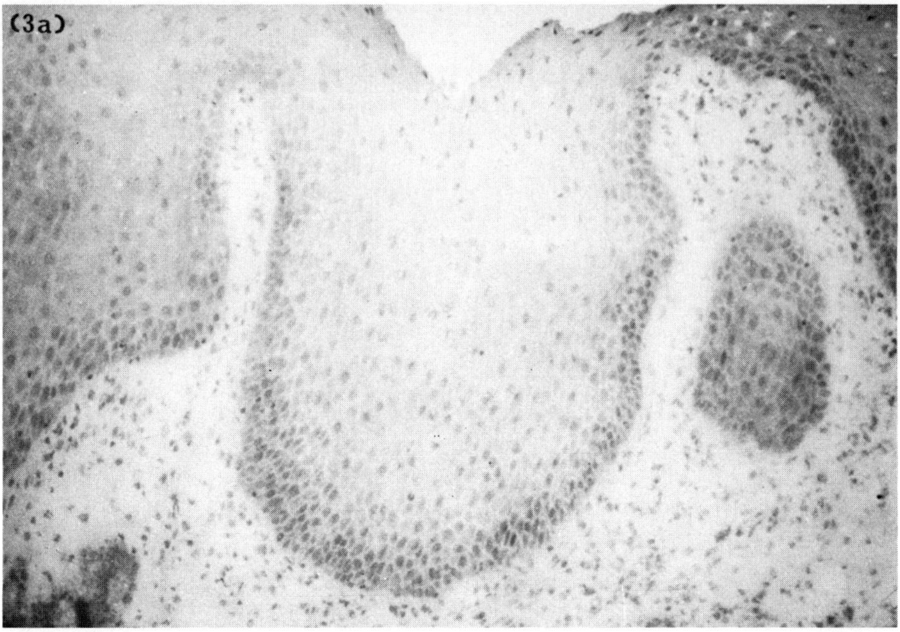

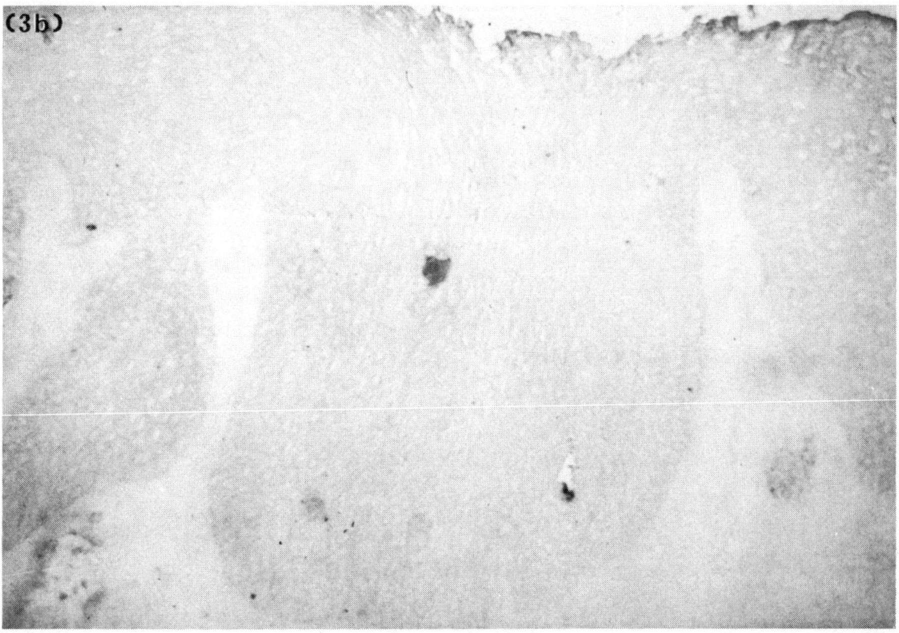

PLATE I (Continued) (3) Epithelium adjacent to the malignant lesion shown in 2a and 2b stained with haematoxylin-eosin and DDD in 3a and 3b respectively.

Free Radicals and Cancer

W. LOHMANN, K.G. BENSCH, H. SAPPER, A. PLEYER, J. SCHREIBER, S.O. KANG, H. LÖFFLER, H. PRALLE, K. SCHWEMMLE and R.D. FILLER

INTRODUCTION

Redox reactions are of importance for biological systems. They are responsible for maintaining normal, optimal biological functions. In the course of these electron transitions organic free radicals might be produced. Since carcinogenic substances might act as electron donors and/or acceptors (Miller, 1970; Szent-Györgyi *et al.*, 1960), they might modify the pathway or the kinetic equilibrium of the electron transitions occurring in healthy tissue. In this way, they might produce free radicals which are not normally present in healthy biological systems and/or modify the spin concentration of the organic free radicals of healthy tissue.

If this working hypothesis is correct, then, differences in the electron spin resonance (ESR) spectra of healthy and neoplastic tissues should be detectable. A number of such investigations have been reported, but they have not led to consistent conclusions (Dodd, 1980; Swartz, 1979). In general, these results provide no evidence of paramagnetic species that are specific for malignancy, although distinct changes in the concentrations of certain radicals occur during malignant development. Real progress can be expected only if, at least in part, an identification of the different ESR peaks is achieved and a suitable interpretation is given.

In this paper we present results obtained with blood and blood constituents from patients with acute lymphatic leukaemia and with bronchial cancer. It will be shown that the spectra obtained are indicative and informative for the disease. They are also cognitive, that is they provide detailed information about the molecular events involved in malignancy whenever their nature is identified.

MATERIALS AND METHODS

One ml of venous blood was drawn without any anticoagulant added, freeze-dried, and 50 mg of each sample was used for measurements at room temperature.

Erythrocytes were obtained from fresh ACD-blood (acid-citrate-dextrose solution used as an anticoagulant) from both healthy and leukaemic donors. The erythrocytes as well as their white ghosts (membranes) were prepared according to methods previously described (Lohmann *et al.*, 1979a; Lohmann *et al.*, 1979e).

The lung samples were obtained immediately following surgical removal from different parts of the lung of 11 patients with bronchial cancer. Details about experimental conditions, e.g. case history and place of excision of the tissue samples, have been published elsewhere (Lohmann *et al.*, 1981b).

Ascorbic acid, H_2O_2, $KMnO_4$ (Merck, Darmstadt), and ascorbate oxidase (EC 1.10.3.3; Boehringer, Mannheim) were added to blood and its constituents or to lung tissue before freeze-drying. Dehydroascorbic acid (DHA) was prepared and kindly donated by Prof. W. Weis, Zentrum für Biochemie, Universität Giessen. D_2O was purchased from Merck, Sharp, and Dohme. The copper containing proteins ceruloplasmin (EC 1.16.3.1; Sigma, Munich) and haemocyanin (Sigma,Munich) were used without further purification.

The electron spin resonance (ESR) spectra of the lyophilised samples were obtained as described elsewhere (Lohmann *et al.*, 1979e).

The ^1H-nuclear magnetic resonance (NMR) spectra were taken with a Varian HA-100 spectrometer operating at 100 MHz in the CW-mode with a probe temperature of 30°C. External TMS (tetramethylsilane) provided the field-frequency lock. The signals were referred to an external *t*-butanol standard with respect to their intensities. All experiments were performed in deuterated acetate buffer (1.0 M, pD 6).

RESULTS AND DISCUSSION

In Fig. 1 the ESR spectra of native blood of healthy volunteers and of patients with acute lymphatic leukaemia are shown. As can be seen, there is an additional peak at g = 2.005 not present in control samples. Furthermore, the spin concentration is increased. It should

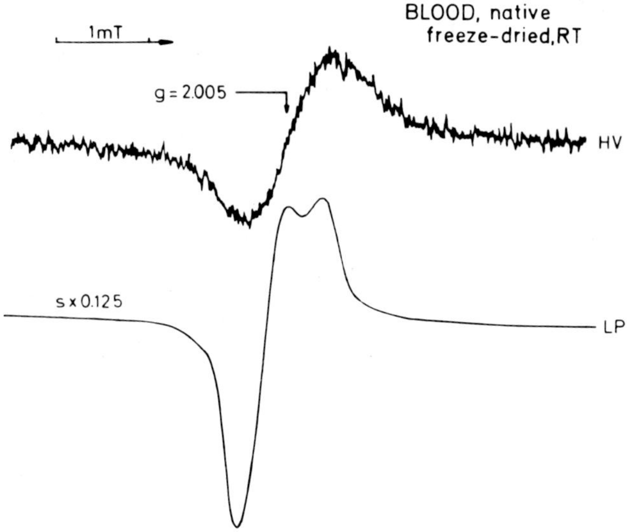

FIG. 1 ESR spectra of native lyophilised blood of healthy volunteers (HV) and of patients with acute lymphatic leukaemia (LP). (s = rel. sensitivity.)

be emphasised that the presence and intensity of the "leukaemic" peak is independent of the leukocyte count, that is patients with a low leukocyte count (1000 - 3000 cells/μl) also exhibit the "leukaemic" spectrum while in cases of non-leukaemic leukocytosis this spectrum is never observed. This is also the case for blood of patients with other types of blood disease or with different types of tumour, e.g. anaemias, lymphomas, plasmocytoma, acute or chronic myeloic leukaemias, spherocytosis, Hodgkin's disease, breast tumour, lung tumour, liver tumour.

The ESR response to therapy in which case patients with acute lymphatic leukaemia have been treated with prednisolone, vincristine, and doxorubicin (Lohmann *et al.*, 1979c) is shown in Fig. 2. The signal amplitude as well as the shape of the signal change with treatment and appear to become almost normal. Concomitantly there is a "normalisation" of the blood count (10 July). It is interesting to note that prolonged treatment again results in an increased spin concentration with a concomitant appearance of an additional peak located slightly downfield (28 July). This latter peak, which has not yet been identified, is probably due to some oxidised state since

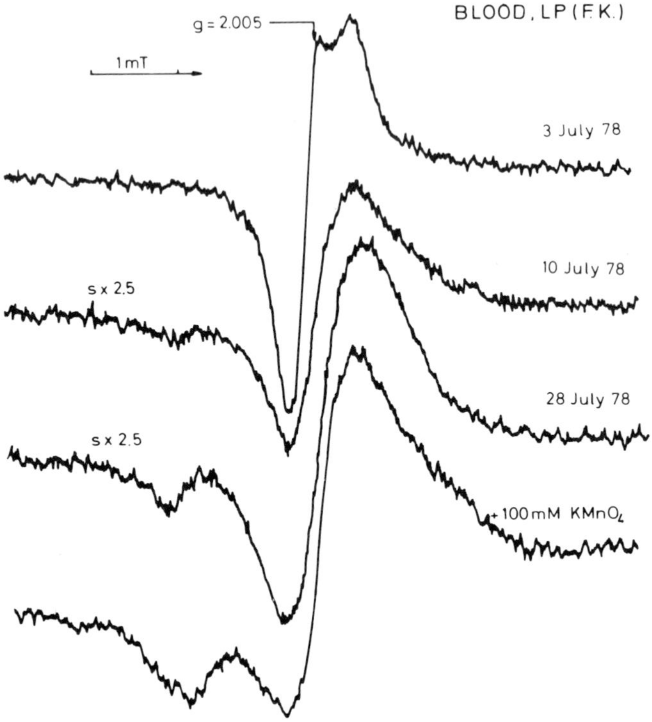

FIG. 2 ESR spectra of native lyophilised blood of a female patient (F.K.) with acute lymphatic leukaemia after treatment with several cytostatic agents (see text). The blood was drawn on the dates given. Upper spectrum: untreated blood. Lower spectrum: 100 mM of $KMnO_4$ added to untreated blood. (s = rel. sensitivity.)

it can also be obtained by adding $KmnO_4$ to the blood of a leukaemic patient (Fig. 2, lower spectrum). It can be assumed, then, that cytostatic agents (at least the ones used) act like oxidising substances. This assumption is further supported by the finding that other oxidising substances, such as H_2O_2 or $CuCl_2$, produce an effect similar to these cytostatic agents (Lohmann *et al.*, 1981c).

The results obtained so far suggest an accumulation of a reducing entity in neoplastic tissue. This agrees well with the generally accepted hypothesis that malignant tissue contains a considerable concentration of antioxidants (Duchesne, 1977; Harrington, 1967; Neish and Rylett, 1963; Neish *et al.*, 1964; Shuster, 1955; Ziegler, 1960).

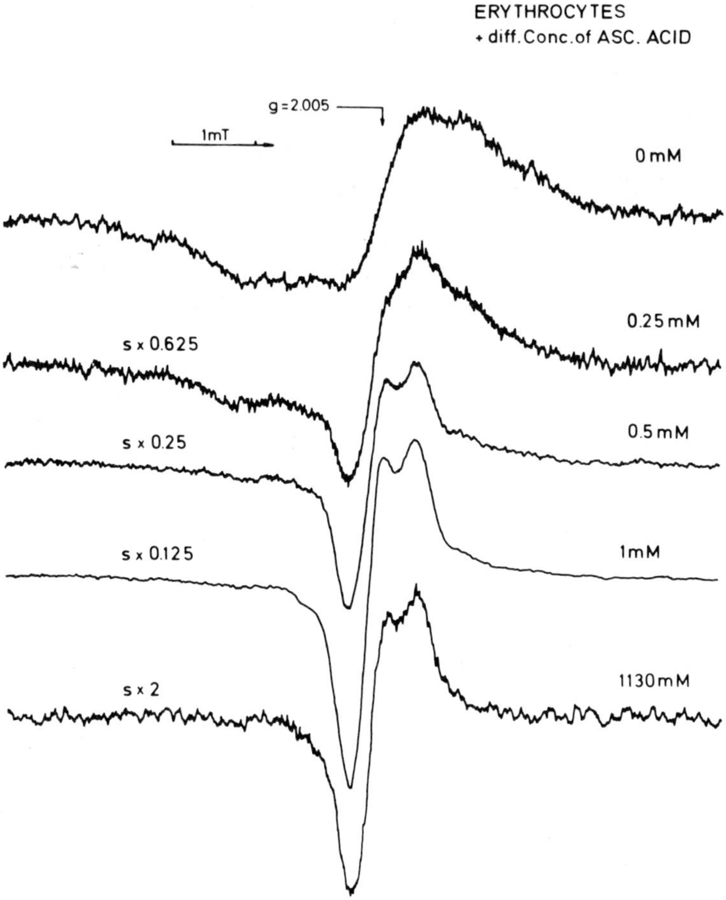

FIG. 3 The effect of different concentrations of ascorbic acid on the ESR spectrum of erythrocytes. (s = rel. sensitivity.)

In order to elucidate the nature as well as the possible origin of the ESR peaks, the effect of different reducing substances on healthy erythrocytes was investigated. Healthy erythrocytes were chosen for simplicity and because the erythrocytes of leukaemic patients already revealed the "leukaemic" peak which is not present in healthy ones.

Of all the antioxidants tested (Lohmann *et al.*, 1979e) only vitamin C produced the "leukaemic" peak when added to healthy erythrocytes (Fig. 3). With increasing concentration of ascorbic acid the spin concentration first increases followed by a decline to near zero

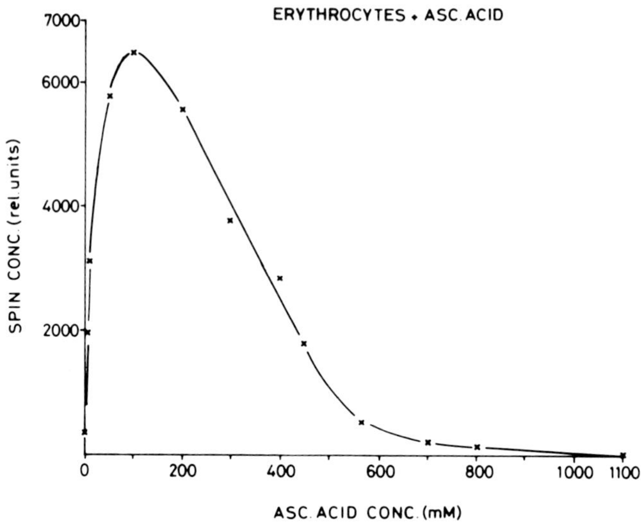

FIG. 4 The effect of different concentrations of ascorbic acid on the spin concentration of the erythrocyte-ascorbic acid suspension.

at about 1 M of ascorbic acid (Fig. 4). Oxidising substances (e.g. $KMnO_4$, H_2O_2) added to erythrocytes reversed the effect produced by ascorbic acid depending, of course, on the concentration used (Lohmann *et al.*, 1979e).

These findings confirm observations that malignant tissue, in a terminal state, exhibits a lower spin concentration and a higher concentration of antioxidants than its corresponding healthy tissue (Duchesne, 1977; Harrington, 1967; Neish *et al.*, 1963, 1964; Shuster, 1955; Ziegler, 1960; Commoner and Ternberg, 1961; Kolomitseva *et al.*, 1960; Mallard and Kent, 1964; Vithayathil *et al.*, 1965).

Because determination of free radical changes during the development of acute lymphatic leukaemia could obviously not be made, samples of different sections of healthy lung and its tumour tissue of patients with bronchial carcinoma were studied on the assumption that they might reflect free radical concentration in the development of a neoplasm (Lohmann *et al.*, 1981b). A characteristic change in shape of the ESR spectrum and in spin concentration could be observed between healthy and tumour tissue. The spin concentration of the peripheral rim of the tumour turned out to be about twice as large as

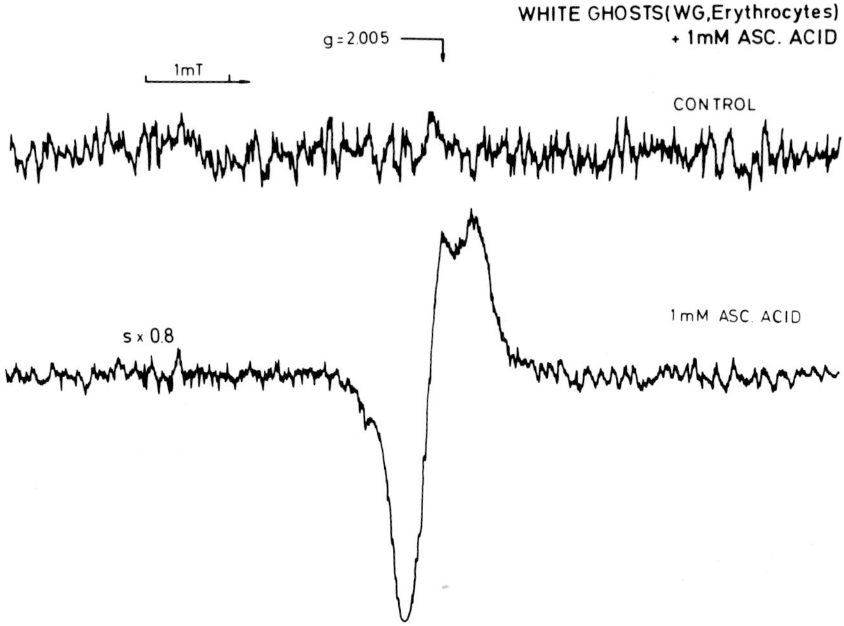

FIG. 5 The effect of 1 mM of ascorbic acid on the ESR spectrum of white ghosts of erythrocytes. (s = rel. sensitivity.)

of healthy tissue and decreased towards the centre of the tumour. This result confirmed the model experiments mentioned above (Fig. 4). The high spin concentration at the surface of the tumour could be due to a high metabolic rate of this region.

In order to determine the nature of the receptor for ascorbic acid, the effect of ascorbic acid on white ghosts of healthy erythrocytes has been investigated. As can be seen in Fig. 5 a spectrum is obtained which resembles the one obtained with leukaemic blood. Therefore, the ascorbic acid receptor(s) ought to be a constituent of the membrane.

There were some indications that certain metal ions or metalloproteins might act as receptor(s). The interaction between Cu^{2+}, Fe^{3+}, or Mn^{2+} and ascorbic acid, as studied by ESR spectroscopy, results in a reduction of the metal ions (Lohmann and Lange, 1979b). None of these metal ion complexes, however, exhibits the ESR spectrum obtained with leukaemic blood.

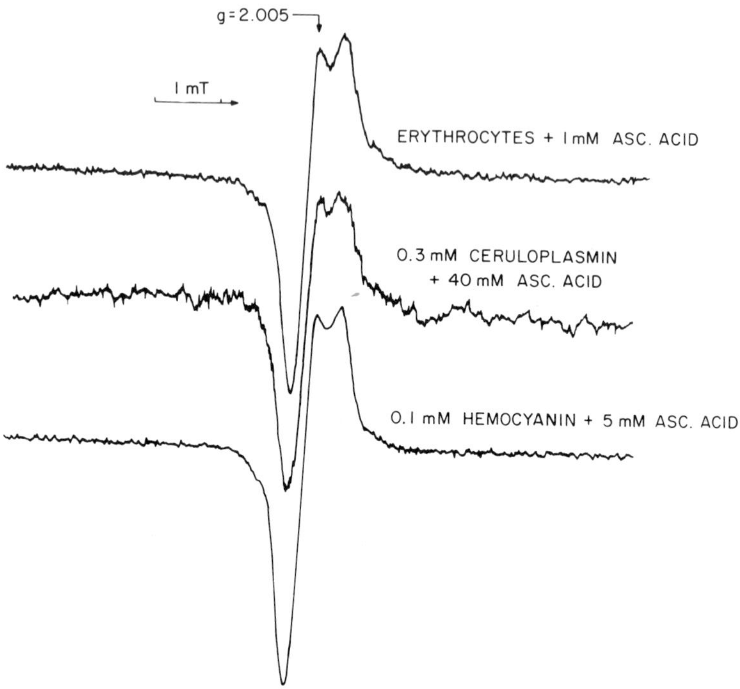

FIG. 6 The effect of ascorbic acid on different copper proteins and erythrocytes.

Since Cu^{2+} exerted the strongest interaction with vitamin C, it seemed quite possible that certain copper-containing proteins might function as receptors for ascorbic acid. The ESR spectra, obtained with lyophilised samples of some copper proteins (ceruloplasmin, haemocyanin) and ascorbic acid are identical to the one obtained with leukaemic blood (Lohmann *et al.*, 1979d) (Fig. 6).

The two peaks located at about g = 2.005 do not belong to the same species. ESR power saturation studies show that the "leukaemic" peak saturates faster indicating a free radical while the relatively non-saturating signal might belong to a metal ion. It could be shown that the low field peak was due to the semidehydroascorbate (SDA) radical (Lohmann *et al.*, 1979d). This radical could act as a pro-oxidant and might, therefore, cause lipid peroxidation. This would lead to structural and functional derangements of lipoprotein membranes. In the case of erythrocytes, this peroxidation would cause haemolysis of the red cells.

From these results it was also concluded that a copper protein should be present in the erythrocyte membrane. Atomic absorption studies revealed that about 3% of the total copper content of the erythrocytes is present in their white ghosts (Lohmann *et al.*, 1979a). This copper protein was either unknown hitherto or its presence in the membrane has not yet been verified.

The studies so far carried out dealt with ascorbic acid added *in vitro* to the different systems under investigation. When 1 g of ascorbic acid was administered intravenously to healthy volunteers the ESR spectrum of native blood was identical to that obtained in the case of acute lymphatic leukaemia (Lohmann *et al.*, 1981a). While the "unhealthy" spectrum prevails in untreated leukaemic patients, it returns to normal within several hours to one day in these healthy volunteers. The ESR spectrum of the erythrocytes was not affected by ascorbic acid. In the plasma of most of the volunteers, the ascorbic acid concentration increased considerably within the first 2 min following injection and decreased gradually to near normal levels within several hours. Ascorbic acid was distributed uniformly all over the body within the first 2 min. In the erythrocytes, a slight increase in ascorbic acid concentration could be observed only within the first few minutes after injection.

It should be pointed out that in two individuals with an increased leukocyte count (11.5 and 16 x 10^3 cells/μl), i.v. administration of 1 g of ascorbic acid resulted in a steady decrease (8.5 and 10.5 x 10^3 cells/μl after 24 h).

In one healthy male volunteer the erythrocytes exhibited the SDA peak and a considerable increase in both spin and vitamin C concentrations. From these results it might be concluded that there is a substance which reacts specifically with ascorbic acid. In patients with acute lymphatic leukaemia it might be present in a diminished quantity only. There were some indications that ascorbate oxidase or an enzyme acting similarly might be the substance in question. Therefore, the effect of this enzyme on erythrocytes treated with ascorbic acid, on blood of patients with acute lymphatic leukaemia

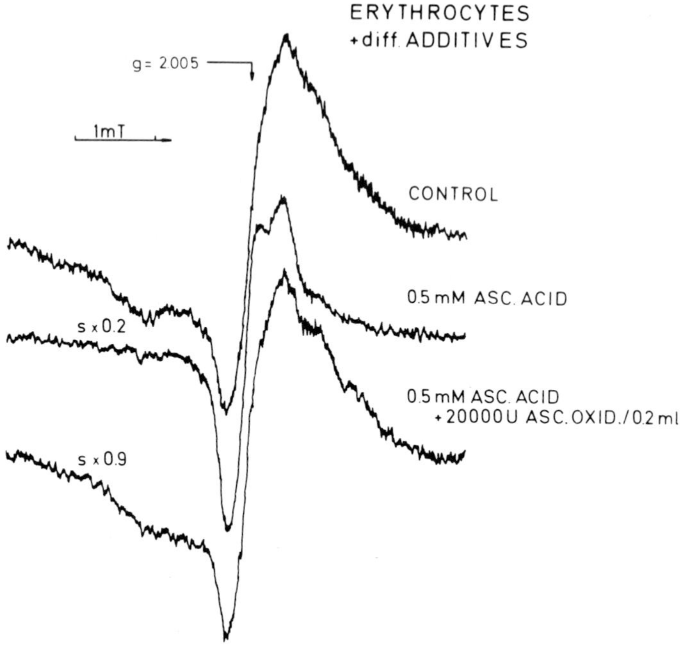

FIG. 7 Effect of ascorbate oxidase on the ESR spectra of erythrocytes treated with 0.5 mM of ascorbic acid. (s = rel. sensitivity.)

and on malignant lung tissue has been investigated (Lohmann, 1981). As can be seen in Fig. 7, the vitamin C effect as expressed by the appearance of the additional peak at g = 2.005 and the increase in spin concentration could be reversed by the addition of ascorbate oxidase. Similar results were obtained when ascorbate oxidase was added to blood of patients with acute lymphatic leukaemia or to malignant lung tissue.

Obviously, this enzyme interacts with ascorbic acid. Many years ago it was proposed that ascorbate oxidase oxidises vitamin C to dehydroascorbic acid (DHA) in the presence of oxygen (Szent-Györgyi, 1928). In order to test whether this happens in our system, nuclear magnetic resonance (NMR) investigations were conducted. In Fig. 8, upper spectrum, the proton resonances of ascorbic acid can be seen. The spectrum of the oxidised form DHA is shown in the third row. All peaks have been shifted down-field due to the reduced charge density of the oxidised form. The down-field shift of the CH_2-6 resonances, however, is larger than would be anticipated from an inductive charge

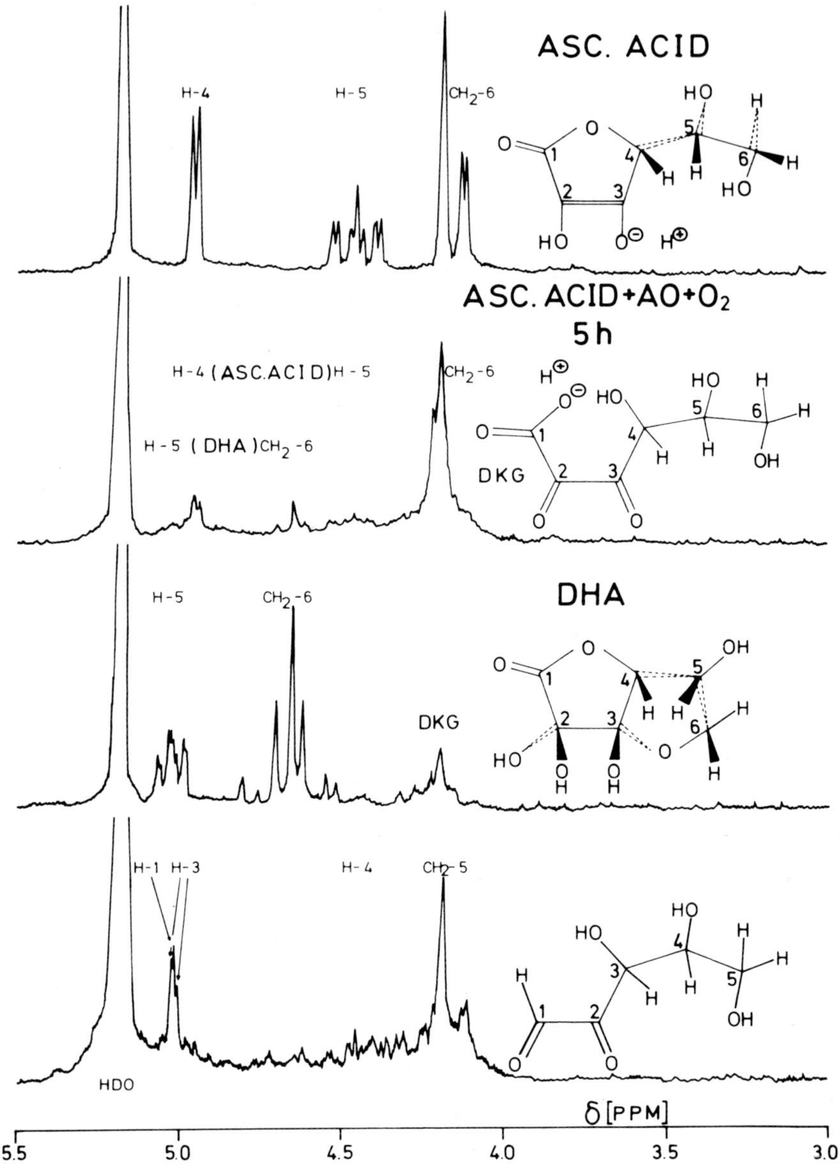

FIG. 8 ^{1}H-NMR spectra of ascorbic acid (0.5 M, top spectrum), dehydroascorbic acid (DHA, 0.5 M, third from top), 1,2,3-tridehydroxypropylglyoxal (bottom spectrum), and of ascorbic acid (0.5 M) treated with ascorbate oxidase (AO, 0.01 mM) in deuterated acetate buffer (1 M, pD 6) and in the presence of O_2 and registered after 5 h.

effect along a free side chain, indicating the existence of a cyclic side chain structure. In this way, CH_2-6 is more receptive to a change in charge density of the C-2/C-3 region. The magnetic non-equivalency of the CH_2-6 protons also confirms this special structure. H-4 is covered by the HDO resonance. A new degradation product (3,4-diketogulonic acid, DKG) appears at a concentration of approx. 4.2 ppm. When ascorbic acid is treated with ascorbate oxidase and oxygen, the proton resonances of ascorbic acid disappear gradually, while those of DHA, which are present in minute quantity only, disappear also after longer reaction times (second spectrum from top, registered after 5 h of reaction time). In this spectrum, the degradation product DKG is well expressed and it seems that the enzyme not only oxidises ascorbic acid but also destroys it. The main mechanism involved seems to be a ring closure of the side chain first (see structural formula in the third row Fig. 8) followed by an opening of the two ring structures of DHA (see structural formula given at the second spectrum from top Fig. 8). One of the successive oxidation products of ascorbic acid seems to be glyoxal, the spectrum of which (1,2,3-trihydroxypropylglyoxal) is also shown in Fig. 8 (bottom spectrum). A more detailed description of the mechanism involved will be published elsewhere.

From the NMR results it can be concluded that the oxidation of ascorbic acid occurs via a ring closure of its side chain. This finding was further supported by ESR measurements. The hf-splitting of the SDA radical, as shown in Fig. 9 (Laroff *et al.*, 1972), can be explained best by assuming the ring closure as indicated in the structural formula given. The splitting parameters are as follows: $a_4 = 1.75 \times 10^{-4}$ T, $a_5 = 0.06 \times 10^{-4}$ T, $a_6 = 0.18 \times 10^{-4}$ T.

If there is a substitution in position 6 by e.g. an acetyl group, preventing a ring closure of the side chain, the spectrum shown at the bottom will be obtained. As can be seen, the hf-structure produced by the 5- and 6-protons is no longer present. This spectrum seems to be composed of two contributions caused by acetylation at different positions. An acetylation occurs, at any rate, at position 6 resulting in a loss of the triplet structure. Details of these investigations will be published elsewhere.

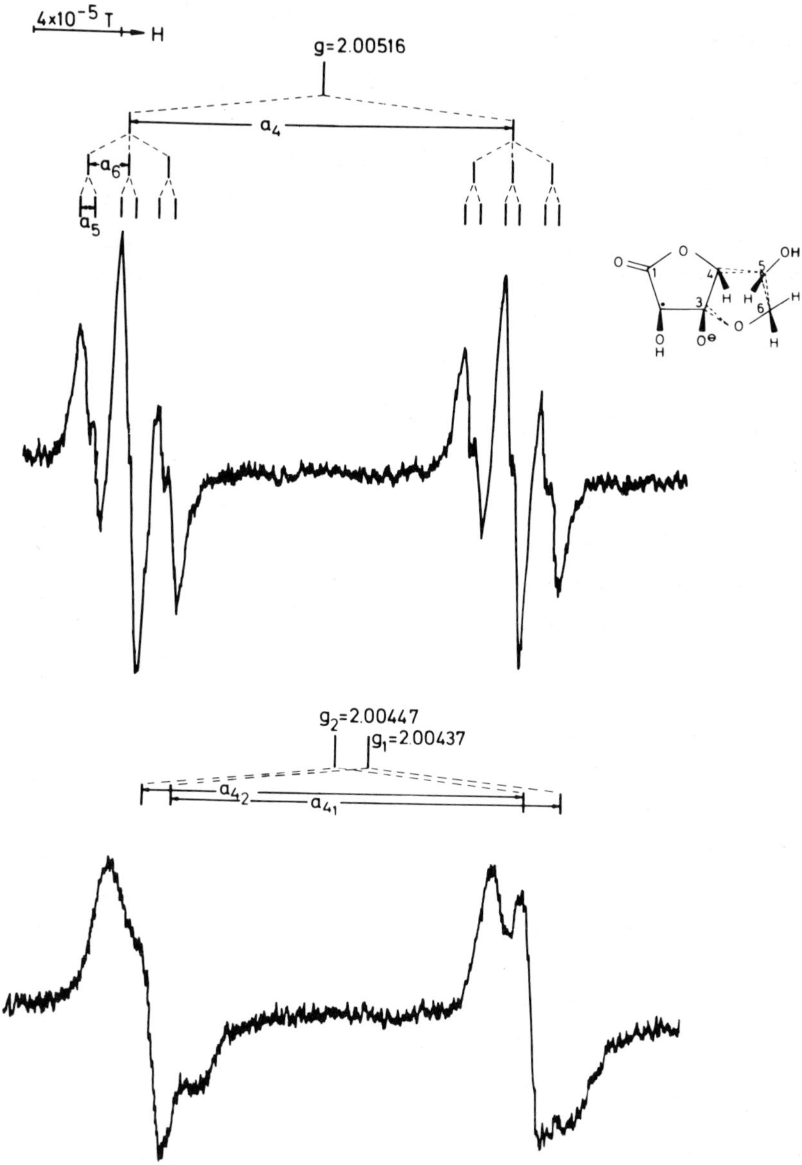

FIG. 9 ESR spectra of the semidehydroascorbate radical without (upper spectrum) and with acetylation at positions 5 and 6 (lower spectrum) measured at room temperature as liquid sample.

SUMMARY

The electron spin resonance (ESR) spectra of lyophilised blood (or of its constituents) from patients with acute lymphatic leukaemia exhibit an increase in spin concentration and a signal at about $g = 2.005$ which is not present in control samples. Systematic changes with time during the treatment of the patients with cytostatic agents show that the method can be used to provide an additional indication of the progress of disease and its response to therapy. Furthermore, it has been possible to identify this signal as being due to the semidehydroascorbate (SDA) radical. Possible receptor(s) for vitamin C are some copper-containing proteins. These are proposed since addition of ascorbic acid to them resulted in identical signals to those obtained in the case of acute lymphatic leukaemia. Since similar results were obtained when vitamin C was added to white ghosts of erythrocytes it can be concluded that there is also a copper protein in their membranes. Atomic absorption studies revealed about 3% of the total copper content of erythrocytes as being present in their membranes.

In *in vivo* experiments, in which 1 g of ascorbic acid was administered intravenously to healthy volunteers, the ESR spectrum of native blood is identical to that obtained in the case of acute lymphatic leukaemia. While the signal is always present in untreated leukaemic patients, it returns to normal within several hours in these healthy volunteers. From these findings it is concluded that a substance which reacts with ascorbic acid specifically exists in healthy individuals but this is present in diminished quantities in patients with acute lymphatic leukaemia. There are some indications that ascorbate oxidase or an enzyme acting similarly might be the substance in question. When ascorbate oxidase was added to healthy erythrocytes treated with ascorbic acid, to blood of patients with acute lymphatic leukaemia, or to tissue samples of lung cancer, the SDA signal disappeared and the spin concentration returned to normal depending, of course, on the concentration used. This favours the idea that ascorbate oxidase might play a decisive role in ascorbic acid metabolism and that this has been modified in the case of certain types of cancer. Its exact mechanism of action has still to be elucidated. It is assumed that ascorbate oxidase oxidises ascorbic acid to dehydroascorbic acid (DHA) in the presence of oxygen. Nuclear magnetic resonance (NMR) investigations reveal, however, a ring closure of the side chain first, followed by an opening of the two ring structures of DHA and the degradation of ascorbic acid. These results have been confirmed by ESR measurements according to which the hf spectrum of the SDA radical, which can be explained by a cyclic side chain, is changed drastically if an acetyl group is substituted at position 6 of the side chain. In this way, no ring closure is possible.

In summary, the ESR changes observed in malignant tissue seem to reflect disturbances of normal metabolism especially of those of ascorbic acid and some copper proteins. They are likely to be of diagnostic value for cancer (tumour marker) and can be used as an additional indication of the progress of disease and its response to therapy.

ACKNOWLEDGEMENTS

The excellent technical assistance of Miss P. Bräunlich, Miss E. Decher, and Miss P. Ferber is greatly appreciated. This work was supported in part by Euratom grant EUR no. 213-76-7 BIO D, by the Bundesministerium des Innern, and by the Fonds der Chemischen Industrie.

REFERENCES

Commoner, B. and Ternberg, J. (1961). *Proc. Natl. Acad. Sci. (USA)* 47, 1374-1384.
Dodd, N.J.F. (1980). *In* "Metal Ions in Biological Systems" (Ed. H. Sigel) Vol. 10, pp.95-128. Marcel Dekker, New York.
Duchesne, J. (1977). *J. Theoret. Biol.* 66, 137-145.
Harrington, J.S. (1967). *Adv. Cancer Res.* 10, 247-310.
Kolomitseva, I., L'Vov, K. and Kayushin, L. (1960). *Biofizika* 5, 636-637.
Laroff, G.P., Fessenden, R.W. and Schuler, R.H. (1972). *J. Am. Chem. Soc.* 94, 9026-9073.
Lohmann, W., Greulich, W. and Döll, G. (1979a). *Blut* 39, 327-332.
Lohmann, W. and Lange, R. (1979b). *Z. Naturforsch. Teil. C* 34, 546-549.
Lohmann, W., Schreiber, J., Gerhardt, H., Breithaupt, H., Löffler, H. and Pralle, H. (1979c). *Blut* 39, 147-151.
Lohmann, W., Schreiber, J. and Greulich, W. (1979d). *Z. Naturforsch. Teil. C* 34, 550-554.
Lohmann, W., Schreiber, J., Strobelt, W. and Müller-Eckhardt, Ch. (1979e). *Blut* 39, 317-326.
Lohmann, W. (1981). *Z. Naturforsch.* (in press).
Lohmann, W., Bensch, K.G., Müller, E. and Kang, S.O. (1981a). *Z. Naturforsch. Teil. C* 36, 1-4.

Lohmann, W., Bensch, K.G., Schreiber, J., Müller, E., Schwemmle, K., Feustel, H. and Filler, R.D. (1981b). *Z. Naturforsch. Teil. C* 36, 5-8.
Lohmann, W., Schreiber, H., Greulich, W., Strobelt, W., Müller, E., Löffler, H., Pralle, H., Feustel, H., Schwemmle, K. and Filler, R.D. (1981c). *Collect. Phenom.* 3, 245-258.
Mallard, J. and Kent, M. (1964). *Nature (London)* 204, 1192-1194.
Miller, J.A. (1970). *Cancer Res.* 30, 559-576.
Neish, W.J.P. and Rylett, A. (1963). *Biochem. Pharmacol.* 12, 893-903.
Neish, W.J.P., Davies, H.M. and Reeve, P.M. (1964). *Biochem. Pharmacol.* 13, 1291-1303.
Shuster, C.W. (1955). *Proc. Soc. Exp. Biol. Med.* 90, 423-426.
Swartz, H.M. (1979). *In* "Submolecular Biology and Cancer" (Eds. G.E.W. Wolstenholme, D.W. Fitzsimons and J. Whelan). Symposium 67, pp.107-130. Excerpta Medica, Amsterdam.
Szent-Györgyi, A. (1928). *Biochem. J.* 22, 1387-1409.
Szent-Györgyi, A., Isenberg, I. and Baird, S. (1960). *Proc. Natl. Acad. Sci. (USA)* 46, 1444-1449.
Vithayathil, A., Ternberg, J. and Commoner, B. (1965). *Nature (London)* 207, 1246-1249.
Ziegler, E. (1960). "Messung und Bedeutung des Redoxpotentials im Blut *in vivo* und *in vitro*." 10. Beiheft der Arzneimittelforschung. Editio Cantor, Aulendorf/Wurtt.

DISCUSSION

Slater: Thank you Professor Lohmann for a very interesting and important presentation. You mentioned in your lecture Szent-Györgyi's discovery of vitamin C; for those of you who don't know, Albert Szent-Györgyi is the Scientific Director of the National Foundation for Cancer Research, based in Bethesda, Maryland. A feature of Szent-Györgyi's recent work has been to emphasise the importance of methyl-glyoxal and related aldehydes as potential inhibitors of cell division. One of the projects within the N.F.C.R. during the last few years has been to combine methyl glyoxal (and other aldehydes) with vitamin C to make a cyclic acetal that has very interesting properties (Fodor *et al.*, 1979). So from the N.F.C.R. point of view we have been putting methyl glyoxal together with vitamin C whilst you, in effect, have actually produced it in the reverse process. I think that is an interesting point.

Lohmann: Most of the results I reported here, I have presented to Professor Szent-Györgyi at Woods Hole about two years ago; I had an interesting discussion with him, in which he made valuable suggestions.

Adams: I am very interested, Wolfgang, in this work. Is your technique sensitive enough to be of useful prognostic value, indicating perhaps increased danger of relapse, because that's what a clinician would like to know, particularly if one were able to do that before the pathology laboratory could? If one could show a change in the kinetics of handling ascorbic acid in patients who are apparently still in remission, then you would have a very good prognostic test.

Lohmann: This is what we are doing at present. Unfortunately, I didn't have the time to elaborate on this. In a few cases with patients in a complete remission, ESR spectrum as well as ascorbic acid concentration were normal. There will be a follow-up of these patients.

The results I have reported are characteristic for ALL. In other types of leukaemia the response is different. In the case of AML, for example, the ESR spectrum of erythrocytes resembles that of erythrocytes of healthy individuals; the vitamin C concentration, however, is lower than in healthy individuals.

In a few instances we have been asked to investigate the blood of patients with a presumably pre-leukaemic state. In one case the methods applied by us revealed values indicating a possible AML very likely to occur.

Adams: Have you ever seen ones that are abnormal and the clinicians told you three months later that this patient has relapsed?

Lohmann: Not yet.

Dianzani: I was interested a lot in your paper. I wonder what is the mechanism by which cancer cells can produce changes in the erythrocyte membranes? Do you think there is any influence on the genetic code of the stem cells? Have you tried to put together leukaemic cells with normal erythrocytes to see if there is any active secretion from leukaemic cells or not? I have now another question. Do you find that there is any difference between different types of leukaemic cells, for instances B cells or T cells or undifferentiated cells?

Lohmann: We have not yet mixed together leukaemic and healthy cells. In regard to your other question concerning the molecular mechanism involved, I repeat what I have already stated in my talk: the appearance of the ascorbyl radical might be a tertiary indicator showing, nevertheless, that, in the case of ALL, the metabolism of ascorbic acid has been modified. The secondary indicator might be, then, the enzyme responsible for regulating the vitamin C metabolism. This is presumably ascorbate oxidase or an enzyme acting similarly. If, like in the case of ALL, the vitamin C concentration in the blood is too high, then, the concentration of this enzyme should be too low and vice versa in the case of AML. In the latter case, vitamin C should be administered, as Linus Pauling has suggested originally. If our working hypothesis is correct, then, a vitamin C treatment, like an insulin treatment in the case of diabetes, will cure secondary or tertiary effects and not the primary damage. The primary damage seems to be a change in the genetic code.

In regard to the ascorbyl radical I have to add some additional information. The double peak shown in the previous slides does not belong to one species alone as power saturation studies have shown. The peak located in the middle saturates faster and belongs to the ascorbyl radical as we have shown. The other peak is a result of the interaction between vitamin C and presumably a copper containing protein resulting in some sort of protein radical. The ascorbate radical causes, then, lipid peroxidation as Dunkley has already shown. It should be pointed out that the relative concentration of vitamin C is very important: if the vitamin C concentration is low compared to an oxidising agent, presumably a copper protein, then it will be oxidised to the ascorbyl radical which, in turn, will act as pro-oxidant and will cause lipid peroxidation. If, however, the vitamin C concentration is too high, then it will act as an anti-oxidant. This is the mechanism we envoked for explaining the shape of the curve shown in Fig. 4. At high vitamin C concentrations no lipid peroxidation can occur, an intermediate concentration is critical for this process. This problem is currently being investigated by us.

I believe there was another question.

Dianzani: My other question concerned the cell types, that is the B and T lymphocytes.

Lohmann: We have just started to do these investigations. In this connection, we became interested in interferon, too. Thus, we determined the effect of interferon on erythrocytes treated with ascorbic acid.

Dianzani: Which type was that? Immunological interferon? You know there are several types of interferon; I suppose yours was lymphocyte interferon?

Lohmann: Yes, I know. We used human fibroblast interferon. Whenever we added increasing concentrations of interferon to our model system, the spin concentration increased first, followed by a decrease; finally the "normal" erythrocyte spectrum was obtained. From this we concluded that the interferon used must contain copper. Atomic absorption studies revealed the presence of copper and there seems to be a correlation between its activity and its copper content.

Dianzani: I think you must do the experiment of mixing the cell types. Interferon acts as a lymphokine and something could be secreted from the cells.

Lohmann: It is generally assumed that interferon is an ingredient of T lymphocytes. Recently we determined, therefore, the influence of T lymphocytes on our model systems. Conclusions cannot be drawn yet. Furthermore, we have not mixed yet the different cell types, a suggestion which is worthwhile to be considered.

Slater: I should like to thank this morning's speakers for getting us off to an extremely stimulating start.

REFERENCES to Discussion

Fodor, G., Mujumdar, R. and Butterick, J. (1979). *In* "Submolecular Biology and Cancer", Ciba Foundation Symposium No.67 new series, pp.165-169. Excerpta Medica, Amsterdam.

Application of Electron Spin Resonance Spectroscopy to Biological Problems

M.C.R. SYMONS

INTRODUCTION

Unlike the related technique of nuclear magnetic resonance spectroscopy (n.m.r.), electron spin resonance (e.s.r.) or electron paramagnetic resonance (e.p.r.) spectroscopy is not a major analytical tool to be found in most chemical or biochemical laboratories. This is because paramagnetic nuclei are ubiquitous, whereas unpaired electrons are rare. They are present in radical intermediates formed during chemical reactions, and these are sometimes sufficiently stable for direct detection by e.s.r. spectroscopy, which is fortunately more sensitive than n.m.r. spectroscopy. They are also present in certain transition-metal complexes, and e.s.r. is then a powerful tool. Essentially, it gives detailed information about the molecular orbital of the unpaired electron, and about neighbouring filled and empty levels, as I indicate below.

THE SPECTROSCOPIC ACT

Most forms of spectroscopy depend upon coupling between the electric vector of electromagnetic radiation and a linear electrical change in the molecule, such as the movement of an electron or a change in dipole moment. In e.s.r. and n.m.r. spectroscopy it is the magnetic component that is involved. Separation between the magnetic states is achieved by the application of a magnetic field (B) as indicated in Fig. 1. The sample is placed in the region of high magnetic field in a microwave cavity sustaining stationary microwaves of relatively low power, and the DC magnetic field is increased (with a superimposed modulation) until resonance is achieved (Fig. 1). The coupling can be thought of as a spin-flip, the precessing electron spin

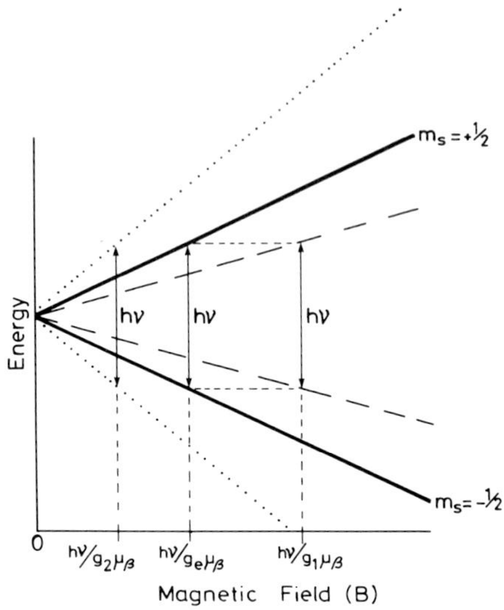

FIG. 1 The effect of an applied static magnetic field (H) on the $M_S = \pm\frac{1}{2}$ levels of an unpaired electron. These are degenerate at zero field. The thick lines represent the spin-only behaviour, the transition ($h\nu$) occurring at a field corresponding to $g_e = 2.0023$. The dashed lines are for a radical having a low-lying vacant excited state, giving $g_1 < 2.0023$, and the dotted lines are for a radical having a neighbouring filled level, giving $g_2 > 2.0023$. (Taken from Symons, 1978).

going from the $+\frac{1}{2}$ to the $-\frac{1}{2}$ state or oritentation in the magnetic field. (Spins are flipped both ways: a nett absorption of microwave power occurs because, at equilibrium, the upper state is populated slightly less than the lower state.)

The g-value

This measures the rate of divergence of the levels indicated in Fig. 1. A rapid divergence gives a low-field resonance and a high g-value, and vice-versa. In systems in which the unpaired electrons are not involved in any orbital motion, the g-value is 2.0023 (the "free-spin" value). It is given by

$$h\nu = g\ \mu_\beta\ B, \qquad \ldots\ldots (1)$$

where ν is the microwave frequency, B the applied DC field and μ_β, the Bohr magneton, is a constant. Orbital motion occurs when there are either low-lying vacant levels, or partially filled levels, which

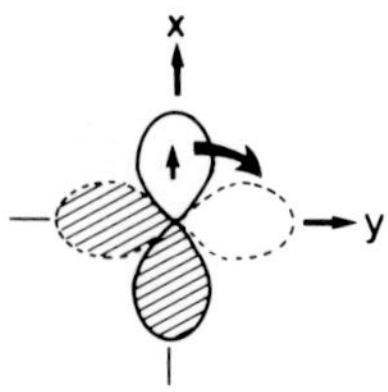

FIG. 2 Movement of the unpaired electron from one *p*-orbital (p_x) into another (p_y) induced by a magnetic field (B_z) gives rise to orbital motion and hence a shift in the *g*-value.

are magnetically coupled (by a rotatory motion, as shown in Fig. 2) to that of the unpaired electron. Hence a measure of Δg, the shift from 2.0023, gives a measure of the proximity of other levels. For most organic radicals, Δg is a very small and not of much significance, but for transition metals it can be large, because of the proximity of other *d* orbitals.

Electron Nuclear Hyperfine Coupling

For those familiar with n.m.r. spectroscopy, it may be helpful to realise that the e.s.r. *g*-shift is comparable with the n.m.r. chemical shift. Similarly, electron-nuclear hyperfine coupling can be compared with nuclear-nuclear spin-spin coupling in n.m.r. (In systems containing more than one unpaired electron per molecule, electron-spin - electron-spin coupling is, of course, important. For doublet-state radicals this coupling does not arise: it is of great importance in triplet-state molecules and in many high-spin transition-metal complexes.)

To understand the origin of hyperfine coupling it must be recalled that many nuclei have nett magnetic moments (these are far smaller than that of the electron). Those with nuclear spin (I) of $\frac{1}{2}$ take up two ($\pm\frac{1}{2}$) orientations in the resultant magnetic field, those with I = 1 have three choices (+1, 0, -1), etc. Consider a radical containing a single nucleus with I = $\frac{1}{2}$. Half thse radicals will have nuclei with $m_I = +\frac{1}{2}$ and the other half will have m_I ; $-\frac{1}{2}$. Hence two resolved features are expected in the e.s.r. spectrum, the separation (in first order) giving the hyperfine coupling (A) (Fig. 3). If I = 1, there are three possible orientations (+1, 0, -1) giving three e.s.r. transitions, the separation again giving the hyperfine coupling.

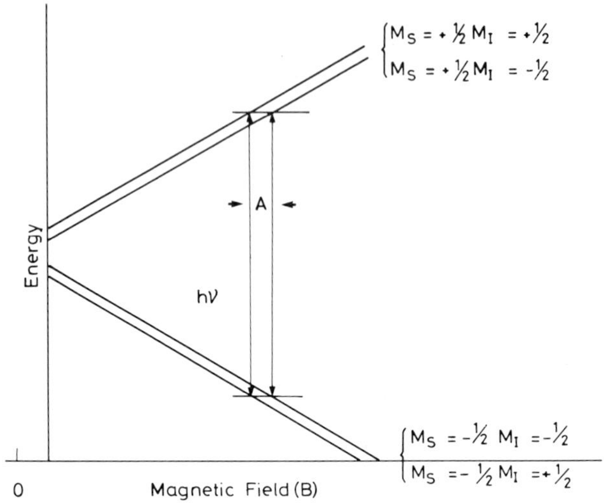

FIG. 3 Divergence with field of the $M_S = \pm\frac{1}{2}$ levels in the presence of a single nucleus having $I = \frac{1}{2}$, in the high-field approximation. Note the two allowed transitions involve no change in M_I. (Taken from Symons, 1978).

Two or more coupled nuclei in the same radical will each contribute to the overall pattern: thus one nucleus with $I = \frac{1}{2}$ and one with $I = 1$ gives 6 components (M_I values of $1 + \frac{1}{2}$, $1 - \frac{1}{2}$, $0 + \frac{1}{2}$, $0 - \frac{1}{2}$, $-1 + \frac{1}{2}$, $-1 - \frac{1}{2}$) from which both hyperfine coupling constants can be derived. Hence the hyperfine pattern acts as a finger-print, just as does the spin-spin coupling in n.m.r. spectroscopy. This is usually the major factor involved in identification of species, arguments from g-shifts being less compelling.

Isotropic Hyperfine Coupling

Solution spectra usually compise narrow components from which the isotropic hyperfine coupling and average g-value can be derived (Fig. 4a).

Anisotropic Hyperfine Coupling

Radicals trapped in solids generally exhibit more complex spectra, as indicated in Figs. 4b and c. This arises because both the g-value and the hyperfine coupling are tensor quantities and have three principle components along three orthogonal axes (x, y, z). In the

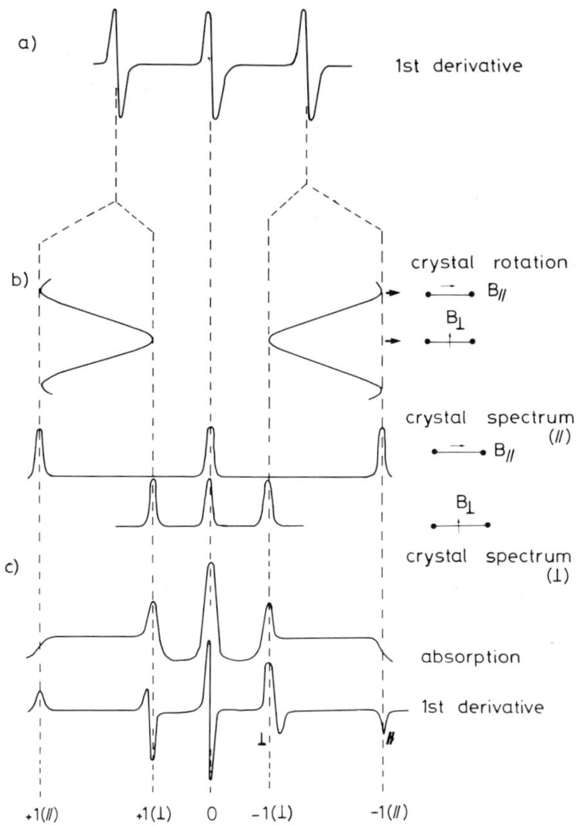

FIG. 4 This figure illustrates the connection between a typical solution spectrum for a radical with a single coupled nucleus with I = 1 (a), and the changes on rotation observed for a single crystal. (b) The rotation is selected such that the parallel and perpendicular orientations are traversed. An isotropic *g*-value has been assumed. The corresponding powder spectrum in absorption and as the first derivative is given in (c).

liquid-phase, rapid averaging occurs, but in the solid three different *g*-values and three different hyperfine coupling constants contribute. In Fig. 4b and 4c a simple system is illustrated in which I have set $g_x = g_y - g_z$ and $A_x = A_y$. The latter condition is frequently encountered in practice, in which case, A_x and A_y are described as $A_\perp$ and A_z as $A_{//}$, as indicated. Figure 4c shows a typical "powder" spectrum such as is obtained from powdered crystals or glasses. Had a single crystal been used the spectrum would have resembled the liquid-phase spectrum except that the parameters would have varied with orientation between the limits given by the powder spectrum (Fig. 4b). There are, in general, sets of such features equal to the number of orientationally distinct radicals per unit cell. Spectra from amorphous solids are generally more difficult to interpret than from the liquid-phase or single crystals because of the asymmetrically broadened sets of lines.

Orbital Hybridisation From E.S.R. Spectra

We have seen that hyperfine coupling parameters have isotropic (A_{iso}) and anisotropic (2B) components. In examples exhibiting axial symmetry, $A_{//}$ and $A_{\perp}$ can be used to extract A_{iso} and 2B, where 2B is the parallel component of the anisotropic tensor components (2B, -B, -B) (Scheme 1). Fairly accurate quantum mechanical calculations have

SCHEME 1

Derivation of A_{iso} and 2B and of orbital populations, $a_{\underline{s}}^2$ and $a_{\underline{p}}^2$	
$A_{//} = A_{iso} + 2B$	$3A_{iso} = A_{//} + 2A_{\perp}$
$A_{\perp} = A_{iso} - B$	
$A_s^2 = A_{iso}/A^o$	$a_{\underline{p}}^2 = 2B/2B^o$

been carried out for atoms to give the expected hyperfine coupling for unit electron population of valence *s* orbitals (isotropic) and *p* or *d* orbitals (anisotropic), usually given the symbols A^o and $2B^o$. A table giving these parameters is given in Symons (1978). Hence "experimental" orbital populations can be estimated, as indicated in Scheme 1.

For a more detailed but not too sophisticated account of e.s.r. spectroscopy see Symons (1978).

BIOLOGICAL APPLICATIONS

These cover a range of quite disparate topics. Thus, **Spin-Labelling** is concerned with using nitroxide radicals ($R_2NO^{\bullet}$) to learn about local environments and relaxation processes such as rotational correlation times. The technique gives information similar to that from the use of fluorescent probes and deuterium n.m.r. spectroscopy. (The ^{2}H n.m.r. technique has the great advantage that the labelled species are chemically unchanged.) In these studies, the unpaired electron itself is of no particular interest.

Spin-trapping is also concerned with nitroxide radicals but, in this case, these are of direct importance, since the technique is a method of converting highly reactive radicals into stable radicals that can be easily studied by liquid-phase e.s.r. spectroscopy. In favourable cases, new hyperfine features are resolved which reveal the nature of the reactive radical intermediate ($R^{\bullet}$): otherwise it may be possible to infer something about the nature of $R^{\bullet}$ from slight changes in the ^{14}N or ^{1}H coupling constants of the nitroxide.

In certain systems, **stable organic radicals**, often aromatic semiquinones or related species, are present, or they may be formed in readily detectable yields during the course of chemical reaction.

Reactive organic radicals are not normally detectable directly, but can be formed and trapped, using photochemical or radiochemical methods, in low-temperature solids, in which case they can be readily studied by e.s.r. spectroscopy. As the temperature is raised, secondary reactions of such radicals can often be detected.

Triplet Excited States can also be studied by conventional e.s.r. spectroscopy. An important area of study is that of chloroplast systems. However, the related technique of optically detected magnetic resonance (ODMR) is probably more useful for such studies. In this method, the emission spectrum is monitored in the presence of magnetic and microwave fields so that the triplet levels are split in a controllable fashion, and population can be changed by the microwave energy. These changes are monitored via the emitted light and the normal e.s.r. spectrum can be obtained (see, for exmaple, El-Sayed, 1971; Hoff *et al.*, 1977).

Transition-Metal Complexes are often paramagnetic, in which case e.s.r. spectroscopy is valuable since it can give information about the number of unpaired electrons, the spin-density on the metal atom, and the nature of the ligands. If the system of interest does not contain paramagnetic metal ions, it may help to add such ions as a form of spin-label. For example, Mn(II) may take the place of Mg^{2+} ions, and e.s.r. spectroscopy can then be used to give details of the binding site and, indirectly, of the binding constant.

I now consider some of these aspects in greater detail.

Spin-Labels

A typical spectrum of a nitroxide radical is given in Fig. 5. The isotropic ^{14}N hyperfine coupling, $A(^{14}N)$, is markedly dependent on the environment, as illustrated in Fig. 6, which shows that water

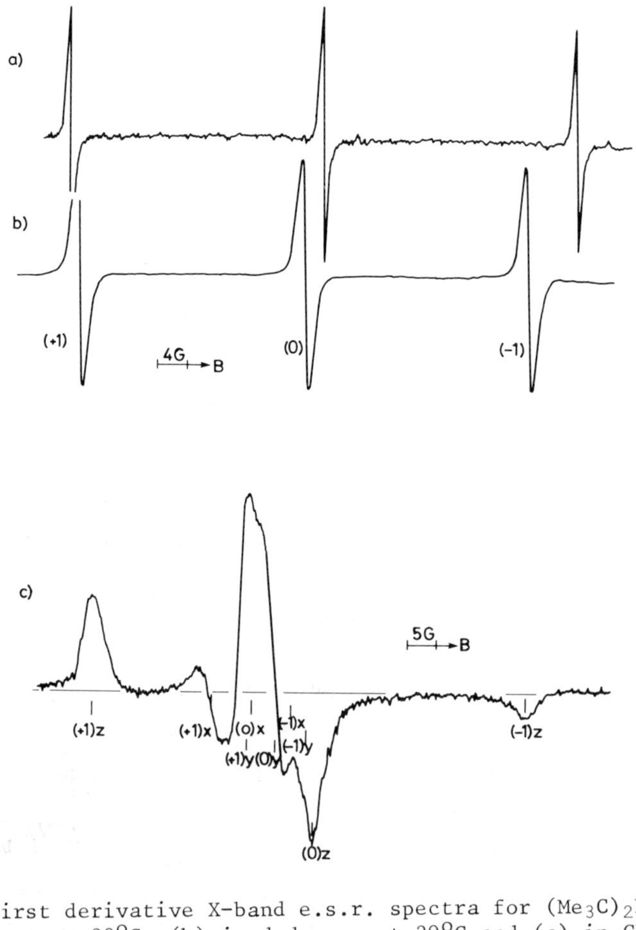

FIG. 5 First derivative X-band e.s.r. spectra for $(Me_3C)_2NO^{\cdot}$ radicals (a) in water at 20°C; (b) in dodecane at 20°C and (c) in CD_3OD at 77 K. In (c) $(CD_3)_3CNO^{\cdot}$ radicals were used to give better definition. (Taken from Symons, 1978).

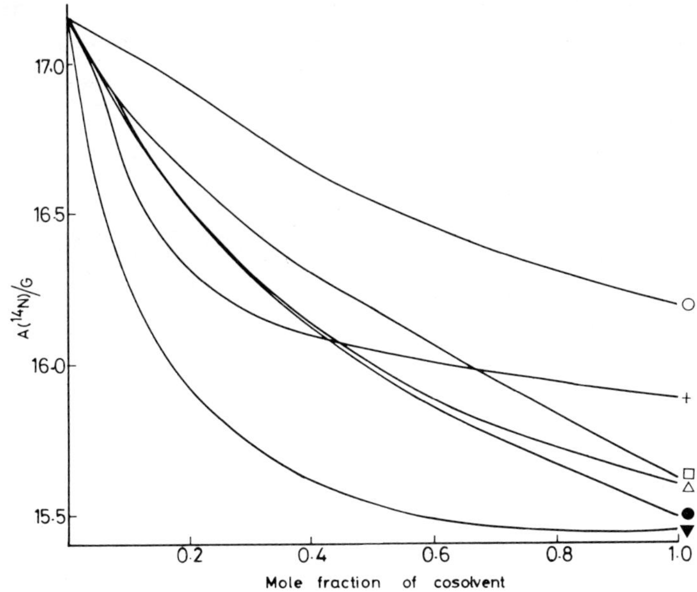

FIG. 6 Hyperfine coupling constants (^{14}N) for DTBN in aqueous solutions as a function of the mole-fraction (M.F.) of added cosolvents. Key: ○ MeOH = methanol; + *t*BuOH = *t*-butyl alcohol; □ MeCN = methylcyanide; △ DMSO = dimethylsulphoxide; ● Me_2CO = acetone; × HMPA = hexamethylphosphoramide; ▼ DMF = dimethylformamide.

produces the largest splitting of all common solvents. This is because water forms two strong hydrogen-bonds to the nitroxyl oxygen atom, which constrains the unpaired electron onto nitrogen because of the antibonding nature of the π*-orbital. In mixed aqueous systems containing aprotic solvents first one and then the second hydrogen-bond is broken with consequent reduction in A(^{14}N).

When probe nitroxides are attached to biomolecules they may be in an aqueous or a non-aqueous, non-hydrogen bonding environment such as a "hydrophobic" pocket or a membrane (hydrocarbon-like) environment, and A(^{14}N) can give this information. Equally informative are trends in line-width: these may arise for a variety of reasons, but for labelled biomolecules the cause of broadening is usually slow rotation. Indeed, if the nitroxide is rigidly held by, for example, a high molecular weight protein, the normal spectrum is almost identical to that for the non-rotating radical, as in Fig. 5c. What is then needed is some method of sampling the spectrum at intervals within which significant re-orientation occurs, and this is, in effect, what is achieved in the technique of "saturation transfer" (Thomas *et al.*, 1976; Thomas and McConnell, 1974).

With conventional e.s.r. spectroscopy, τ_2, the rotational correlation time of the spin-label, can be estimated within the range $10^{-11} \lesssim \tau_2 \lesssim 10^{-7}$s. Using the saturation transfer (ST) method this is extended to the range $10^{-7} \lesssim \tau_2 \lesssim 10^{-3}$s. This is a vital range for many biological systems, including large proteins, and large assemblies such as membranes, contractile systems, chromosomes, etc. The essence of the technique is to use a high microwave power, so that there is partial saturation, and then to exploit the fact that the rate of spin relaxation varies across the spectrum. Thus the spectrum is most sensitive to the transfer of saturation in those regions in which the rate of change is large: that is, half-way between the turning points. Normal spectral display picks out the turning points specifically, so such spectra are not very sensitive to saturation transfer. However, second harmonic or dispersion modes exaggerate the regions in-between the turning points and are therefore far more sensitive. In practice, therefore, in addition to using high microwave powers, modulation periods are chosen that are comparable with but less than the spin-lattice relaxation time and the correlation time (so that in-between detection times the molecule has rotated and the signal has changed), and second harmonic or dispersion mode display is used. The method is very powerful and is being used widely.

When the $>NO^{\bullet}$ group is attached to some peripheral group that has significant motional freedom, the spectrum may be truly isotropic, but with a broad-narrow-very broad trend in the widths of the +1, 0, and -1 lines that clearly reflects the overall widths of the anisotropic solid-state features. As the molecule rotates, there is an uncertainty in the position of resonance that is directly reflected in the widths of the averaged features. Hence an effective rotational correlation function can be calculated.

Another use to which $R_2NO^{\bullet}$ radicals can be put is based on the phenomena of spin-spin coupling and spin-exchange. In the simple case of two nitroxide groups held at a fixed distance by some rigid molecular cage the following modes of interaction are expected. In the solid-state the normal through-space dipole-dipole coupling occurs, giving rise to a zero-field splitting (D) that has the form 2D, -D, -D if the point-charge model is appropriate. If the interaction is non-axial the perpendicular coupling (-D) is split into D_x and D_y features, the splitting being usually set equal to E. This interaction clearly averages to zero and is lost in the liquid-phase. Nevertheless, unless the diradical tumbles very rapidly, the lines are greatly broadened by the zero-field splitting.

In addition to this dipolar coupling, which falls off with $\langle r^{-3} \rangle$ where r is the mean separation of the spins, electron-exchange will occur. If there is good overlap of wave-functions this will be rapid on the e.s.r.-hyperfine time-scale, and each electron will "see" both ^{14}N nuclei. If these are equivalent, the five features with M_I values of +2, +1, 0, -1 and -2. If overlap is poor, the electrons remain effectively localised, and only three features (+1, 0, -1, coinciding with the +2, 0 and -2 lines of the quintet) will be observed (Fig. 7).

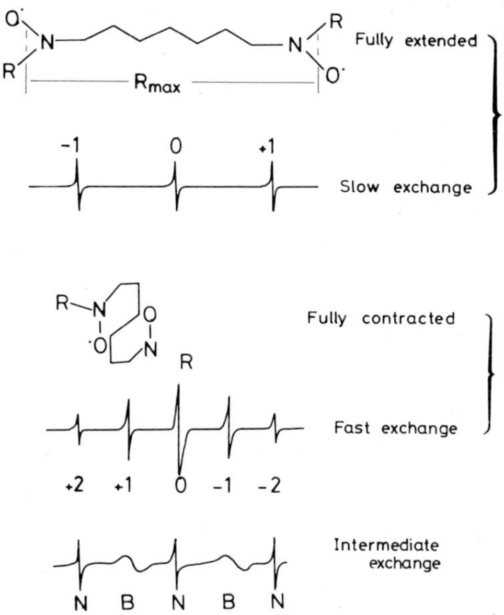

FIG. 7 This shows how coiling of a dinitroxide radical can change the e.s.r. spectrum from that for a normal radical (triplet) to that for a diradical with fast electron exchange (quintet). If this coiling occurs at intermediate rates a marked alternation in linewidths is observed. (Taken from Symons, 1978).

If, as is normally the case, the link between the two >NO$^{\bullet}$ groups is not rigid, the groups can move in and out relative to each other thus moving from of these extremes to the other. This has the effect of introducing an uncertainty into the +1 and -1 features of the quintet so that these lines are often selectively broadened. These extra modes of broadening can be put to good use in biological studies (see, for example, Rey and McConnell, 1977).

If the two components differ, then in slow exchange individual sets of hyperfine lines should be detected, and in fast exchange each electron samples both sets of nuclei for 50% of the time. When these extremes are modulated, there is frequently an overall broadening. This can be put to good use when a spin-label is bound in a site close to a paramagnetic transition-metal ion, or when such an ion is introduced into a site close to a nitroxide label. An example of this approach is included in a recent study of divalent metal binding in the regulatory light-chain sub-units of myosin. Manganese(II) ions were used to replace Ca^{2+} at the divalent metal sites, and cysteine residues were spin-labelled with a nitroxide (Bagshaw and Kendrick-Jones, 1980). In the case of clam myosin, for example, a 25% reduction of intensity of the nitroxide signal was observed. This confirmed that the two centres are close together, thereby establishing which of the possible binding sites is used by Ca^{2+} ions.

Spin-Trapping

The advantages of this method are clear, since nitroxide e.s.r. spectra comprise narrow, isotropic features that are long-lived and usually easy to analyse. The disadvantages are, perhaps, less frequently stressed. One obvious problem is that radicals trapped may not be the significant intermediates in the process studied, but may simply be formed in unimportant side reactions. Another is that different radicals may give rise to extremely similar adduct spectra. One example is that ROO$^{\bullet}$ adducts and RO$^{\bullet}$ adducts of PhCH=NO(CMe_3) (PBN) (I) are expected to give similar spectra and it may be difficult to make a clear distinction between them. Yet another difficulty arises when several different nitroxides are formed together, giving overlapping spectra. However, recent elegant experiments have shown that it is possible to separate such radicals using HPLC techniques and then to study each radical separately (see, for example, Morlya *et al.*, 1980).

Sometimes one can converge on a firm identification by using two alternative types of traps, typified by PBN (see Insert I) and

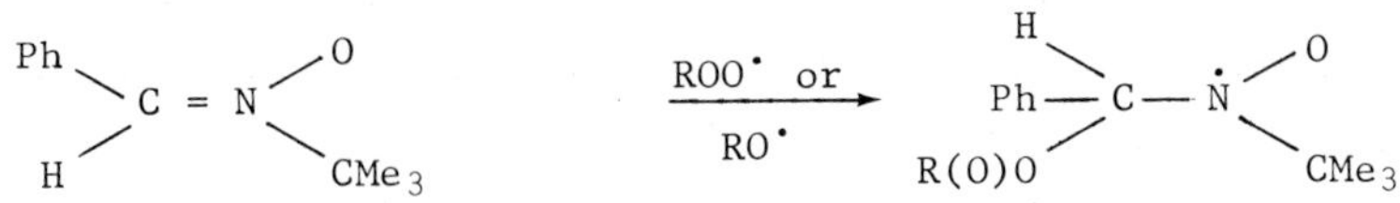

PBN

(I)

Me_3C-NO (MPN). The former is expected to display well-defined hyperfine coupling to directly bonded nuclei, which are β- to the unpaired electron on nitrogen and interact by σ-π overlap (hyperconjugation). More distant nuclei are not normally expected to give detectable hyperfine coupling. In contrast, adducts of MPN should show coupling to both α- and β-atoms, with the latter often greater than the former. A good example is that of the $CCl_3^{\bullet}$ adducts (Leaver *et al.*, 1969). The PBN adduct shows normal coupling to ^1H and ^{14}N, and no resolved coupling to chlorine (^{35}Cl and ^{37}Cl have $I = 3/2$, giving two sets of four components which are often superimposed). However, $^{13}CCl_3^{\bullet}$ displays a well-defined doublet splitting from ^{13}C (Tomasi *et al.*, 1980). In contrast, the $CCl_3^{\bullet}$ adduct of MNP gives well resolved coupling to three equivalent chlorine atoms (10 hyperfine components). One conclusion is that it is probably wise to try both types of spin-trap in the hope that one may give a characteristic extra splitting. An important example of the biological application of spin-traps is in the detection of $^{13}CCl_3^{\bullet}$ radicals formed from $^{13}CCl_4$ in liver extracts (Tomasi *et al.*, 1980).

Another important example of the use of spin-traps is the detection of $OH^{\bullet}$ radicals (see, for example, Okolow-Zubkowska and Hill, 1980; Nohl *et al.*, 1981). These radicals cannot be detected directly in fluid solutions because of rapid spin-relaxation, but they do add to spin-traps, and it seems to be agreed that the data can be taken as being diagnostic of $OH^{\bullet}$ radicals. An important discovery based on the use of spin-traps is that $OH^{\bullet}$ radicals are one of the highly reactive species that are called up in emergencies such as oxygen dependent killing by phagocytes (Okolow-Zubkowska *et al.*, 1980; Nohl *et al.*, 1981).

Stable Organic Radicals

Many delocalised "aromatic" structures are involved in one or two electron redox processes usually coupled to proton transfer reactions, the intermediate one-electron species being relatively stable and hence detectable by e.s.r. spectroscopy. In most cases the spectrum is simply a broad singlet, and ENDOR spectroscopy is needed to give useful structural information (see below). Systems frequently studied by e.s.r. spectroscopy include NAD^+-$NAD^\bullet$-NADH, FAD-FADH-$FADH_2$, and the ubiquinones involved in the photosynthetic process.

Reactive Organic Radicals

In principle, *in situ* photolysis, or reactions involving flow-systems, should be able to give stationary concentrations of radicals in detectable concentrations. In practice, this approach has only been useful in the biological field in the study of small molecules such as amino acids or sugars. Most photochemical work has centred around the photo systems of chloroplasts, and e.s.r. has certainly been of some use in helping to understand these remarkably complex and efficient light-harvesting systems. Unfortunately, the e.s.r. spectra are mainly singlet features but ENDOR and spin-echo spectroscopy together with ODMR have greatly helped in elucidating structural parameters. Unfortunately, space does not permit a review of this field.

A main problem is that, for the study of transient radicals narrow features are required, but high polymer radicals are usually rotating too slowly and give rise to features that may be undetectably broad. Hence low-temperature solid-state studies have much to commend them, since it is then possible to accumulate radicals to well above normal stationary liquid-phase concentrations.

Two methods are used for generation, photolysis and radiolysis. Indeed, much of the photolytic work on chloroplast systems has, in fact, been done at very low temperatures. In these, and in most radiolyses, electrons are lost and gained: in photo ionization both processes are selective, but in radiolysis electron-ejection is usually indiscriminate, although electron capture is often remarkedly selective. It could be argued that the only reason for studying the effects of ionizing radiation on biological systems is for its own sake - that is to probe the way radiation damage occurs. This is, in fact, an extremely important problem since all living systems run a risk of excessive exposure, and very low levels can do enormous damage especially to eucaryotic cells. Any work that can shed light upon radiation processes may point towards chemical methods of protection. Also, since radiotherapy is so widely used, such studies also help in the search for radio-sensitisers.

In fact, however, the use of ionizing radiation should be of more general interest, since it provides a method of injecting electrons into a biological system at very low temperatures. Not only can e.s.r. spectroscopy show where the electrons add initially but, in favourable cases, it can also show which electron-transfer processes can then occur on annealing.

The study of radioprotection has centred around damage to DNA since this seems to be implicated at least for low dose levels. E.s.r. spectroscopy has been most informative in the study of concentrated aqueous systems frozen to 77 K (Bertinchamps and Gregoli, 1981). Under the conditions used, phase separation occurs so that the DNA phase is highly concentrated. Remarkably, damage to this phase at 77 K is shown to be extremely selective, the major electron-loss occurring at the guanine bases (G), the electrons being trapped exclusively at the thymine bases (T). This result is unexpected since electron loss is usually indiscriminate. It implies the operation of an efficient electron-transfer route allowing the "hole" to migrate to give G^+ which is then deeply trapped. It is interesting to note that even with pure mononucleosides or -tides, electron loss centres at low temperatures are predominantly $RO^{\bullet}$ (formed from $ROH^{\bullet +}$ in the sugar moiety). For DNA there are no free OH groups, and hence e^--loss centres cannot be "fixed" by proton loss. Just how the formation of these centres leads to strand-breaking, which is strongly implicated as being the most lethal form of damage, is not clear. However, e.s.r. studies have clearly shown that the T^- units are rapidly protonated, and that the resulting TH radicals react readily with oxygen to give $RO_2^{\bullet}$ radicals.

I stress that, interesting though these results are, they may not be the significant pathway for strand-breaking *in vivo*. There can be no doubt that indirect attack by $OH^{\bullet}$ radicals on DNA can lead to breakage by a well-established pathway (Von Sonntag and Schulte-Frohlinde, 1978), and the fact that this path is not followed under the conditions used may simply be because the conditions are too far removed from *in vivo* conditions. This remains to be seen.

Transition-Metal Complexes

For S = ½ complexes the considerations are just the same as for radicals except that g-value variation is usually far greater. As indicated above, this arises because the orbital containing the unpaired electron is usually close to other filled or empty orbitals with which it can be magnetically coupled. (For example, field along z will couple d_{xy} and $d_{x^2-y^2}$ orbitals: if the structure approaches $d^1_{xy}\ d^0_{x^2-y^2}$ Δg will be negative, but if it is $d^2_{xy}\ d^1_{x^2-y^2}$ it will be positive.) There are two consequences, one is that signals are usually well removed from the free spin (g = 2.0023) region, and the other is that spectra are often too broad to detect in the liquid-phase, or even in frozen systems except at very low temperatures. For example, temperatures in the region of 10 K are usually optimum for studies of many iron-sulphur clusters. This arises largely because the magnitude of the g-shift is governed by the ligand field, and this is readily modulated by thermal motions and variable solvation. These changes broaden the lines and provide better opportunities for electron-spin relaxation.

When liquid-phase spectra can be detected, the line-widths reflect the form of the solid-state spectra, as outlined for $R_2NO^{\bullet}$ radicals. This is illustrated in Fig. 8 for the well-known case of vanadyl ions, VO^{2+}. There is no doubt that e.s.r. spectroscopy is one of the most powerful methods for studying S = ½ complexes, and there are hundreds of examples of significant studies in the biological field. These include many studies of Cu(II) complexes. The most common configuration is the so-called "square-planar" arrangement comprising four relatively strongly bound in-plane (xy) ligands. The $d(\pi)$ orbitals are filled together with the d_{z^2} orbital, the unpaired electron being in the σ*, $d_{x^2-y^2}$ orbital. If there are one or two ligands weakly bonded along z the configuration will be $d^6(\pi)\ d^2_{z^2}\ d^1_{x^2-y^2}$. Usually $g_z \gg g_x \approx g_y > 2.0023$, and $|A_z| \gg |A_x| \approx |A_y|$.

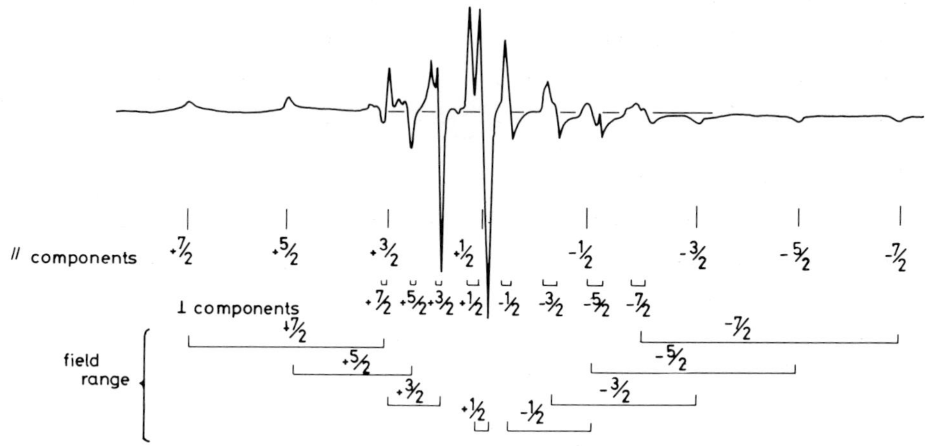

FIG. 8 First derivative e.s.r. spectrum for a rigid solution containing VO^{2+} ions, showing parallel and perpendicular components of the ^{51}V hyperfine coupling. (^{51}V has $I = {}^{7}/_{2}$ and hence there are 8 components: note the small splitting of some perpendicular features into x and y components.)

If the in-plane atoms directly bonded to copper have magnetic nuclei, each copper hyperfine component ($^{63/65}Cu$ have $I = {}^{3}/_{2}$, giving four lines) will be split into characteristic multiplets. For example, four equivalent ^{14}N nuclei give nine components in powder spectra. An important semi-empirical result is that as $g_{//}$ increases in a series of square-planar complexes, so $A_{//}$ ($^{63/65}Cu$) decreases (Symons *et al.*, 1975). Provided, as is usually the case, $g_{\perp}$ is fairly close to the free-spin value (2.0023), this variation is linear, being due to the onset of orbital magnetism which gives an extra contribution to the hyperfine coupling, thereby augmenting the spin-only coupling (Fig. 9). The lines (a,b) drawn in this figure are for square-planar complexes with hyperfine coupling to copper after correction, corresponding to $3d$-orbital populations in the range 75 ± 5%.

Many complexes show marked deviations from this behaviour, and analysis of the corrected hyperfine parameters show that this arises primarily because of a decrease in the magnitude of the isotropic component. For symmetrical square-planar complexes, there can be no direct mixing of $3d_{x^2-y^2}$ and $4s$ orbitals and the isotropic coupling of *ca.* −100 G arises from spin-polarisation of inner s electrons.

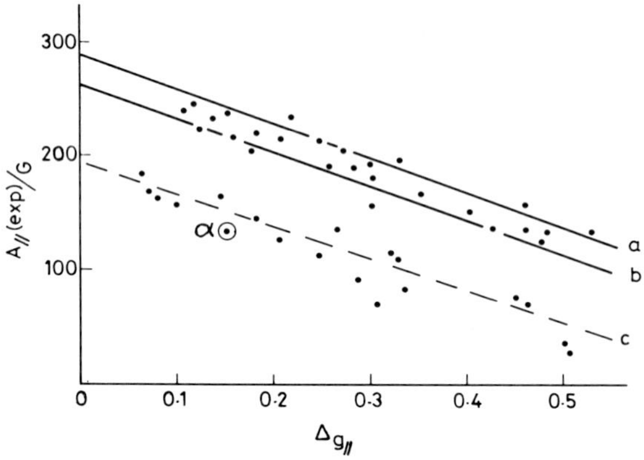

FIG. 9 Correlation between $A_{//}$ (experimental, in Gauss) and $\Delta g_{//}$. Lines a and b are for a range of square-planar complexes whilst c correlates data for complexes having distorted tetrahedral symmetry. The point α is for Cu(II) in a copper-zinc superoxide dismutase.

However, distortion towards a tetrahedral configuration allows these orbitals to mix, and the 4*s* contribution, being positive, causes $|A_{iso}|$ to fall. This is, therefore, a good measure of such distortions, which are often found for Cu(II) complexes in biological systems. A typical example is for Cu(II) in superoxide dismutases having Cu-Zn units (see Fig. 9). An important aspect of the action of this enzyme is the Cu(II) $\rightleftharpoons$ Cu(I) interconversion. Since Cu(I) prefers a tetrahedral co-ordination, its formation will be greatly facilitated by a ligand environment that tries to impose such a configuration on Cu(II). The e.s.r. results confirm that there is a large distortion from the normally preferred square-planar configuration.

Another example, taken at random, is for low-spin Co(II) complexes, typified by the cobalamin complexes including B_{12r}. In Fig. 10 the spectra for the normal B_{12r} complex shows well-defined parallel features to ^{59}Co ($I = {}^{7}/_{2}$, giving 8 lines) each parallel feature being split into triplets by coupling to one ^{14}N nucleus. The results show unambiguously that the unpaired electron is in the d_{z^2} orbital on the metal atom and hence the ^{14}N coupling stems from the nitrogen *s-p* hybridised orbital of the benzimidazole base. The other spectrum was obtained after treatment with $^{13}CN^-$ ions: the results show clearly the loss of coupling to ^{14}N, and the gain of a ^{13}C doublet ($I = \frac{1}{2}$), showing that the cyanide has displaced the benzimidazole ligand.

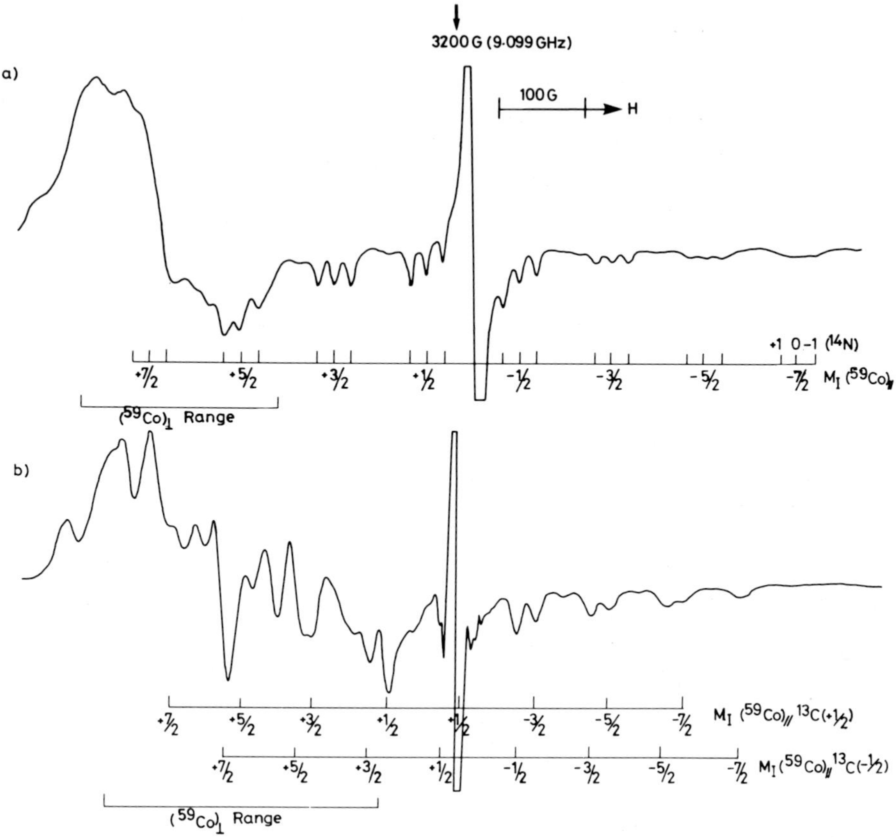

FIG. 10 First derivative X-band e.s.r. spectra at 77 K for (a) vitamin B_{12r} and (b) cyanocobalamine (^{13}CN). (M.C.R. Symons and R.K. Rao, unpublished results.)

In our own work, we have exploited the *g*-shifts exhibited by S = ½ complexes by studying the effect of ionizing radiation on metallo proteins (Symons and Petersen, 1978a,b,c,d). Our results show that it is possible to establish and study specific electron addition to metal ions even when the signals in the *g* = 2 region are large and too ill-defined for interpretation. For example, when whole-blood samples are irradiated at 77 K (after addition of ethylene glycol to prevent phase-separation), two well-defined paramagnetic centres are formed, one associated with the β-chains (g_z = 2.24, g_y = 2.14, g_x = 1.95) and the other, in *ca.* $^1/_3$ of the yield, with the α-chains (g_z = 2.20,

g_y = 2.11, g_x = 1.96). Added electron-scavengers greatly reduce the yields, and the large g-shifts establish that the centres have low-spin Fe(III) character. Use of $^{17}O_2$ enriched samples show that at least 50% of the unpaired electron is on dioxygen.

By raising the temperature above 77 K various changes in the e.s.r. spectra can be followed kinetically. For the $(FeO_2)^-$ unit, we postulate protonation and loss of HO_2^- (or H_2O_2) to explain these changes. This is a powerful method for following the mechanisms of electron-transfer reactions which complements the use of time-resolved spectroscopic methods. Another example of its utility is xanthine oxidaze (Symons and Petersen, 1978a,b,c,d). This enzyme contains Mo(VI) and two different Fe-S clusters, all of which are involved in electron-transfer processes when the enzyme reacts with its substrates. Various paramagnetic entities formed during reaction have been studied by e.s.r. spectroscopy after reaction with electron donors using rapid-mixing and rapid-freezing techniques developed by Bray and co-workers (Bray, 1963). Our results show that on exposing glassy solutions to ^{60}Co γ-rays at 77 K, the major centre formed is the Mo(V) species commonly described as "very rapid" (Bray, 1963). This converts to a different (rapid) centre on slight annealing, presumably as a result of ligand re-arrangement, possibly including protonation since well-defined ^1H hyperfine coupling is then observed. Later, this centre decays by electron-transfer to one of the (Fe-S) clusters, and finally this decays as a result of electron-transfer to the second (Fe-S) cluster. One limitation of this work is that we cannot follow changes in the concentrations of stable organic radicals which are probably also involved in these electron-transfer reactions, because of the large g = 2 signal caused by other radiation induced radicals.

Many Electron Systems

Some reference has already been made to triplet-state species. In many cases, S = 1 and S = 2 transition-metal complexes cannot be studied by conventional e.s.r. spectroscopy because the unpaired electrons are on the same atom and zero-field splitting (D) can be very large or rapidly modulated by the ligand-field. However, S = $^3/_2$ and S = $^5/_2$ systems usually have well-defined and characteristic e.s.r. features.

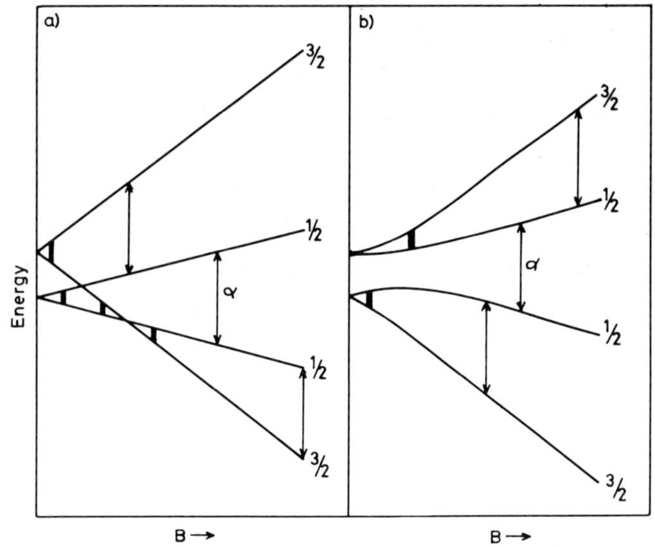

FIG. 11 Ways in which the energy levels of a complex with $S = {}^3/_2$ and $E = 0$ diverge with increasing magnetic field, B. (a) $B \| z$ and (b) $B \| x$ or y. The short, thick vertical lines represent transitions if $D > h\nu$ and the long, thin lines are for $D < h\nu$. Note that in the latter case (small zero-field splitting) the $\pm\frac{1}{2}$ transition (α) is almost isotropic. (Taken from Symons, 1978.)

For complexes with fairly symmetrical environments the zero-field splitting is small, and the $\Delta S = \pm\frac{1}{2}$ transition is almost isotropic, as indicated in Fig. 11. Usually the g-tensor components and any metal hyperfine coupling are also fairly isotropic for such complexes, and hence well-defined features in the $g = 2$ region are commonly observed in fluid and rigid systems. Typical examples are Mn(II) complexes which frequently exhibit six almost isotropic lines (^{55}Mn has $I = {}^5/_2$) in the free-spin region. This is so common that such features are taken as diagnostic of Mn(II) complexes. This is not the case, of course, since large distortions will lead to the changes outlined below, leading to signals far removed from the $g = 2$ region.

As the ligand bonding becomes less symmetrical, zero-field splitting increases, the $\Delta S = \pm {}^3/_2$ or $\pm {}^5/_2$ features become increasingly anisotropic (and hence weaker in powder spectra) and the $\Delta S = \pm\frac{1}{2}$ features split, as indicated in Fig. 11. Fortunately, various limiting situations are rapidly reached, leading to characteristic and quite intense singularities in e.s.r. spectra. Thus for S = $^3/_2$ complexes with axial ligand-fields "perpendicular" features are observed in the g = 4 region and for similar S = $^5/_2$ complexes comparable features are seen in the g = 6 region. Small deviations from axial symmetry result in characteristic splittings of these features into two components. For S = $^5/_2$ complexes there is a limiting rhombic distortion leading to a strong "cross-over" feature at g = 4.3. These limiting cases are frequently encountered for Fe(III) complexes and again are often taken as being diagnostic. I stress, however, that Fe(III) complexes can well have g = 2 features comparable with those for Mn(II), and vice versa.

If the ligand-field gets too large, spin-pairing is induced: for d^5 complexes such as Fe(III) this may lead to S = $^3/_2$ OR S = $\frac{1}{2}$ complexes, but the intermediate d^5, S = $^3/_2$ complexes are rarely encountered. Met-myoglobin and met-haemoglobin complexes are examples in which the S = $^5/_2 \rightleftharpoons$ S = $\frac{1}{2}$ equilibrium is frequently encountered. When the sixth position is vacant or occupied by weakly co-ordinated ligands such as water molecules or fluoride ions S = $^5/_2$ is favoured, but for ligands such as hydroxide or azide both forms are populated whilst for cyanide complexes the S = $\frac{1}{2}$ form is favoured. Our work shows that when O_2^{2-} is the ligand (in the formal sense), the S = $\frac{1}{2}$ structure is favoured.

ENDOR AND SPIN-ECHO SPECTROSCOPY

These are both modifications of the normal e.s.r. technique which are very useful under certain circumstances but are still not widely used, possibly because of the extra cost of commercial instruments. Space does not permit more than a brief mention of these techniques which are well covered in recent books (Kevan and Kispert, 1976; Kevan and Schwartz, 1979). The ENDOR (electron-nuclear double resonance) technique involves the use of saturating microwave fields coupled with a radio-frequency sweep which speeds up relaxation at resonance, leading to an induced e.s.r. signal. The outstanding utility of this technique is its ability to simplify complex spectra (any one type of coupled nucleus gives only one significant pair of features) and to pick out hyperfine interactions within features that are merely broadened by such coupling in the e.s.r. spectra. Thus, for example, the proton hyperfine coupling for $(Me_3C)_2NO^{\cdot}$ radicals can be accurately monitored by ENDOR spectroscopy even when it is completely unresolved in normal e.s.r. spectra.

An interesting new development in single crystal ENDOR spectroscopy is the very accurate pin-pointing of nuclear co-ordinates relative to a transition-metal ion in complex molecules (Hutchinson and McKay, 1977). If the coupling is purely or largely dipolar the sites of such nuclei can be mapped with very high accuracy, and this is proving to be especially useful in the detection and citing of water molecules close to paramagnetic ions, which are often difficult to locate using diffraction methods.

The spin-echo technique can be compared with F-T n.m.r. spectroscopy. As well as providing important relaxation information in a direct sense (T_1), it can also be useful for very rapid detection and is complementary to ENDOR in its ability to pick up weak, "hidden" hyperfine interactions.

CONCLUSIONS

I hope that in this brief Review I have succeeded in imparting some idea of the utility of e.s.r. spectroscopy when applied to biochemical problems. Having used the technique extensively to study purely chemical problems during the past 27 years, it has been a revelation for me on turning towards biochemistry to find how widely and effectively it has been applied to biochemical problems. It certainly seems to have a bright and extensive future in this broad area.

ACKNOWLEDGEMENT

I thank Professor Trevor Slater for encouraging me to write this Review.

REFERENCES

Bagshaw, C.R. and Kendrick-Jones, J. (1980). *J. Mol. Biol.* 140, 411-433.

Bertinchamps, A.J. and Gregoli, S. (1981). (in press).

Bray, R.C. (1963). *In* "The Enzymes" 2nd Ed., Vol. 7, pp.533-546.

El-Sayed, M.A. (1971). *Acc. Chem. Res.* 4, 23-29.

Hoff, A.J., Govingjie and Romija, J.C. (1977). *FEBS Lett.* 73, 191-192.

Hutchinson, C.A. and McKay, D.B. (1977). *J. Chem. Phys.* 66, 3311-3319.

Kevan, L. and Kispert, L.D. (1976). *In* "Electron Spin Double Resonance Spectroscopy". Wiley-Interscience, New York.

Kevan, L. and Schwartz, R.N. (1979). *In* "Time Domain Electron Spin Resonance". Wiley-Interscience, New York.

Leaver, I.H., Ramsey, G.C. and Suzuki, E. (1969). *Aust. J. Chem.* 22, 1891-1899.

Morlya, F., Maklno, K., Suzuki, N., Rokushika, S. and Hatano, H. (1980). (1980). *J. Phys. Chem.* 84, 3085-3090.

Nohl, H., Jordan, W. and Hegner, D. (1981). *FEBS Lett.* 123, 241-244.

Okolow-Zubkowska, M.J. and Hill, H.A.O. (1980). *Dev. Biochem.* 11B, 201-212.

Rey, P. and McConnell, H.M. (1977). *J. Am. Chem. Soc.* 99, 1637-1642.

Sonntag, C. von and Schulte-Frohlinde, D. (1978). *In* "Effects of Ionizing Radiation on DNA" (Eds. J. Huttermann, W. Kohnlein, R. Teouls and A.J. Bertinchamps). Springer-Verlag, Berlin.

Symons, M.C.R., West, D.X. and Wilkinson, J.G. (1975). *J. Chem. Soc. Dalton Trans.* 1696-1700.

Symons, M.C.R. (1978). "Chemical and Biochemical Aspects of Electron Spin Resonance Spectroscopy". Van Nostrand Reinhold Company Ltd., London.

Symons, M.C.R. and Petersen, R.L. (1978a). *Proc. Roy. Soc. London Ser. B.* 201, 285-298.

Symons, M.C.R. and Petersen, R.L. (1978b). *Biochim. Biophys. Acta* 535, 241-246; 537, 70-76.

Symons, M.C.R. and Petersen, R.L. (1978c). *J. Chem. Res.* (S) 382; (M) 4572-4576.

Symons, M.C.R. and Petersen, R.L. (1978d). *Biochim. Biophys. Acta* 535, 247-252.

Thomas, D.D. and McConnell, H.M. (1974). *Chem. Phys. Lett.* 25, 470-474.

Thomas, D.D., Dalton, L.R. and Hyde, J.S. (1976). *J. Chem. Phys.* 65, 3006-3011.

Tomasi, A., Albano, E., Lott, K.A.K. and Slater, T.F. (1980). *FEBS Lett.* 122, 303-305.

DISCUSSION

Ts'o: A quick question in terms of sensitivity in the procedure of freezing a solution, particularly a tissue sample, to become a solid state in order to look at the superoxide radical: do you know the sensitivity of this procedure as compared to a spin trap? Which one is likely to be more sensitive?

Symons: The spin trap will be much more sensitive provided trapping is efficient. If 100% of your radicals were trapped by the spin trap then it would be much more sensitive.

Ts'o: Let's say it's 5%, then what happens?

Symons: I would have to do the sums. The reason why it is more sensitive of course is because your solid state spectrum of the $O_2^{\cdot-}$

is spread over a wide field range, whereas the nitroxide is giving very narrow lines. I don't know where it would break even.

Swartz: It would be complex also because you could use much bigger samples and so it really would be a complex calculation indeed. From a small sample to a big sample, from a narrow line to a wide line.

Symons: The sensible thing to do is to try both.

Slater: I regret that this discussion is curtailed because of lack of time.

Aldehydic Products of Lipid Peroxidation

H. ESTERBAUER

INTRODUCTION

Lipid derived aldehydes and other carbonyl compounds have in the past mainly attracted the interest of food chemists because these secondary autoxidation products are among the most important substances responsible for the flavour and flavour defects of many foodstuffs and beverages. Schauenstein and colleagues (Schauenstein *et al.*, 1977) have shown that some aldehydic breakdown products of polyunsaturated fatty acids are highly cytotoxic and can bring about a wide variety of inhibitory effects on cell functions. Although it was not clear at that time whether such aldehydes were of importance in biological systems, this work now appears in a new light.

Recent findings have shown that aldehydes, in particular 4-hydroxyalkenals, are also produced during stimulated microsomal lipid peroxidation and that such aldehydes might be responsible, at least in part, for the deleterious effects of lipid peroxidation on cells and cell constituents (Benedetti *et al.*, 1980; Esterbauer *et al.*, 1981b). The mechanisms by which lipid peroxidation causes subsequent cellular alterations are very complex and not completely understood, but basically three major events must be considered. Firstly, the alteration of membrane lipids can lead to a loss of membrane function and to an impairment of membrane bound enzymes. Secondly, various highly reactive free radicals generated by the process of lipid peroxidation can attack and inactivate enzymes and other cell constituents. Thirdly, reactive aldehydes and possible other compounds, which are cytotoxic themselves, can be formed through the peroxidative degradation of the membrane lipids. It is clear that all three mechanisms are of equal importance and act in a concerted fashion simultaneously or consecutively. Nevertheless, the formation of cytotoxic aldehydes with relative long life times, at least in comparison with free radicals, could explain some "long distance" effects promoted by lipid peroxidation. It is therefore of importance to study in more detail both the generation of aldehydes during lipid peroxidation as well as their chemical reactivity and biochemical effects. This contribution is intended to give, for those not familiar with this subject, a short survey of mechanisms of aldehyde formation, the methods and some of the difficulties of aldehyde analysis, the chemical reactivity of aldehydes and their biochemical properties. Some of the work reported here has already been published (Schauenstein *et al.*, 1977; Schauenstein and Esterbauer, 1979; Benedetti *et al.*, 1980) or is in press (Esterbauer and Slater, 1981a; Esterbauer *et al.*, 1981b). In addition, many new results, especially concerning peroxidation in model systems and analysis of aldehyde mixtures are included in this paper.

LIPID PEROXIDATION AND POSSIBLE MECHANISMS OF ALDEHYDE FORMATION

It is generally accepted that the peroxidation of polyunsaturated fatty acids proceeds through a free radical chain reaction. The process needs an initiation through the formation of an initial radical which is able to attack α-methylene groups (CH_2 groups adjacent to one or two C-C double bonds) of the intact lipid chain leading to formation of a lipid radical $L^\bullet$. In many cases of lipid peroxidation, especially those occurring in biological systems, the identity of this initial free radical is unknown and many possible candidates, including semiquinones, $O_2^{\bullet-}$, $OH^\bullet$, have been suggested (Vladimirov *et al.*, 1980). The lipid radical $L^\bullet$ combines with ground state oxygen to give the peroxiradical $LOO^\bullet$, which in turn attacks another α-methylene group yielding a lipid hydroperoxide and a new lipid radical which propagates the chain reaction. The monohydroperoxides LOOH, which are the first products of peroxidation, are rather unstable and easily decompose into other products. Moreover, their catalytic decomposition by metal ions such as bivalent iron may produce new free lipid radicals which can initiate new chains of peroxidation (chain branching) and thus enhance the rate of peroxidation in an autocatalytic way.

$$LOOH + Fe^{2+} \longrightarrow LO^{\bullet} + OH^{-} + Fe^{3+}$$

It is assumed that these chain branchings promoted by ferrous ions play an important role in determining the rate, control and extent of peroxidation in biological systems. Depending on the complexity of the system the unstable lipid hydroperoxides LOOH may be converted in consecutive scission, fission, rearrangement and oxidation reactions into a great diversity of products containing various oxygen functional groups such as the aldehydo-, keto-, hydroxy-, epoxi-, carboxy-, and peroxi-. The scheme in Fig. 1 gives a summary of the classes of substances which have been shown to be formed either by enzymatic or non-enzymatic oxidation of polyunsaturated fatty acids.

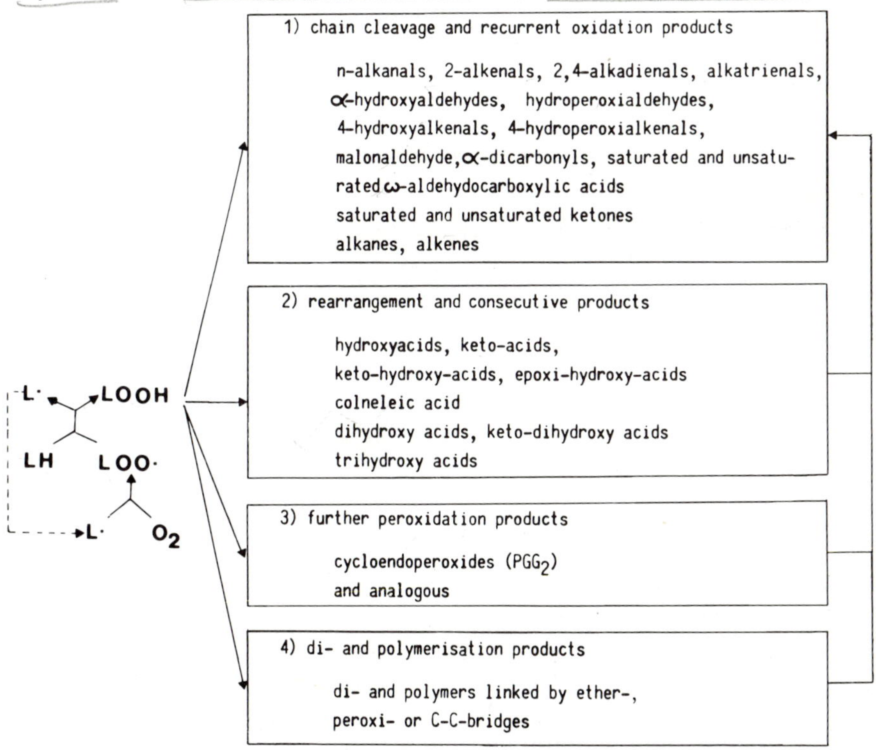

FIG. 1 Schematic presentation of the aldehyde classes and other products derived from peroxidised lipids. Note that aldehydes are formed by chain cleavage reactions from both the fatty acid monohydroperoxides and the secondary substances listed under 2, 3 and 4.

Lipoxidase type reactions, catalysed by enzymes of plant seeds may convert linoleic acid into oxygenated C-18 fatty acids (Graveland *et al.*, 1972; Esterbauer and Schauenstein, 1977a,b) as for example hydroxy- and keto-octadecadienoic acids, keto-hydroxy-, dihydroxy-, trihydroxy-, epoxi-hydroxy-, and keto-dihydroxy octadecenoic acids.

Prostaglandins and numerous other related compounds are specific products of high biological activity generated from arachidonic acid by enzyme catalysed peroxidation reactions. Prostaglandin analogues are also produced from γ-linolenic acid by the action of soybean lipoxidase (Porter and Funk, 1975).

In some peroxidation systems fission reactions leading to dimers and polymers, in which the chains are linked by C-C, -O- or -O-O- bonds seem to be a main process. If, for example, methyl-linoleate (mol. weight: 294) is autoxidised in aqueous emulsion at 37°C for 80 h, two molecules of oxygen are taken up per mole of parent methyl-linoleate and the reaction product has an average molecular weight of 500 (Esterbauer and Schauenstein, 1967).

In respect to lipid derived aldehydes most important are the chain cleavage reactions. The production of saturated and unsaturated aldehydes and other carbonyl compounds is an inevitable event associated with lipid peroxidation. Although the complexity of the peroxidation reactions has not yet permitted unambiguous identification of the pathways of production of all aldehydes found in various peroxidised samples, it is reliable to assume that most of the aldehydes are formed by one or more of the chain scission reactions shown by the equations of Fig. 2. After the oxidative cleavage of the lipid chain the aldehyde function can be present either in the moiety derived from the methyl chain end or in the moiety derived from the carboxyl end. Therefore the oxidative alterations of phospholipids contained in biomembranes, as they occur in microsomes during the course of stimulated (ADP/Fe^{++}, CCl_4, $BrCCl_3$) peroxidation, produce in addition to the short chain carbonyls containing no lipid phosphorus also altered phospholipids which contain acyl residues possessing an aldehyde function in the ω-position (Poyer and McCay, 1971).

The homolytic cleavage of the C-C bond(s) next to the hydroperoxigroup (dismutation) proceeds most probably via the alkoxiradical,

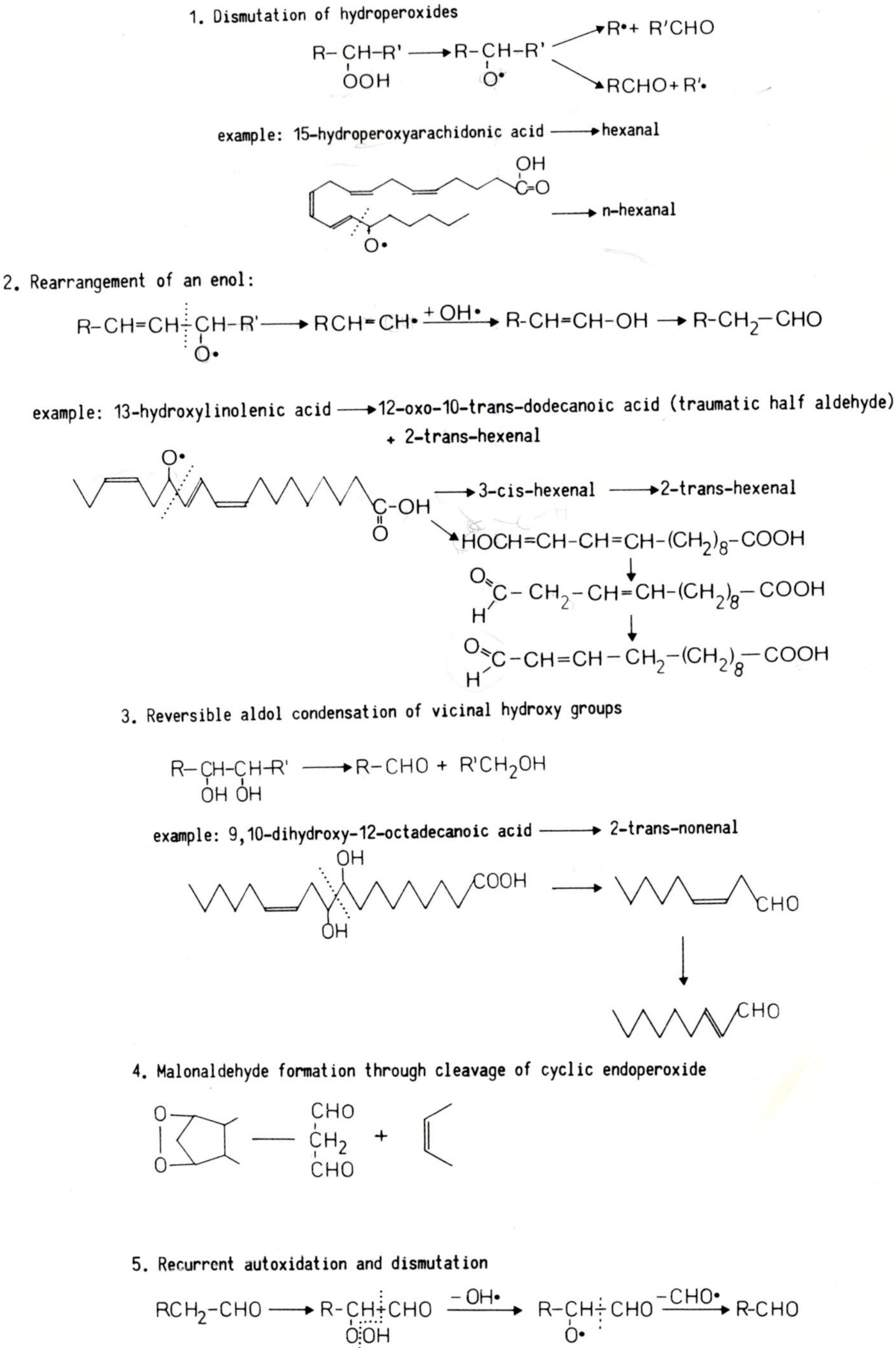

FIG. 2 Possible mechanisms for chain cleavage reactions leading to aldehydes.

TABLE 1 Amounts of 4-hydroxynonenal, alkanals, 2-alkenals, and 2,4-alkadienals produced during the course of peroxidation of fatty acids or microsomes respectively

	nmole aldehyde/mg fatty acid					aldehydes in microsomes, ADP/Fe
	18:1	18:2	18:3	γ-18:3	20:4	
Alkenals (total)	1.52	205.7	1.02	54.6	194.2	++++
Pentanal	0.11	6.7	0.47	1.6	5.2	+
Hexanal	0.25	199.0	0.55	53.0	189.0	++++
Heptanal	0.19	0	0	0	0	0
Octanal	0.36	0	0	0	0	0
Nonanal	0.51	0	0	0	0	0
Decanal	0.10	0	0	0	0	0
2-alkenals (total)	1.95	25.8	12.3	24.1	30.9	++
Pentenal	0	0	2.5	0	0	+
Hexenal	0	1.1	9.8	0.6	0	+
Heptenal	0	10.1	0	4.1	6.2	+
Octenal	0	13.1	0	7.7	15.4	+
Nonenal	0.08	1.5	0	11.7	9.3	0
Decenal	0.90	0	0	0	0	0
Undecenal	0.97	0	0	0	0	0
2,4-alkadienals	0	0.44	7.8	14.9	10.6	+
Heptadienal	0	0	4.6	0	0	
Nonadienal	0	0.36	3.2	0	4.6	
Decadienal	0	0.08	0	14.9	6.0	
4-hydroxynonenal (-Fe)	-	2.8	-	-	37.5	-
4-hydroxynonenal (+ 20 μM Fe^{++})	0	10.3	trace	26.9	103.8	++++

The values for alkanals, 2-alkenals, and 2,4-alkadienals were estimated by the method described in Fig. 4. The flask contained 320 ml H_2O, 20 ml 0.2 M acetate buffer pH 4.0 and 20 mg of the fatty acid and was gassed with air (60 ml/min) at 50°C for 24 h. The volatile aldehydes recovered in the DNPH trap were then analysed. The peroxidation experiments, in which 4-hydroxynonenal was estimated and the microsomal peroxidation were performed are described in Table 2.

which decomposes into an aldehyde and an alkylradical (Badings, 1970). Many of the aldehydes, the formation of which might be predicted theoretically from dismutation of the primary monohydroperoxides of the fatty acids have been actually identified (Badings, 1970; Rachelsperger, 1979). Hexanal, for instance, which is the main *n*-alkanal produced by peroxidising microsomes, is the dismutation product of

13-OOH-linoleic-, 13-OOH-γ-linolenic-, and 15-OOH-arachidonic acid (Table 1). Linolenic acid (18:3 Δ9,12,15) on the other hand produces mainly propanal (not shown in Table 2, but see Fig. 8) through dismutation of the 16-OOH-linolenic acid.

The combination of an OH• radical with an alkyl radical produced by dismutation is another pathway which can lead via the intermediate enol to aldehydes. This mechanism has been used to explain the formation of traumatic half aldehyde from linolenic acid (Kajiwara *et al.*, 1977).

There are of course many aldehydes other than those expected on theoretical grounds from the dismutation of the fatty acid monohydroperoxides present in peroxidised lipid samples. Schauenstein *et al.* (1977), for example, found among the autoxidation products of methyl-linoleate 4-hydroxyoctenal, 4-hydroperoxi-nonenal and a ω-carbmethoxy-4-hydroxy-alkenal. We have found recently 4-hydroxynonenal as one of the major aldehydes formed during the course of peroxidation of linoleic, γ-linolenic and arachidonic acid and liver microsomes (see Table 1).

Many of the rearrangement products and most probably also the prostaglandin analogues and the fission products listed in the scheme of Fig. 1 may be aldehyde precursors and cleavage of their carbon chains could yield a great diversity of aldehydes including 4-hydroxyalkenals. It has been demonstrated that trihydroxy- and dihydroxyoctadecanoic acids break down even under mild conditions (pH 4-6, 30-50°C) to many different carbonyl compounds (Esterbauer, Rachelsperger and Schauenstein, unpublished work; Tressl *et al.*, 1979).

Malonaldehyde, which is a common product of lipid peroxidation is formed, according to Pryor and Stanley (1975), from cyclic endoperoxides produced by autoxidation of fatty acids containing three or more double bonds. Recent experiments (Esterbauer *et al.*, 1981b) have shown that peroxidising microsomes (ADP/Fe) produce only free malonaldehyde and no other substances which can act as malonaldehyde precursors in the thiobarbituric acid (TBA) test. Finally, it must be considered that all aldehydes are unstable themselves and can undergo consecutive peroxidation reactions leading to a complete new set of compounds including peracids and aldehydes (Loury, 1973).

α-Peroxidation of a saturated aldehyde can give an intermediate α-hydroperoxyaldehyde which then decomposes to formic acid (or formaldehyde) and an aldehyde with one less carbon atom, which in turn can start a new reaction.

ANALYSIS OF COMPLEX ALDEHYDE MIXTURES

From what was said above, it is clear that lipid peroxidation results in a very complex pattern of carbonyl compounds. Since these carbonyls possess very different molecular structures and chemical properties (volatile short chain aldehydes, aldehydes bound to phospholipids, aldehyde-carboxylic acids, etc.) it is clear that in their complete analysis one encounters many difficulties, which are amplified in many cases by the lack of proper reference compounds. According to the experience of our laboratory it is appropriate to convert the carbonyls, by reacting with 2,4-dinitrophenyl hydrazine, into the corresponding hydrazone derivatives and to analyse the hydrazone mixture by a combination of thin layer chromatography and high performance chromatography as shown schematically in Fig. 3. The method can, of course, be modified and simplified if only a few classes of the total carbonyls present in the sample under investigation are of interest. Thus, for example, the fraction of volatile aldehydes, i.e. alkanals, 2-alkenals, 2,4-alkadienals, with 11 or less carbon atoms can be separated from all other compounds and recovered as DNPH derivatives by the simple equipment shown in Fig. 4 (Rachelsperger, 1979). If preformed volatile aldehydes contained in a sample are going to be analysed, nitrogen is used to carry the aldehydes from the sample solution into the DNPH trap. If, on the other hand, the formation of the aldehydes during peroxidation is going to be followed, the sample to be peroxidised is gassed with air. In this case the aldehydes are removed as they are formed, thus a secondary alteration of the aldehydes is avoided. In this procedure the recovery is excellent (greater than 90%) and proportional to concentration down to aldehyde concentrations of 0.3 μg/ℓ. All values for alkanals, 2-alkenals and 2,4-alkadienals given in Table 1 were estimated by this procedure. If information about all carbonyls (volatile, non volatile, polar and non polar, etc.) is needed, the complete sample is derivatised with DNPH and all hydrazones are

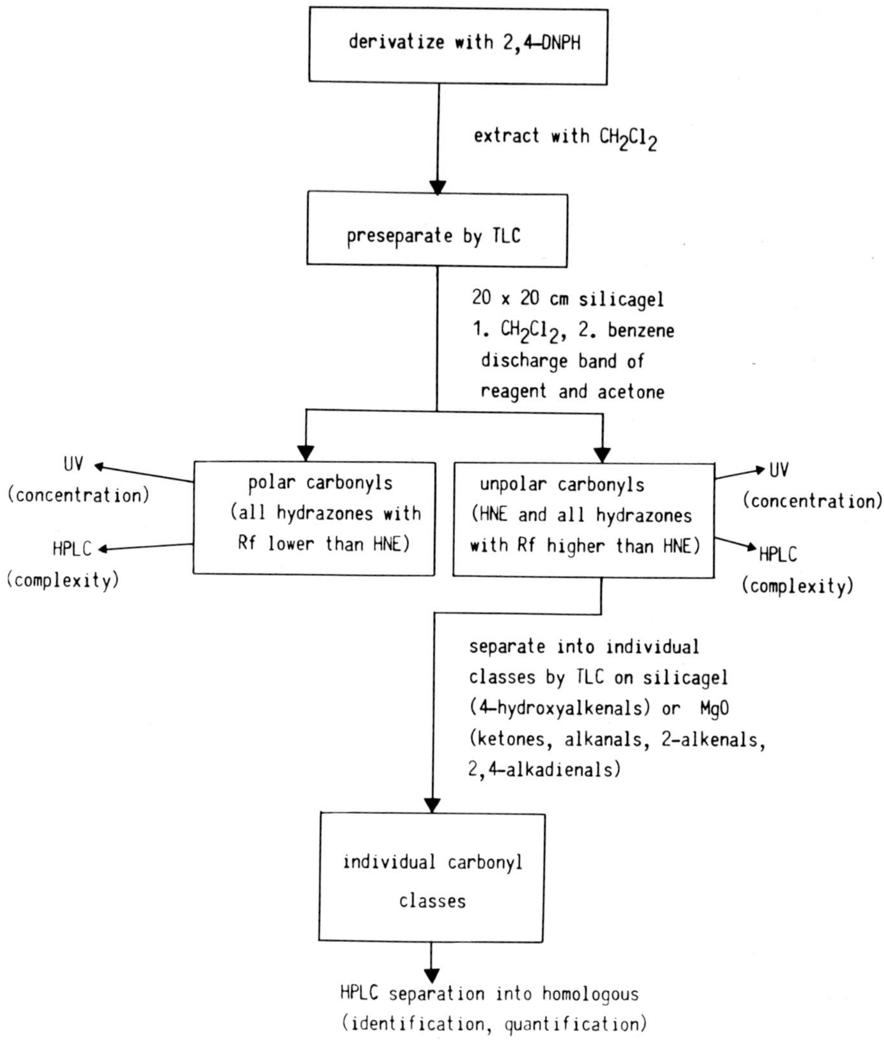

FIG. 3 Schematic presentation of the analysis of complex aldehyde mixtures.

removed by extraction with a suitable solvent such as dichloromethane. It was found to be of advantage in the subsequent HPLC analysis to preseparate the carbonyl hydrazones by TLC into two fractions, i.e. polar and non polar carbonyls (Fig. 3). The hydrazones give characteristic UV-vis spectra as shown in Fig. 5 and the amount of carbonyls contained in each fraction can be calculated approximately from the

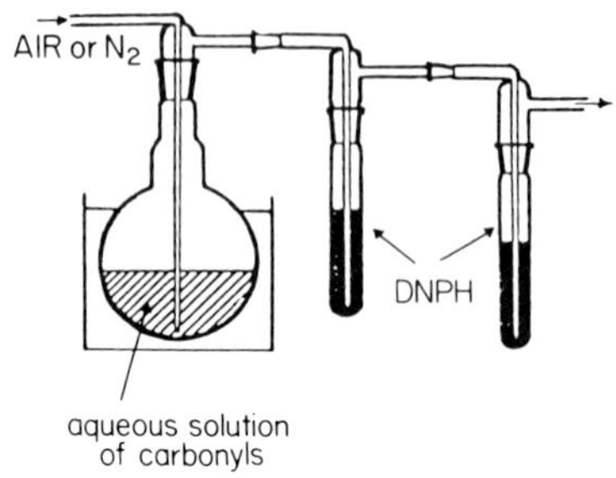

FIG. 4 Method for the separation of preformed volatile aldehydes (gas with N_2) or aldehydes produced during the course of peroxidation (gas with air) from other constituents. The gas stream is adjusted to above 60 ml/min, the temperature of the bath is between 30 and 50°C. The trap contains 10 ml of saturated DNPH reagent in 1 N HCl.

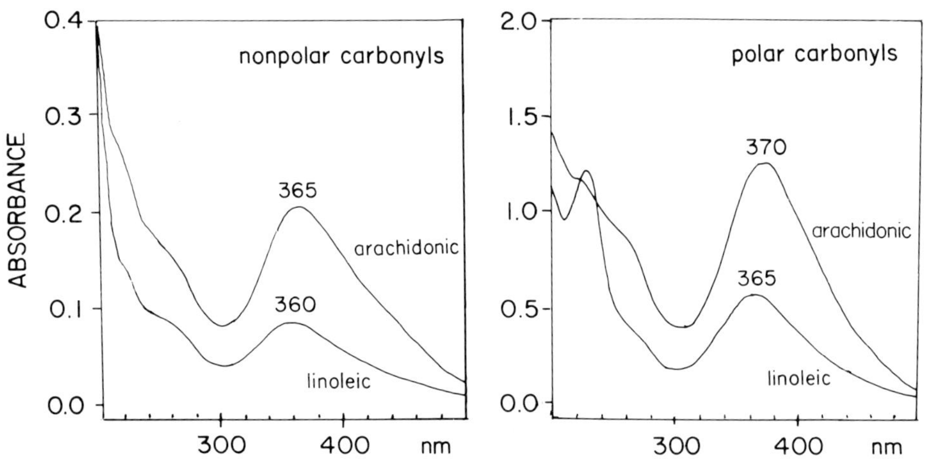

FIG. 5 UV-vis spectra of the non polar and polar carbonyls recovered as dinitrophenylhydrazones (see method in Fig. 3) from arachidonic and linoleic acid peroxidised 18 h in the presence of 20 μM Fe^{++}. The measured solution (2.5 ml) contained the carbonyls produced from either 0.08 mg arachidonic acid or 0.2 mg linoleic acid.

maximum absorbance at 365-370 nm using a molar extinction coefficient of ε = 26 000. This value is an average of the molar absorbtivity (solvent: methanol) estimated in our laboratory for *n*-alkanals (ε = 22 000-26 000), 2-alkenals (ε = 28 000-29 000), 2,4-alkadienals (ε = 36 000-38 000), ketones (ε = 22 500) and 4-hydroxy-2-alkenals (ε = 27 800-29 300).

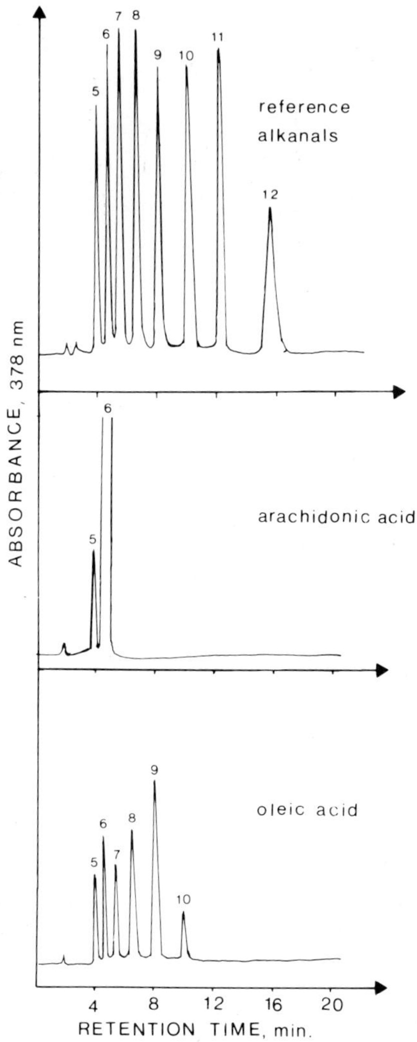

FIG. 6 HPLC separation of reference n-alkanal-dinitrophenylhydrazones and the n-alkanals produced during the peroxidation of arachidonic and oleic acid. The numbers indicate the chain length of the aldehyde: 5:pentanal, 6:hexanal, etc.) For peroxidation conditions see Table 2. Separation conditions: Zorbax ODS, 4.6 x 250 mm; methanol/water 92.5/7.5, 1.2 ml/min, detector wave length 378 nm.

The separation of the non polar or polar carbonyl fraction obtained from model peroxidations of PUFA or from peroxidised microsomes by HPLC yields highly complex chromatograms (see for example Fig. 8

later) which do not permit definite identification of the peaks, even if reference compounds are available. For an unequivocal identification of the individual aldehydes contained in the non polar carbonyl fraction it is essential to preseparate the mixture into the various carbonyl classes by TLC on magnesium oxide (Schwarz and Packs, 1963) and silicagel and to analyse the individual classes so obtained separately by HPLC using the appropriate standards for peak identification and quantification. Figure 6 shows as an example the analysis of alkanals from oleic acid and arachidonic acid together with the reference chromatogram. It is evident from the peak pattern, that arachidonic acid produced mainly hexanal, together with small amounts of pentanal, while oleic acid produced during the peroxidation pentanal, hexanal, heptanal, octanal, nonanal and decanal. From the peak heights the amount of each individual aldehyde can be assessed in the usual way. The values found are given in Table 1. Figure 7 shows as

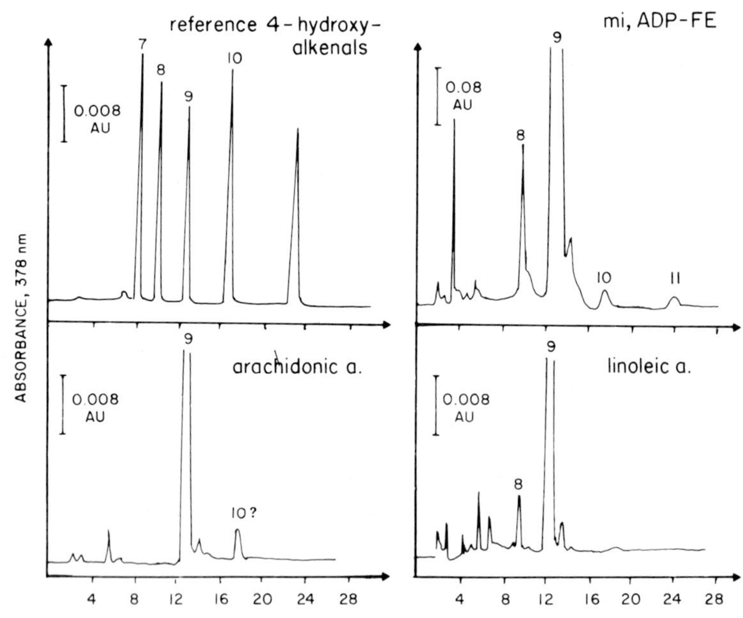

FIG. 7 HPLC separation of reference 4-hydroxy-2-alkenal dinitrophenylhydrazones and the 4-hydroxyalkenals produced by peroxidising microsomes and by peroxidation of arachidonic and linoleic acid. The numbers indicate the chain length of the aldehyde (7:4-hydroxy-2-heptenal, 8:4-hydroxy-2-octenal etc.) For peroxidation conditions see Table 2. Separation conditions: Lichrosorb 5-RP-18, 4.6 x 200 mm, methanol/water 80/20; 1.0 ml/min; detector wave length 378 nm.

a further example the HPLC separation of the class of 4-hydroxyalkenals contained in a sample of peroxidised (ADP/Fe^{++}) microsomes and in peroxidised arachidonic and linoleic acids. From the comparison with the corresponding reference chromatogram it is evident that the major 4-hydroxyalkenal in each case is 4-hydroxynonenal. In addition, the microsomes also produce some minor amounts of 4-hydroxyoctenal (also present to a small extent in oxidised linoleic acid), 4-hydroxydecenal and 4-hydroxyundecenal. It should be emphasised here that the identification of 4-hydroxynonenal as a peroxidation product of liver microsomes was achieved not only by chromatographic methods but also by various spectroscopic analyses performed with the underivatised aldehyde as well as with its dinitrophenylhydrazone (Benedetti *et al.*, 1980). Similarly the presence of 4-hydroxynonenal in the autoxidised samples of arachidonic acid and linoleic acid was also established by the identification of the aldehyde in its underivatised form.

The aldehydes and carbonyls contained in the fraction of the polar carbonyls (see scheme in Fig. 3) have not been analysed up to now. From preliminary HPLC separations it is evident that the mixture is even more complex than the mixture of the non polar carbonyls, but we are confident that future experiments will enable us to identify at least the major compounds.

COMPARISON OF ALDEHYDE PRODUCTION BY VARIOUS PEROXIDATION SYSTEMS

In model autoxidation experiments we have compared the capacity for aldehyde production of oleic, linoleic, linolenic, γ-linolenic and arachidonic acid by measurement of the amount of non polar and polar carbonyls present after 18 h incubation at 37°C in the presence (20 μM) and absence of $FeSO_4$ (Table 2). The values for microsomes (ADP/Fe, 37°C, 30 min) were also included in this comparison. As expected the highest productivity was obtained with arachidonic acid, which gave 1728 nmole carbonyls per mg parent fatty acid. Expressed on a molar basis, this value corresponds 0.54 mole carbonyl per mole arachidonic acid, indicating that carbonyl formation is indeed a major event during the course of peroxidation. The capacity for aldehyde formation decreases in the order arachidonic, γ-linolenic, linolenic, linoleic, oleic acid. The catalytic effect of bivalent iron is clearly

TABLE 2 Total carbonyls, polar and unpolar carbonyls, and malonaldehyde produced by various unsaturated fatty acids and rat liver microsomes

System	$FeSO_4$	Rel. rate of O_2 uptake	Malonaldehyde nmole/mg	Carbonyls as hydrazones[1)]		
				nmole/mg	% unpolar	% polar
Oleic acid, 18:1,Δ9	0	1	-	-	-	-
Oleic acid	20 μM	-	0	62	69.3	30.6
Linoleic acid, 18:2,Δ9,12	0	30	0	98	29.3	70.7
Linoleic acid	20 μM		12	317	16.3	83.7
Linolenic acid, 18:3,Δ9,12,15	0	72	-	-	-	-
Linolenic acid	20 μM	-	13	562	21.3	78.6
γ-linolenic acid, 18:3,Δ6,9,12	0	-	-	-	-	-
γ-linolenic acid	20 μM	-	37	999	23.0	77.0
Arachidonic acid, 20:4Δ5,8,11,14	0	144	19	588	15.6	84.3
Arachidonic acid	20 μM	-	45	1728	16.6	83.4
Microsomes[2)]	0	-	5	10	30	70
Microsomes	20 μM	-	60	104	42.6	57.3

[1)] Malonaldehyde does not give a 2,4-dinitrophenylhydrazone, these values therefore include all carbonyls other than malonaldehyde. [2)] Malonaldehyde and carbonyl values expressed as nmole/mg microsomal protein. The peroxidation of the fatty acids was carried out in tris/KCl buffer pH 7.4 at 37°C for 18 h in shaken flasks in the absence and presence of $FeSO_4$ (20 μM final). The fatty acid concentration was 1 mg/ml. The ADP/Fe^{++} stimulated peroxidation of microsomes was performed for 30 min at 37°C (Slater and Sawyer, 1971). The peroxidised samples were derivatised with 2,4-DNPH and the hydrazone mixture was separated into polar and non-polar hydrazones by TLC, the amount of carbonyl hydrazone in each fraction was estimated from the UV-absorbance at 370 nm using an average molar absorptivity of $\varepsilon = 26{,}000$. Malonaldehyde was estimated by the TBA assay. The relative rates of oxidation were calculated from the figures (moles O_2 taken up per mole of fatty acid or fatty acid methyl ester per hour) given by Badings (Badings, 1970).

by arachidonic acid, which forms under comparable conditions about 10 times more of this aldehyde than linoleic and four times more than linolenic acid (Table 1). Many years ago 4-hydroxyoctenal (Schauenstein *et al.*, 1964) and 4-hydroperoxinonenal (Esterbauer and Schauenstein, 1966) were isolated from the water soluble products produced during the course (70-100 h, 37°C, stirred) of autoxidation of methyl linoleate in water. According to the new results presented here it seems more likely that the hydroxyalkenal isolated from oxidised methyl linoleate was in fact 4-hydroxynonenal or a mixture of hydroxyoctenal and hydroxynonenal).

Some quantitative data concerning the amounts of alkanals, 2-alkenals, 2,4-alkadienals and 4-hydroxynonenal produced during the peroxidation of the fatty acids are given in Table 1. The corresponding values for microsomes are given only as symbols (0 not present; + low amounts; ++++ high amounts) since the absolute values have so far proved difficult to reproduce. Though, microsomes obtained from different laboratories always show a similar aldehyde pattern, the absolute peak intensities and to some extent the distribution show a considerable variation.

THE CHEMICAL REACTIVITY OF ALDEHYDES AND THEIR INHIBITORY EFFECTS ON BIOLOGICAL SYSTEMS

Long chain saturated aldehydes show a low reactivity towards molecules of biological interest, i.e. amino acids, proteins, nucleic acids, etc. The only reaction which readily takes place is the reaction with cysteine to give thiazolidine carboxylic acids. This reaction could be responsible for the inhibitory effect of some saturated aldehydes on protein biosynthesis in liver slices and hepatoma cells (Guidotti *et al.*, 1965). If used in high concentration, alkanals can produce inter- and intramolecular crosslinking in proteins. Most reactive in this respect are highly hydrated aldehydes such as formaldehyde, acetaldehyde and other shorter chain aldehydes. In contrast to the alkanals the 2-alkenals and 4-hydroxyalkenals are highly reactive substances which readily react even at neutral pH and at low concentrations with biomolecules, especially those possessing sulphydryl groups as for example cysteine, glutathione, coenzyme A and proteins or enzymes containing SH groups (Esterbauer *et al.*, 1975; Esterbauer *et al.*, 1976; Schauenstein *et al.*, 1971). Under physiological conditions the main reaction appears to be a 1,4-addition to the conjugated system leading to saturated aldehydes which have the sulphydryl compound by a thio ether linkage at carbon 3.

$$\text{R-CH = CH-CHO + R'SH} \longrightarrow \text{R-CH(SR')-CH}_2\text{-CHO}$$

The main difference between 2-alkenals and 4-hydroxyalkenals lies in the reaction rate and in the stability of the products formed. On average 4-hydroxyalkenals react about five times faster with thiols and the formed adducts are about 500 times more stable (Esterbauer *et al.*, 1975). The higher stability of the 4-hydroxyalkenal reaction products results from the fact that cyclic hemiacetals are formed.

$$\text{R-CH(OH)-CH = CH-CHO + R'SH} \longrightarrow \text{R-CH(OH)-CH(SR')-CH}_2\text{-CHO} \longrightarrow$$

$$\longrightarrow \underbrace{\text{R-CH-CH(SR')-CH}_2\text{-CHOH}}_{\text{O}}$$

Under extreme conditions (i.e. pH 9-10 and high concentrations of the reactants) 2-alkenals and 4-hydroxyalkenals also react with the NH_2 group of amino acids (Suyama *et al.*, 1979; Napetschnik, 1981) and most probably also with those of proteins. The reaction products are probably a mixture of Schiff bases and Michael addition products (Suyama *et al.*, 1979). Figure 9 shows for comparison the time dependence of the reaction of 4-hydroxynonenal with low molecular weight thiols (cysteine and glutathione), proteins possessing SH groups (human serum albumin and bovine serum albumin) and with glycine. The high reactivity of hydroxynonenal towards molecules with SH groups is evident from the rapid disappearance of the aldehyde. With glycine, on the other hand, under comparable conditions there is only an insignificant decrease in the amount of the aldehyde. The relative rates calculated from the half life-times show that the reactivity of the amino group of glycine is 2 to 3 orders of magnitude less than the reactivity of the SH group. It can therefore be concluded that 4-hydroxynonenal formed in biological systems, such as peroxidising microsomes, will preferentially attack molecules with SH groups. Reactions with amino groups in proteins and other biomolecules on the other hand would require either high concentrations of the

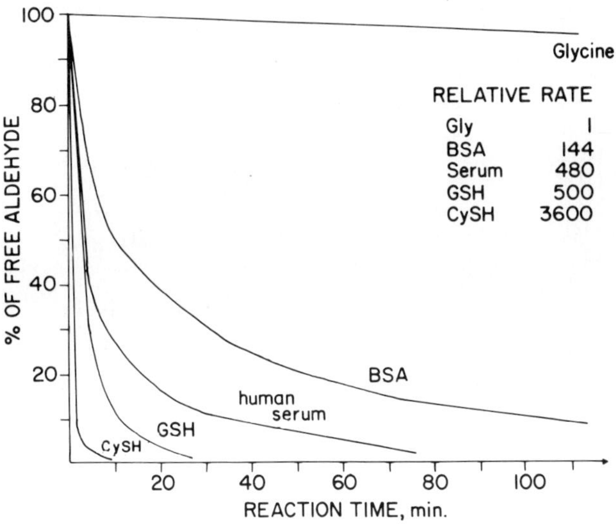

FIG. 9 Time dependence of the reaction of 4-hydroxynonenal (0.1 mM) with cysteine (1 mM), glutathione (1 mM), human serum (60 mg protein/ml), bovine serum albumin (66 mg/ml = 1 mM) and glycine (1 mM) in tris buffer pH 7.4. The decrease of the hydroxynonenal concentration was followed by HPLC (Spherisorb ODS, 80% methanol, 222 nm).

aldehyde (about 1 mM) or amino groups which are extremely reactive due to the effect of neighbouring groups. All biological inhibitory effects of 4-hydroxyalkenals investigated so far can be explained, however, by the inactivation of functional SH groups. Furthermore, if isolated SH-proteins or SH-enzymes are incubated with 4-hydroxyalkenals the number of aldehyde molecules bound to the protein equals the number of SH groups lost during the incubation (Schauenstein *et al.*, 1971).

Malonaldehyde, an aldehyde that is formed in the free form in large amounts (Esterbauer *et al.*, 1981b) during iron stimulated peroxidation of microsomes is much less reactive than 4-hydroxynonenal (Fig. 10). With glycine or glutathione there is virtually no reaction at all within 5 h reaction time. Human serum, bovine serum albumin and cysteine do react with malonaldehyde, however, at rates which are considerably slower than with hydroxynonenal. In the case of cysteine the ratio of reaction rates is 1:780.

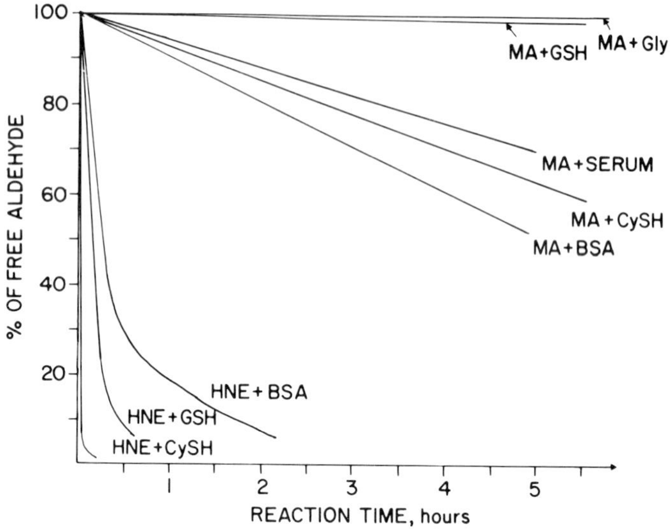

FIG. 10 Time dependence of the reaction of malonaldehyde (0.1 mM) with glycine, cysteine, glutathione, human serum and bovine serum albumin. Reaction conditions as in Fig. 9. The curves for hydroxynonenal were taken from Fig. 9. The decrease of the malonaldehyde concentration was followed by HPLC (Esterbauer *et al.*, 1981).

It is beyond the scope of this article to describe even briefly the various biological effects including the anti-cancer activities of 4-hydroxyalkenals and their derivatives which have been reported in the literature. The reader is therefore referred to several review articles (Schauenstein *et al.*, 1977; Schauenstein *et al.*, 1979) and some original articles (Tillian *et al.*, 1976; Benedetti *et al.*, 1980; Conroy, 1979; Dianzani, 1979).

CONCLUDING REMARKS

From the new data presented here and from what was already known several conclusions can be drawn regarding the biological importance of lipid derived aldehydes:

1. Nonenzymatic and enzymatic (iron stimulated) peroxidation of polyunsaturated lipids leads to the formation of a great diversity of aldehydes.
2. *n*-Hexanal and 4-hydroxynonenal are major aldehydes produced by peroxidising microsomes and by nonenzymatic oxidation of arachidonic,

linoleic, and γ-linolenic acid. The formation of these aldehydes can be explained from the decomposition of the 13- and 15-monohydroperoxides.

3. Each individual unsaturated fatty acid (oleic, linoleic, linolenic, γ-linolenic, arachidonic acid) on peroxidation gives a typical and characteristic pattern of aldehydes.
4. Microsomal, iron stimulated peroxidation can be distinguished from nonenzymatic peroxidation by the different rate of carbonyl formation and by malonaldehyde production. The enzymatic system reaches a maximum level of aldehyde concentration within 30 min, while in the nonenzymatic systems the carbonyl production continues to increase even after 20 h. Microsomes produce 1.6 mole carbonyls (other than malonaldehyde) per mole of malonaldehyde, the nonenzymatic systems on the other hand produce about 30-40 mole carbonyls per mole of malonaldehyde.
5. From the aldehydes identified so far only 4-hydroxynonenal shows high reactivity towards important biomolecules and therefore this aldehyde is the only known possible candidate which could be responsible for cytopathological effects associated with lipid peroxidation *in vitro* and *in vivo*.
6. Large amounts of aldehydes including 4-hydroxynonenal are also formed during non enzymatic peroxidation. In working with biological samples it is therefore extremely difficult to ascertain and unequivocally prove the true "biogenic" nature of aldehydes. For this very reason the work on biogenic aldehydes remains a difficult but challenging problem for the future.

ACKNOWLEDGEMENTS

The author is grateful to the National Foundation for Cancer Research for financial assistance, and to Professor Dr. E. Schauenstein (University of Graz), and Professor T.F. Slater (Brunel University) who have initiated and stimulated this work.

The author dedicates this paper to Professor Dr Erich Ziegler with best wishes on the occasion of his 70th birthday.

REFERENCES

Badings, T.H. (1970). Thesis, Wageningen, and Verslag Nr.124 van het Nederlands Instituut voor Zuivelonderzoek (NIZO) te Ede.

Benedetti, A., Comporti, M. and Esterbauer, H. (1980). *Biochem. Biophys. Acta* 620, 281-296.
Conroy, P.J. (1979). *In* "Submolecular Biology of Cancer" Ciba Foundation Symposium 67, pp.271-300. Excerpta Medica, Amsterdam.
Dianzani, M.U. (1979). *In* "Submolecular Biology of Cancer" Ciba Foundation Symposium 67, pp.245-270. Excerpta Medica, Amsterdam.
Esterbauer, H. and Schauenstein, E. (1966). *Fette. Seifen. Anstrichm.* 68, 7-14.
Esterbauer, H. and Schauenstein, E. (1967). *Nahrung* 11, 607-621.
Esterbauer, H., Zollner, H. and Scholz, N. (1975). *Z. Naturforsch. Teil. C* 30, 466-473.
Esterbauer, H., Ertl, A. and Scholz, N. (1976). *Tetrahedron* 32, 285-289.
Esterbauer, H. and Schauenstein, E. (1977a). *Monatch. Chem.* 108, 963-972.
Esterbauer, H. and Schauenstein, E. (1977b). *Z. Lebensm. Unters. Forsch.* 164, 255-259.
Esterbauer, H. and Slater, T.F. (1981a). *IRCS Med. Sci.* 9, 749-750.
Esterbauer, H., Cheeseman, K., Dianzani, M.U., Poli, G. and Slater, T.F. (1981b). The separation by high pressure liquid chromatography of the aldehydic products of microsomal lipid peroxidation. To be published.
Graveland, A., Pesman, L. and van Eerde, P. (1972). *Master Brewers Assn. Amer. Tech. Quarterly* 9, 98-104.
Guidotti, G.G., Loreti, L. and Ciaranfi, E. (1965). *Eur. J. Cancer* 1, 23-32.
Kajiwara, T., Sekiya, J., Kido, Y. and Hatanoka, A. (1977). *Agric. Biol. Chem.* 41, 1793-1794.
Loury, M. (1973). *Lipids* 7, 671-675.
Napetschnik, St. (1981). Thesis, University of Graz, Austria.
Porter, N.A. and Funk, M.O. (1975). *J. Org. Chem.* 40, 3614-3615.
Poyer, J.L. and McCay, P.B. (1971). *J. Biol. Chem.* 246, 263-269.
Pryor, W.A. and Stanley, J.P. (1975). *J. Org. Chem.* 40, 3615-3617.
Rachelsperger, M. (1979). Thesis, University of Graz, Austria.
Schauenstein, E., Esterbauer, H., Jaag, G. and Taufer, M. (1964). *Monatch. Chem.* 95, 180-183.
Schauenstein, E., Taufer, M., Esterbauer, H., Kylianek, A. and Seelich, Th. (1971). *Monatch. Chem.* 102, 517-529.
Schauenstein, E., Esterbauer, H. and Zolner, H. (1977). "Aldehydes in Biological Systems" Pion Limited, London.
Schauenstein, E. and Esterbauer, H. (1979). *In* "Submolecular Biology of Cancer" Ciba Foundation Symposium 67, pp.225-244. Excerpta Medica, Amsterdam.
Schwartz, D.P. and Parks, O.W. (1963). *Microchem. J.* 7, 400-406.
Slater, T.F. and Sawyer, B.C. (1971). *Biochem. J.* 123, 805-814.
Tillian, H.M., Schauenstein, E., Ertl, A. and Esterbauer, H. (1976). *Eur. J. Cancer* 12, 989-993.
Treesl, R., Bahri, D. and Silwar, R. (1979). "European Brewery Convention, Proceedings of the 17th Congress". Berlin (West) 1979, pp.27-41.
Suyama, K., Tachibana, A. and Adachi, S. (1979). *Agric. Biol. Chem.* 43, 9-14.
Vladimrov, Yu.A., Olenev, V.I., Suslova, T.B. and Cheremisina, Z.P. (1980). *Adv. Lipid Res.* 17, 173-249.

DISCUSSION

Slater: Thank you very much for a most helpful survey of the area of lipid peroxidation chemistry and biochemistry.

Willson: I was very interested, Professor Esterbauer, in the mechanisms that you proposed for the production of these unsaturated aldehydes, but I didn't see in the mechanism any involvement of metal ions. In another part of the mechanism I think you showed the combination of a hydroxyl radical with an alkyl radical.

Esterbauer: Yes, I showed an unsaturated alkyl radical which forms by the addition of a hydroxyl radical an enol.

Willson: This type of mechanism seems to me a rather unlikely reaction because as you know the hydroxyl radical is a very reactive species and would react more readily with the lipid itself rather than with an alkyl radical in low concentration. On another point, have you considered the possibility that the hydroxyl radical, which can easily be formed in this type of system, adds on to the double bond of the fatty acid rather than abstracting a hydrogen atom. If you form the adduct you could then form malondialdehyde by a mechanism similar to that in which muconaldehyde is formed during the oxidation of benzene in the presence of ferric iron.

Esterbauer: Do you mean an adduct between the hydroxyl radical and an alkyl radical?

Willson: No, I mean the addition of the hydroxyl radical directly to the unsaturated bond of the lipid and then this OH adduct adding on oxygen and then through a sequential set of reactions forming malondialdehyde. It is very difficult, of course, to evaluate the reaction details exactly since we are looking at products that are formed a long time after very rapid early events.

Esterbauer: I believe that in addition the environment of these reactions is of importance. I am sure you are right about the reactivity of the hydroxyl radical in solution, but I don't know what actually would go on in the complex environment of a biological membrane. The hydroxyl radical could certainly also be formed in such a lipid environment but whether the reactivity would be the same there as in aqueous solution is something that I'm not sure about. But if the alkyl radical is formed in the lipid environment and at the same time hydroxyl radical is formed - are you saying that you feel it unlikely that these two would combine together?

Willson: Yes, I think it is rather unlikely.

Asmus: I had almost the same question as Dr Willson because I was also puzzled by this reaction between two radicals. Such a bi-molecular radical-radical interaction, I would think, is not the most likely reaction to occur on this time scale. I would certainly support the view put forward by Dr Willson in the sense that you wish to involve hydroxyl radicals at this stage. It will certainly do something to the neighbouring molecules by addition, for example, to a double bond or by reacting with some other site on the molecule, and then by consecutive reactions yielding products such as the aldehydes, but at the initial stage not through a radical-radical interaction. I think that such a radical-radical interaction is just not possible from the time scale point of view. If I can now make an additional remark on Professor Esterbauer's paper I was very impressed by the analytical chemistry involved in these separations of products from peroxidation of lipids. Would this not be a very good system in which to use for example compounds labelled with ^{14}C in order to clarify the reaction sequence leading to the products? I saw many question marks still on your analysis diagrams - maybe with labelled compounds one could obtain further information on how the molecules break up.

Esterbauer: Well, this in fact relates to a project that is now in progress between our group in Graz and Professor Comporti's group in Sienna. In fact, using ^{14}C labelled arachidonic acid we are beginning to evaluate the reaction pathway that results in the formation of 4-hydroxy nonenal. But perhaps Dr Benedetti who is here from Siena can give us more details on this specific point.

Slater: Perhaps before we hear from Dr Benedetti I could add that almost all of the reference compounds you saw on the slides of Professor Esterbauer were, in fact, synthesised by him, so that it is really a colossal project to consider synthesising and separating upwards of 100 different products from the peroxidising lipids of the microsomal membrane. But they are making progress with ^{14}C-labelling to help identify the reaction pathways as suggested by Professor Asmus.

Benedetti: Concerning the origin of 4-hydroxynonenal from the microsomal NADPH-Fe dependent lipid peroxidation, I will mention the results of very recent experiments done in cooperation between my institute in Sienna and Professor Esterbauer.

In these experiments we used rat liver microsomes pre-labelled *in vivo* with [^{14}C(U)] arachidonic acid; the incorporated radioactivity was almost entirely associated with arachidonic acid of phospholipids and neutral lipids.

The data (Table 1) showed that the specific radioactivity of 4-hydroxynonenal released from microsomes is nearly the same as that of the phospholipid-arachidonic acid; while it is disimilar to that from neutral lipids-arachidonic acid.

It seems possible, therefore, to assess that 4-hydroxynonenal is created almost entirely from arachidonic acid of membrane phospholipids.

TABLE 1 Specific radioactivity of evolved 4-hydroxynonenal and of arachidonic acid bound to polar and neutral lipids of liver microsomes containing [^{14}C(U)] arachidonic acid and incubated in the NADPH-Fe dependent system

Incubation time (min)	Arachidonic acid bound to polar lipids specific activity dpm/mg ($\times 10^{-3}$)	Arachidonic acid bound to neutral lipids specific activity dpm/mg ($\times 10^{-3}$)	4-hydroxynonenal specific activity dpm/mg ($\times 10^{-3}$)
0	91.6	2783.0	-
10	87.5	2483.0	89.7
60	87.2	2305.0	92.5

Slater: Do you think Professor Esterbauer, that this very rapid reaction with cysteine that you showed with 4-hydroxyalkenals yield a thiazolidine-carboxylic acid would occur when such reactive aldehydes are injected directly into animals. If so, would this help to produce a slow release of the reactive aldehyde from the thiazolidine derivative since this type of reaction is essentially reversible.

Esterbauer: Yes, in fact the adducts are not very stable and they can certainly release the aldehyde (and also of course the cysteine or any thiol) again, slowly and gradually, to the same extent as it is consumed by another, more aldehyde-affinitive SH compound. But of course, the mechanism we suggest for the biological effects of free aldehydes when injected into animals is a direct attack of essential SH groups in proteins and not an indirect effect via the liberation of the aldehyde from primarily formed thiol adducts. On the other hand, the inhibition of protein synthesis in hepatoma cells by saturated aldehydes (acetaldehyde, propionaldehyde, α,β-dihydroxybutyraldehyde, and others) has been explained (Guidotti *et al.*, 1965) by the disturbance of the balanced amino acid pool through the reaction of the aldehydes with cysteine to thiazolidine carboxylic acids.
Magee: I would like to follow up the question of Professor Slater. You showed a general slide where aldehydes react with thiol compounds. Would this also apply to formaldehyde in particular if the formaldehyde was taken in by inhalation, because as you know, there is considerable concern at the moment that formaldehyde may be carcinogenic?
Esterbauer: Yes, indeed, formaldehyde will give all the reactions that I show in the following figure (Fig. 1) and it is the most reactive aldehyde.

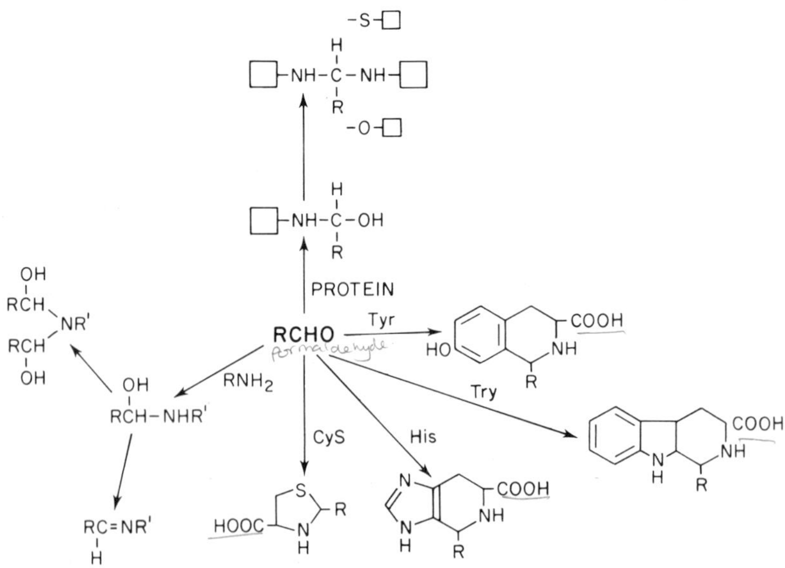

FIG. 1

Formaldehyde will give cross links in proteins, it will react with cysteine and tryptophan, tyrosine and other amino acids. Rosenkranz (1972) has reported that formaldehyde preferentially inhibits the growth of a strain of *E. coli* which lacks the enzymes involved in DNA repair and it was assumed that it alters the amino groups of DNA bases (Haselkom and Doty, 1961; see also Schauenstein *et al.*, 1977).

Magee: Can I follow up with another question? As you know, a number of drugs are metabolised by the cytochrome P_{450} system especially in the liver with the liberation of formaldehyde. A specific drug, for example, would be aminopyrene which does not seem to produce in the liver any of the sorts of reactions that carbon tetrachloride does and yet it is known to produce formaldehyde. Do you think that formaldehyde would be formed intracellularly in such cases and would it go into the sorts of reactions that you described?

Esterbauer: Well, it is difficult to answer, of course, that specific point. I know, for example, in the metabolism of cyclophosphamide that acrolein was claimed to be produced when liver microsomes were incubated with the drug, but then other groups have disputed that the so-formed acrolein is the active principle. Acrolein would react similarly to 4-hydroxyalkenals and preferentially attack SH groups. Using aldehyde precursors it seems generally possible to liberate aldehydes directly inside the cell but it will depend very much on the type of the aldehyde and on the experimental conditions which sorts of reactions are then given by the aldehyde. I really cannot answer your precise question in this sense.

Slater: I think Professor Magee's question may be answered, at least partially, by the results of Professor Dianzani who is going to speak next, because there is no doubt that the different groups of aldehydes like the saturated aldehydes, or the alkenals, or the hydroxyalkenals have different reactivities in relation to important biological systems, and what Professor Esterbauer said just now was that formaldehyde falls basically into the group of the saturated aldehydes as opposed to the much more reactive 4-hydroxyalkenal group. In addition, of course, the release of formaldehyde by the oxidative metabolism of substances like aminopyrene mentioned by Professor Magee, would produce rather small amounts of formaldehyde in unit time and these could be removed by aldehyde metabolising systems as well as combination locally with thiols and amino groups.

Riley: I should like to ask a rather general question that emerges from the discussion so far. Is it correct to assume that now the major emphasis in lipid peroxidation as a damaging or a cytotoxic process has shifted from the damage that is done to membrane constiu-ents, as we considered, for example, in our work on photosensitisation reactions (Slater and Riley, 1966) to the formation of compounds that can have cytotoxic actions at a distance from the original lesion?

Esterbauer: I don't believe that tissue injury caused by lipid per-oxidation can be attributed to a single cause like reactive free radicals, or membrane damage, or reactive diffusible factors (as alde-hydes are). I think we have to consider that all of them act together, maybe there are some pathological phenomena where one aspect is more important than the others, but I certainly cannot envisage that there is a situation, for example, where only free radicals are important, or even only just damage to the membrane structures. I also believe, of course, that tissue damage cannot be explained only on the basis of aldehydes, because there must be many other compounds that are also formed during the breakdown of these unsaturated lipids, which could be biologically highly active and highly cytotoxic.

Slater: I think the outcome of that answer is that Professor Esterbauer, like myself and Professor Dianzani, doesn't believe in the principle of unicausality for cellular damage.

REFERENCES to Discussion

Casini, A., Benedetti, A., Ferrali, M. and Comporti, M. (1979). *Chem. Biol. Interact.* 25, 211-227.

Guidotti, G.G., Loreti, L. and Ciaranfi, E. (1965). *Eur. J. Cancer* 1, 23-32.

Haselkom, R. and Doty, P. (1961). *J. Biol. Chem.* 236, 2738-2745.

Rosenkranz, H.S. (1972). *Bull. Environ. Contam. Toxicol.* 8, 242-251.

Schauenstein, E., Esterbauer, H. and Zolner, H. (1977). *In* "Alde-hydes in Biological Systems". pp.20-21, Pion, London.

Slater, T.F. and Riley, P.A. (1966). *Nature (London)* 209, 151-154.

Biochemical Effects of Saturated and Unsaturated Aldehydes

M.U. DIANZANI

INTRODUCTION

Our approach to the problem of the biochemical effects of aldehydes was originally derived from the knowledge that these substances are end products of lipid peroxidation. Whilst CCl_4-derived free radicals and lipoperoxides are short-lived and so are expected to produce direct damage only in the cell structures where they are produced (i.e. the liver smooth endoplasmic reticulum, or SER), aldehydes are more diffusible and long-lived, so have to be considered as possible agents in cell damage occurring in "far" sites in CCl_4-treated animals. A first survey of the effects of the aldehydes on several cell functions has already been published (Dianzani, 1979).

During our investigations, however, new interest arose in the possible biological functions of aldehydes derived from other directions. In fact, it has been reported that lipid peroxidation is very low in tumour tissues, and especially in hepatomas (Lash, 1966; Fonnesu *et al.*, 1966; Ugazio *et al.*, 1968, 1969; Utsumi *et al.*, 1965; Player *et al.*, 1977; Bartoli and Galeotti, 1979). Notwithstanding the fact that in our recent investigations using either ascites or solid hepatomas, or also hepatoma cell lines cultivated *in vitro*, we were able to find tumour cells clearly able to display lipid peroxidation (Rossi and Dianzani, unpublished results), it seems certain that very undifferentiated tumours have very low peroxidative capacities. Our previous work on the action of aldehydes *in vitro* has shown that these substances are able to decrease the mitotic index both in normal and in hepatoma cells (Dianzani, 1979). In addition, they are able to inhibit tubulin, the main functional protein of microtubules which are involved in the formation of the mitotic spindle (Gabriel *et al.*, 1977). Furthermore, Albano *et al.* (1981a,b) found that aldehydes can act as inhibitors *in vitro* of putrescine-activated S-adenosylmethionine decarboxylase (SAMD), the enzyme producing spermidine from S-adenosylmethionine. Spermidine, as well as other polyamines, is thought to play a regulatory role in cell multiplication. These facts suggest the working hypothesis that lipid peroxidation and polyamine metabolism may be involved in an integrated mechanism for the regulation of cell multiplication. This paper is a summary of a number of experiments that were done by my group in Turin during the last few years on this topic.

MATERIALS AND METHODS

Male rats of the Wistar strain (200-300 g body wt.), fed *ad libitum* on a semisynthetic diet (Fratelli Piccioni, Brescia) and fasted 15-18 h before killing by decapitation, were used. Homogenates were prepared using a Potter-Elvehjem apparatus. They were submitted, when necessary, to differential centrifugation in a Spinco-Beckman Model L centrifuge, according to the procedure described by De Duve *et al.* (1955). Mitochondria were isolated according to Feo *et al.* (1973). The polarographic measurements of the respiratory rate and of the acceptor control ratio, as well as of the ADP/0 ratio, were done according to Feo *et al.* (1973). All other techniques regarding mitochondria are those as indicated by Feo *et al.* (1975). Aldehyde dehydrogenase activity was measured according to Lebsack *et al.* (1977).

Lysosomal acid phosphatase was measured according to De Duve *et al.* (1955). Its "total" activity was assayed in the presence of 0.1% Triton X-100, whereas "free" activity was measured on preparations protected by 0.25 M sucrose. "Residual latent" activity (RLA), i.e. the fraction of activity remaining latent after extensive hypo-osmotic shock and requiring the addition of Triton X-100 to be unmasked, was measured according to Zuretti *et al.* (1980). Plasma membranes were isolated from liver homogenates according to Paradisi *et al.* (1981). Their purity was assessed by electron microscopy. Adenylate cyclase activity was measured according to the modifications suggested by Paradisi *et al.* (1981) of the method of Keirns *et al.* (1974). 5'-Nucleotidase was assayed by the method of Gerlach and Hiby (1974).

Amino acid incorporation into liver post-mitochondrial supernatant was assayed by the method adopted by Dianzani *et al.* (1976). Protein was determined in samples used for enzymatic analysis by the method of Lowry *et al.* (1951). Hepatocytes were isolated from normal liver as described by Gravela *et al.* (1977). Protein and lipoprotein secretion from isolated hepatocytes was assyed according to the pre-labelling and analytical procedures described by Poli *et al.* (1979). Glucose-6-phosphatase activity in isolated hepatocytes was measured according to Poli *et al.* (1981b); Cytochrome P_{450} was measured in intact cells according to the procedure adopted by the same authors.

Putrescine-activated S-adenosylmethionine decarboxylase (SAMD) activity was measured according to Poli *et al.* (1981a).

Tubulin activity was studied as described elsewhere (Gabriel *et al.*, 1977). Polymerised and soluble tubulin were differentiated and quantitated according to Pipeleers *et al.* (1977).

Effects on the cell cycle were studied on ascites AH-130 Yoshida hepatoma cells maintained by weekly intraperitoneal inoculation in tumour adapted male Wistar rats weighing 130-150 g. Each recipient rat received about 10^8 tumour cells i.p. These cells were withdrawn from donor rats on the fifth day of tumour growth. All animals received on the fourth day of tumour growth a single dose i.p. of 1 mCi /Kg body wt (b.w.) of [^{3}H]thymidine (specific activity 25 Ci/mmol).When used, aldehydes (25 or 50 mg/Kg b.w.) were injected i.p. dissolved in saline 30 min after [^{3}H]thymidine to allow its incorporation into DNA. Samples of the ascitic fluid from each rat were taken off at various intervals. Smears of ascites cells were fixed in Carnoy liquid and autoradiographed with Ilford K2 emulsion. The slides were stored in light-tight boxes at 4^oC for about one month, developed in Kodak 19D developer and stained with May-Grümwald-Giemsa stain. The percentage of labelled mitoses for each specimen was determined after examining about 1000 mitoses.

The following aldehydes were used: methylglyoxal (MG), maleylaldehyde (MA), hexanal (HEA), 2-oxo-pent-2-enal (KPA), trans-4-hydroxy-non-2-enal (HNE), trans-4-hydroxy-pent-2-enal (HPE), malonaldehyde (MDA), acetaldehyde (AA), acrolein (ACR), trans-4-hydroxy-tetradecen-2-al (H-14-E), trans-4-hydroxy-pentadecen-2-al (H-15-E) and trans-4-hydroxy-heptadecen-2-al (H-17-E). All the 4-hydroxy-alkenals were gifts of Professor Esterbauer, University of Graz, Austria. The other aldehydes with the exception of MDA and MLA, were Merck products. They were redistilled before use. MDA was freshly prepared from malonaldehyde-bis-dimethylacetal, as described by Poli *et al.* (1981a). MLA was prepared from 2,5-dihydro-2,5-dimethoxyfuran, according to Poli *et al.* (1981a). All chemicals used were Sigma, Merck, or Boehringer products, when not stated differently.

RESULTS

Influence of the Aldehydes on Mitochondria

Previous experiments (Dianzani, 1979) showed that the respiratory stimulation induced by addition of ADP or dinitrophenol (DNP) to mitochondria is strongly decreased by MLA and HPE; the ADP/O ratio remains unaffected but the acceptor control ratio is strongly decreased. Furthermore, the aldehydes were able to stimulate mitochondrial swelling in the absence of added ions, whereas they decreased both Ca^{+}-induced and K^{+}-plus valinomycin-induced swelling. The active concentrations of the aldehydes were 1 mM in the case of MLA and 2 mM for HPE. These concentrations are biochemically high, but the possibility exists that this fact may be related to the presence of mitochondria of aldehyde dehydrogenase which decreases the effective aldehyde concentration. New experiments have been done on this subject. A first part consisted of comparing the effect of MLA and HPE with that of HNE, an aldehyde produced during lipid peroxidation and possessing high toxicity (Benedetti *et al.*, 1980). Figure 1 shows that in the case of liver mitochondria 0.2 mM HNE produced more than a 40% decrease in the acceptor control ratio, whereas 1 mM and 2 mM concentrations produced decreases respectively of about 60% and about 76%. Under the same conditions, 1 mM MLA inhibited by about 48% and 2 mM HPE by about 67%. So, it is clear that HNE is much more effective than the aldehydes used previously on this parameter. Figure 1 shows that HNE is much more effective on hepatoma samples than on normal liver mitochondria. In fact, an 0.1 mM concentration of the aldehyde decreased the tumour acceptor control ratio by about 40%.

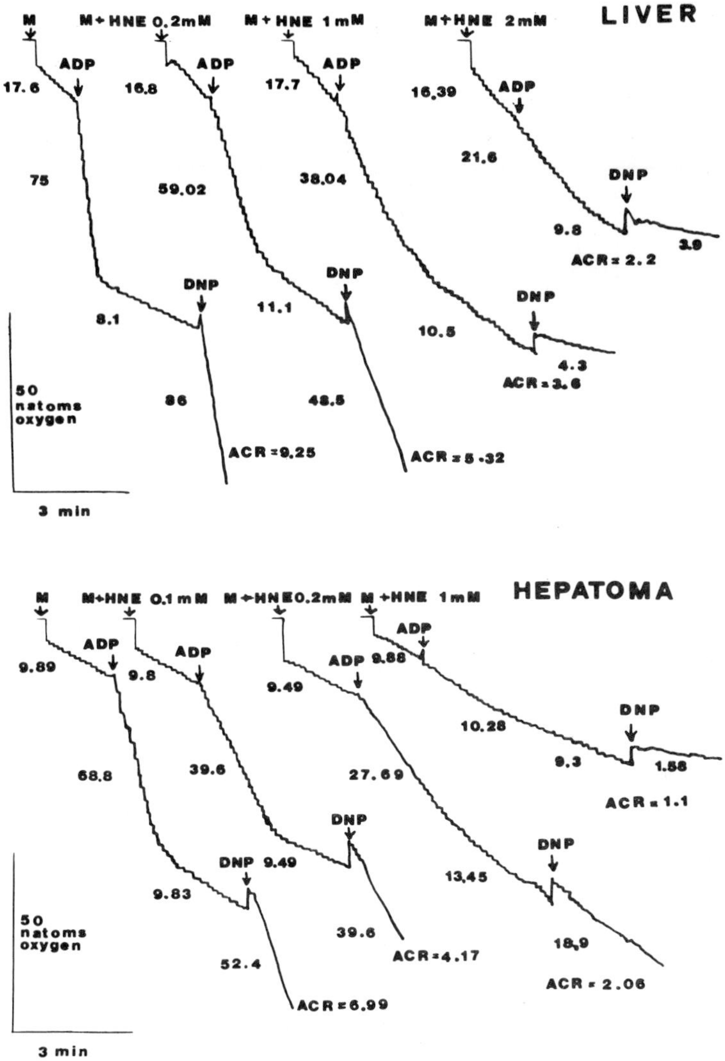

FIG. 1 Respiratory control of mitochondria from normal liver and from AH-130 Yoshida hepatoma. Inhibition by different concentrations of HNE. Glutamate (10 mM) plus malate (5 mM) plus inorganic orthophosphate (5 mM) were added as substrate. Adenosine diphosphate and dinitrophenol additions were done according to Feo *et al.* (1973). Oxygen uptake was measured polarographically.

In other experiments, the presence and distribution of aldehyde dehydrogenase in both normal liver and AH-130 hepatoma were studied. Table 1 shows that both normal liver and hepatoma homogenates display

TABLE 1 Aldehyde dehydrogenase activity in the homogenate of normal liver and of AH-130 Yoshida ascite hepatoma

Substrate	Aldehyde dehydrogenase (units/g wet tissue)	
	Liver	Hepatoma
Formaldehyde	618	178
Acetaldehyde	2911	923
Maleylaldehyde	852	244
Methylglyoxal	812	205
Malonaldehyde	1151	448
Glutaraldehyde	983	232

Aldehyde concentration was 10 mM. Standard deviation values are not indicated, but they never exceeded 10% of the average. The differences between liver and tumour values are highly significant, with a P value lower than 0.005.

aldehyde dehydrogenase activities. Among the aldehydes used as substrates, the most easily attacked was acetaldehyde (AA). The enzyme activity is in any case much higher in normal liver than in hepatoma, the difference ranging from about 2.5 times with MDA to about 4 times with MG or glutaraldehyde. With AA, the activity in liver is about three times higher than in the hepatoma. This lower aldehyde dehydrogenase activity may be at least partially responsible for the higher sensitivity to aldehyde toxicity displayed by tumour cells in comparison to normal ones. Deeper study of the activity of the enzyme towards different AA concentrations showed that at least two different aldehyde dehydrogenases are present in the homogenate, the first one having high affinity for AA and a low Km for the aldehyde, the second one having a low affinity and a high Km. Fractionation experiments showed that aldehyde dehydrogenase activity in normal liver cytosol has a Km of 0.5 mM, whereas the Km is 0.8 mM in hepatoma cytosol. No difference in the specific activity was found between both cytosols (Fig. 2). Figure 3 shows that in microsomes the specific activity is much lower in hepatoma than in normal liver, the enzyme Km being respectively 0.53 mM and 0.99 mM. In normal liver mitochondria two different enzymes exist (see Lebsack *et al.*, 1977), with different

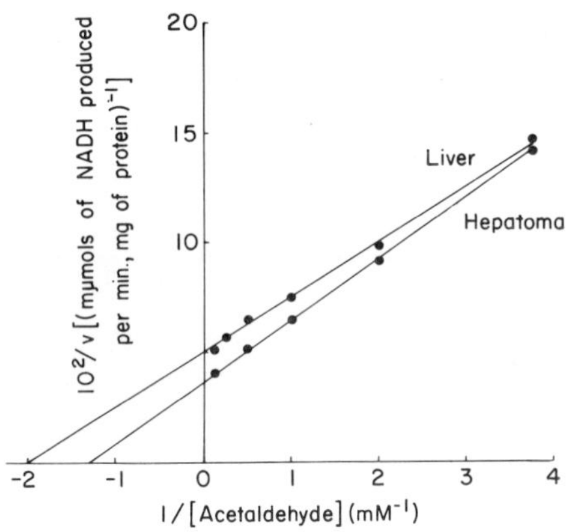

FIG. 2 Changes in aldehyde dehydrogenase activities in cytosol of normal liver and AH-130 Yoshida hepatoma provoked by using different acetaldehyde concentrations. Calculated Km is 0.8 mM in hepatoma, 0.5 mM in normal liver.

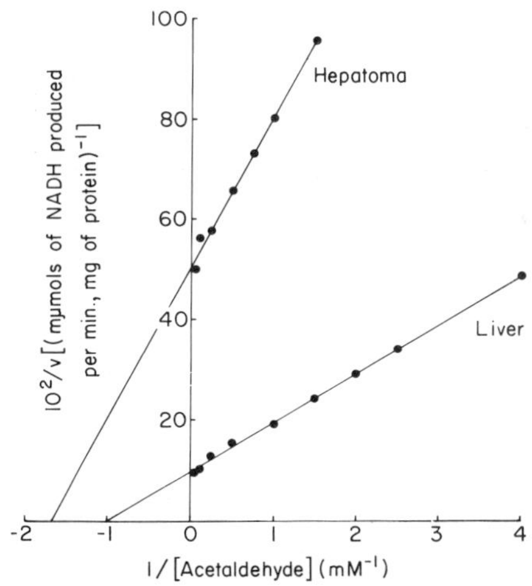

FIG. 3 Activity of aldehyde dehydrogenase with varying substrate concentration in liver and hepatoma microsomes. Calculated Km is 0.53 mM in hepatoma, 0.99 mM in the liver.

substrate affinities and different Kms, whereas in hepatoma mitochondria only one enzyme, with high affinity and low Km (0.03 mM) is present. The two normal liver mitochondria enzymes have respectively low affinity and high Km (2.2 mM) and high affinity and low Km (0.05 mM) (Fig. 4).

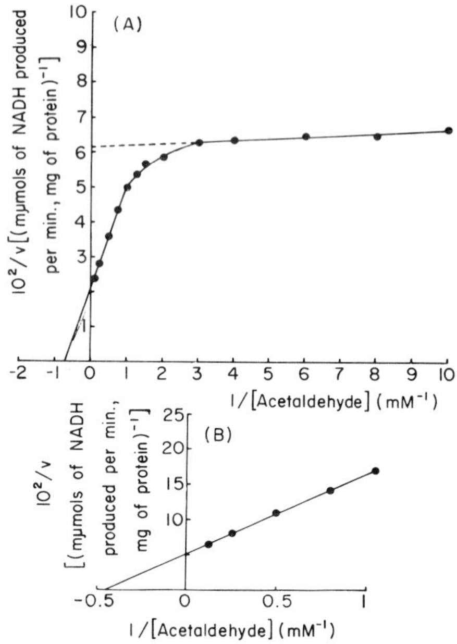

FIG. 4 Activity of aldehyde dehydrogenase with varying substrate concentration in liver mitochondria. The upper figure refers to the high affinity and low Km enzyme, sited in the inner membrane and in the matrix. Calculated Km is 0.05 mM. The lower figure refers to the slow affinity and high Km enzyme, sited in the outer membrane. Calculated Km is 2.2 mM.

Mitochondria subfractionation experiments showed that the high affinity and low Km enzyme is located on the inner membrane and in the matrix, whereas the low affinity and high Km enzyme is located in the outer membrane. This localisation does not change in hepatoma, whose mitochondria contain, however, only the matrix and inner membrane enzyme. Table 2 shows the results of experiments done to study the distribution of aldehyde dehydrogenase activity, as studied with 10 mM AA as substrate, among the different homogenate fractions. It is clear that in normal liver the activity is practically equally distributed among "heavy" mitochondria, microsomes and cytosol, the "light mitochondrial" fraction containing only about 10% of total activity. In hepatoma, however, about 80% of the activity is sited in the cytosol. With 10 mM MLA as substrate, about 48% of the activity is present in the cytosol in the case of normal liver, the same value amounting to 87% in that of hepatoma.

TABLE 2 Effect of MG administration on lysosome-vacuolar apparatus of the liver

Treatment	Acid phosphatase		Osmotic fragility index[a]
	basal free activity	residual latent activity	
Controls	16.23 ± 1.53	19.46 ± 4.34	24.84 ± 3.54
MG, 1 h	14.96 ± 2.08	10.88 ± 4.62**	33.74 ± 2.28*
MG, 2 h	13.86 ± 1.79	13.94 ± 4.07	32.32 ± 5.42+
MG, 6 h	14.27 ± 1.61	18.78 ± 2.87	27.91 ± 4.14

Free activity is always expressed as % of total activity. See the text for full explanation. Results are mean ± S.D. of five animals.
[a]Free activity after "partial" hypo-osmotic shock - basal free activity.
*$P < 0.005$; +$P < 0.05$; **$P < 0.025$.

All these peculiarities of tumour aldehyde dehydrogenases may help to explain the higher sensitivity of tumour cells towards aldehyde toxicity.

Influence of the Aldehydes on Lysosomes

Previous experiments (Dianzani, 1979) showed that lysosomes are rather resistant to aldehyde action *in vitro*. In present experiments we investigated the effect of MG administration to rats *in vivo* on the lysosome-vacuolar apparatus. MG (100 mg/Kg body wt.) was administered intraperitoneally; the rats were killed by decapitation at times ranging from 1 to 6 h after injection and two different homogenates were prepared, the first in 0.25 M sucrose, the second in distilled water. "Free" and "total" activities of acid phosphatase were measured on 0.25 M sucrose homogenate, either immediately ("free" activity = basal "free" activity) or after preincubation at 0°C for 30 min of the homogenate diluted with distilled water to a final 0.15 M sucrose concentration ("partial" hypo-osmotic shock). In the case of the water homogenate, the enzyme measurements were done after preincubation at 0°C for 30 min ("total"-"free" activity = "residual latent" activity).

Results in Table 2 show that MG did not cause any change in lysosomal integrity, as revealed by unmodified values of "basal free" activity. On the other hand, lysosomal osmotic fragility appears to be greatly increased, the increment of "free" activity after "partial" hypo-osmotic shock being almost two times that displayed by control homogenates. As osmotic fragility is taken as a suitable index of autophagic activity (Deter and De Duve, 1967), we considered the possibility that the changes induced by MG could be related to enhancement of autophagy. Therefore we measured the "residual latent" activity i.e. the enzymatic activity remaining masked after hypo-osmotic shock, but still detectable by Triton X-100 addition. This parameter has been recently proposed as a possible measure for autophagy (Zuretti *et al.*, 1980). In fact, these authors have shown that "residual latent" activity (RLA) increases when autophagy is depressed and decreases when it is stimulated, in concomitance with an opposite behaviour of the osmotic fragility. Table 2 shows that MG treatment produces a significant decrease in RLA (the inverse correlation between osmotic fragility) and this parameter is highly significant. Pretreatment of rats with 1 mg/Kg body wt. cycloheximide 20 min before MG prevents the increase in osmotic fragility, as well as the decrease in RLA. Cycloheximide has been shown to be able to prevent both glucagon-induced (Rumpelt and Weisbach, 1978) and D-galactosamine-induced autophagy (Rumpelt *et al.*, 1974). The present results, therefore, favour an increase in autophagy in MG-treated rats. Protein synthesis seems not to be required for autophagy (Kovaks and Rez, 1979). So, the blocking effect of cycloheximide may have an explanation different from its influence on protein synthesis. As it acts as a freezer of polyribosomal profiles, it seems possible that its effect may be related to some stabilisation of the rough endoplasmic reticulum membranes (Rez *et al.*, 1976).

Influence of the Aldehydes on Protein Synthesis

Previous experiments have shown that aldehydes are inhibitory for protein synthesis, the most effective among the tested substances being MLA (Dianzani, 1979). This aldehyde blocked amino acid incorporation into postmitochondrial supernatant proteins by 50% at 1 mM concentration. An 18% decrease was observed at 0.5 mM. The inhibition was stronger when polyphenylalanine synthesis was studied in the presence of poly-(U), about 70% decrease being already present at 0.5 mM. Valine incorporation into proteins of isolated hepatocytes was inhibited by about 30% in the presence of 1.25 mM MG, about 70% inhibition being reached at 2.5 mM. In the present experiments, HNE, the recently isolated aldehyde, was compared with MG and with HPE for inhibitory activity. It was seen that [^{14}C]valine incorporation into isolated hepatocyte proteins was inhibited by 30% at 0.1 mM and by 70% at 0.25 mM by HNE added in the incubation medium; its activity being about 10 times more efficient than those of MG and HPE.

Influence of Aldehydes on Protein and Lipoprotein Secretion from Isolated Hepatocytes

In previous experiments it was seen that 1 mM MG is able to decrease protein secretion from isolated hepatocytes by about 30-40% in conditions where new protein synthesis had been blocked by previous addition of 0.7 μM cycloheximide. MG (2.5 mM) decreased the secretion by about 50%. This concentration is not very far from that able to block colchicine-binding to tubulin (Dianzani, 1979). Protein and lipoprotein secretion from isolated hepatocytes has been previously shown to be partially tubulin-dependent (Gravela *et al.*, 1977). So, the hypothesis might be advanced that an MG-induced block in protein secretion from hepatocytes is related to an influence of MG on tubulin. In the present experiments, we studied the influence of HNE and of hexanal, another aldehyde abundantly produced during lipid peroxidation, on triglyceride secretion from isolated hepatocytes. (Gravela *et al.*, 1977; Poli *et al.* 1979). Figure 5 shows that both aldehydes are strongly inhibitory on triglyceride secretion in cycloheximide-pretreated hepatocytes. HNE blocks by about 40% at 0.1 mM concentration, the inhibition reaching more than 90% at 1 mM. Hexanal is less active, as it blocks by about 50% at 1 mM and by about 25% at 0.5 mM. In other experiments, the effect of the same aldehydes was studied on the isolated hepatocyte microsomal enzymes, cytochrome P_{450} and glucose-6-phosphatase. Figure 6 shows that HNE decreased cytochrome P_{450} by about 50% at an aldehyde concentration of 0.25 mM, the inhibition being about 30% at 0.1 mM. Glucose-6-phosphatase is less affected; hexanal inhibits cytochrome P_{450} by about 20% at 1 mM (Fig. 6). The MG-induced inhibition of cytochrome P_{450} is 17% at 0.1 mM and 24% at 0.25 mM; MLA blocks respectively by 13% and by 45% at the same

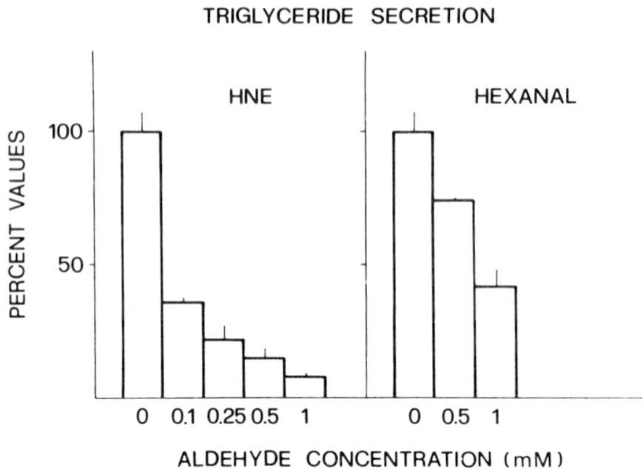

FIG. 5 Effect of 4-hydroxynonenal and hexanal on lipoprotein triglyceride secretion by pre-labelled rat hepatocytes. Triglycerides in hepatocytes were prelabelled *in vitro*, after which the hepatocytes were incubated at 37°C for 30 min in the presence or absence of different concentrations of the two aldehydes. After incubation, the hepatocyte suspension was centrifuged and the supernatant processed for radioactivity measurement as described in the Materials and Methods section. Vertical bars denote the S.D.

concentrations. Even in this case, the inhibition of glucose-6-phosphatase is not more than 12% at the highest concentration.

Influence of Aldehydes on Tubulin

Previous experiments (Gabriel *et al.*, 1977; Dianzani, 1979) showed that several aldehydes are able to decrease colchicine-binding to tubulin *in vitro*. The active aldehyde concentrations were rather high, remaining within millimolar ranges for most tested substances. The most effective were MG and HPE. In the present experiments, the study was extended to HNE. This was found to be much more effective than MG on soluble tubulin. In fact, a high degree of inhibition was obtained with an HNE concentration of 0.05 mM, whereas only a slight inhibition was observed at 0.5 mM in the case of MG. In preliminary expeirments, it was observed, however, that MG is more active than HNE on polymerised tubulin. If these results can be confirmed, they might suggest a different target or mechanism of action on tubulin by these two aldehydes.

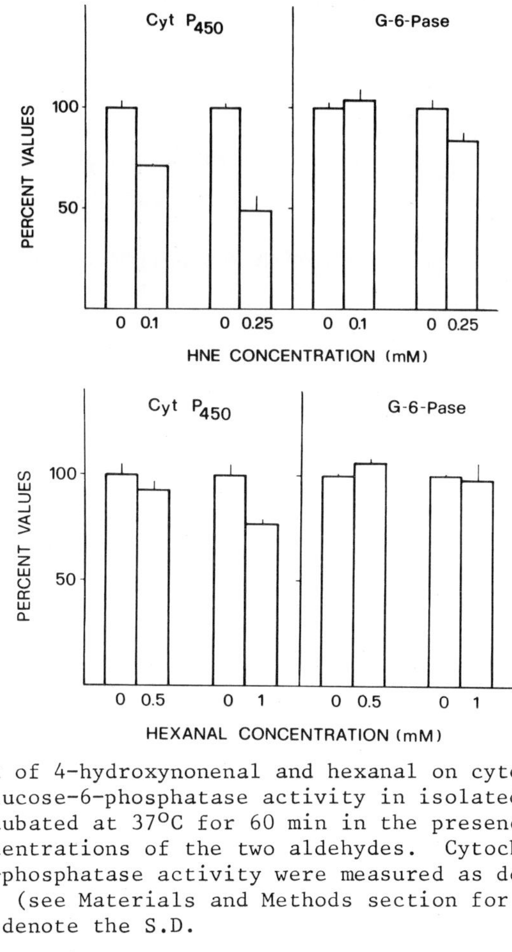

FIG. 6 Effect of 4-hydroxynonenal and hexanal on cytochrome P_{450} content and glucose-6-phosphatase activity in isolated rat hepatocytes. Cells were incubated at 37°C for 60 min in the presence or absence of different concentrations of the two aldehydes. Cytochrome P_{450} level and glucose-6-phosphatase activity were measured as described by Poli *et al.* (1981b) (see Materials and Methods section for further details). Vertical bars denote the S.D.

Influence of Aldehydes on Plasmamembrane Adenylate Cyclase and 5'-Nucleotidase

The experiments were done with MG, HPE and HNE. All these aldehydes were strongly inhibitory for adenylate cyclase of isolated plasma-membranes, the most effective being HNE. This inhibited by about 20% at an extremely low concentration (0.67 μM), the block reaching 50% at 2.68 μM. HPE inhibited by about 18% at 1.34 μM and by about 45% at 5.36 μM. MG inhibited by about 20% at 12.5 μM and by about 55% at 50 mM. The action on 5'-nucleotidase was much less: HNE inhibited by 50% at 2.68 mM, HPE at about 5.36 mM, MG inhibited by about 45% at 50 mM.

When the effect of HNE on adenylate cyclase was studied after incubation for different times, it was seen that after 5 min incubation, 0.67 μM HNE produced a 100% increase in the activity. This was substituted by strong decreases after 15 and 30 min incubation. The big increase in activity observed during the first minutes may be interpreted as an allosteric activation preceeding enzyme damage.

Influence of Aldehydes on Polyamine Metabolism in Normal Hepatocytes and in Hepatoma Cells

Polyamines are considered as stimulators of cell growth and proliferation. Albano *et al.* (1981a,b) have shown that MG interferes with polyamine metabolism, by inhibiting SAMD activity. At the same time, MG impairs RNA synthesis and stimulates RNA degradation. The effect of MG on SAMD was greater in hepatoma than in normal liver cells. In the first part of the present experiments, the effect of MG, MDA, MLA, ACR, HPE, HNE, H-14-E, H-15-5 and H-17-E was studied on SAMD activity of Yoshida hepatoma cells. No inhibition at all was seen with MDA, as well as with the long-chained liposoluble hydroxy-unsaturated aldehydes. Table 3 shows that HNE is, in this case, less effective than

TABLE 3 Effect of aldehydes on putrescine-actived S-adenosylmethionine decarboxylase (SAMD) activity in Yoshida hepatoma cells

Aldehyde	Concentration		
	0.25 mM	0.5 mM	1 mM
HNE	95	70	28
MG	100	92	22
MLA	100	87	37
ACR	92	66	19
HPE	79	49	16

Data are expressed as % of control values and represent means of 4-8 measurements.

HPE, which decreased SAMD activity by about 20% at 0.25 mM and by about 84% at 1 mM. MG was active only at 1 mM (78% inhibition), MLA inhibited by 63% at 1 mM and by about 13% at 0.5 mM; ACR inhibited by 80% at 1 mM and by 34% at 0.5 mM.

In other experiments, the incorporation of [^{14}C]thymidine into DNA of hepatoma cells was studied in the presence of MG. It was seen that 1 mM produced 98% inhibition, whereas 0.5 mM concentration inhibited by 71% and 0.25 mM inhibited by 29%.

It is noteworthy that, according to Poli *et al.* (1981a,b) the influence of the aldehydes on SAMD activity strongly increases if partially purified SAMD is used instead of whole homogenates or cytosols. SAMD activity is inhibited by about 30% in the presence of 50 mM HPE and by about 50% with 100 μM HPE when a partially purified SAMD preparation is used.

Influence of the Aldehydes on the Cell Cycle

In these experiments, the influence of both HPE and MG on the cell cycle of ascites AH-130 Yoshida hepatoma cells was studied *in vivo* during the exponential phase of growth. Serial samples of ascitic fluid containing cells labelled with [^{3}H]thymidine were withdrawn and submitted to autoradiography. The percentage of labelled mitoses *vs.* time is plotted in Fig. 7, while Table 4 summarises the kinetic parameters derived from these curves (analysis of the first mitotic wave). No attempt was made to calculate the time intervals for G_2,M or G_1

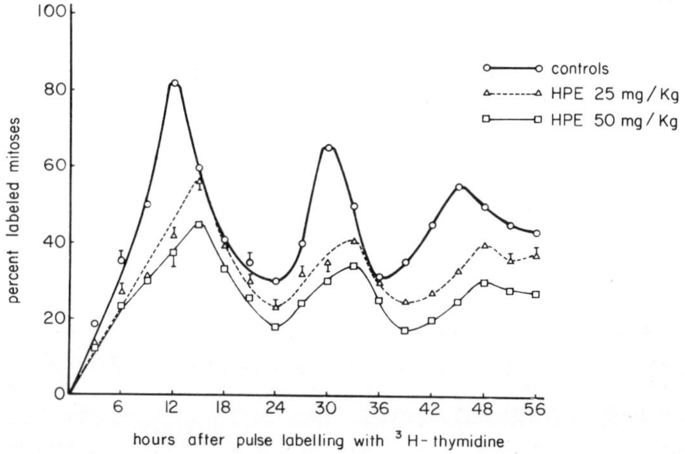

FIG. 7 Effect of HPE on the cell cycle of Yoshida ascites hepatoma (AH-130), as measured by % labelled mitoses. Each point represents the mean of data from four rats.

TABLE 4 The effect of HPE on *in vivo* cell cycle pf AH-130 hepatoma cells. Fourth day of tumour growth in the peritoneal cavity of recipient rats

Treatment	Conc. (mg/Kg)	T_c (h)	T_s (h)	$T_{(G_2 + 1/2)M}$ (h)	GF
Control	0	18	10.5	7.5	0.99
HPE	25	18	13.8	7.5	0.70
HPE	50	18	15.6	6	0.72

T_c is the time interval between the midpoint of the two phases of labelled mitoses. T_s is calculated from the 50% points of the ascending and the descending limbs of the curve. $T_{(G_2+1/2)M}$ is calculated as the time between the 0 and 50% points. GF (growth fraction) is calculated by dividing % labelled cells by % labelled mitoses. Each value represents the average of measurements done in four rats. S.D. is not given, but differences between control and treated groups are significant.

phases, because of the gross method of measurement. The cell cycle for the second mitotic wave of tumour cells is shorter (15 h) than for the first one, probably due to the fact that paracentesis may influence tumour growth resulting in a more sustained exponential growth rate. Two doses of HPE (25 mg/Kg and 50 mg/Kg respectively) were used. Both doses significantly increase the mean DNA synthetic period (S-phase) without apparently modifying the mean cell cycle time, as estimated from the time interval between the midpoints of the two peaks of labelled mitoses (Table 4). This discrepancy probably results from some degree of inaccuracy in the adopted procedure, due to the relatively long (3 h) interval between two successive paracenteses. The growth fraction (GF) of AH-130 cells, calculated, according to Mendelsohn *et al.* (1962) by dividing the percentage of labelled cells by the percentage of labelled mitoses, approaches a figure of 1. HPE significantly decreases the number of cells participating in the cell cycle, especially at the lower dose (Table 4). Moreover, HPE decreased the peak of the mitotic wave, suggesting an impairment of the S-phase (Fig. 7). HPE has been reported to interfere with all the macromolecular synthetic pathways, although the primary effect on the cell has been suggested to be inhibition of

DNA synthesis (Conroy, 1979). Although the technical limitations of the method used may hinder accurate estimates of the component of the cell cycle, the present observations seem to indicate that HPE affects the S-phase, as shown by the reduced percentage of labelled mitoses as well as by the higher T_s values. Experiments done with MG, at the same doses, showed substantially similar results.

DISCUSSION

The results described in this paper extend our knowledge of the action of aldehydes on the biological activities of liver and hepatoma cells. It seems evident now that carbonyls may display not only toxic activities, but are possible candidates for regulatory functions in the cells. Their high reactivity with both -SH and $-NH_2$ groups may be the chemical reason for their mechanism of action. The fact that most aldehyde actions, including those described in this paper, are inhibited by the previous addition of thiols in the incubation medium, whereas amino acids are generally inactive, points in favour of -SH groups as the most common target for aldehydes in the cells.

In this present discussion I shall especially examine two main questions. Are the present results in favour of a role of lipid peroxidation in the regulation of cell proliferation, or not? Why are tumour cells more sensitive to aldehydes than normal cells?

As regards the first question, it is clear that the present results in no way demonstrate a physiological role of lipid peroxidation. However, they add new arguments for continuing the discussion. The fact that tumour cells display little or no lipid peroxidation is, of course, an important point. We know at present, however, that this is not an absolute statement, as we have evidence for an almost normal rate of lipid peroxidation in some of the hepatomas studied so far in my laboratory. We can, however, state that the rate of lipid peroxidation in hepatomas parallels the degree of differentiation of tumour cells. In fact, the least differentiated tumour studied, i.e. AH-130 Yoshida hepatoma, has an extremely low rate of lipid peroxidation with a different aldehyde pattern compared with normal liver, whereas minimal deviation hepatomas display practically "normal" lipid peroxidation. Moreover, Gravela *et al.* (1975) have found that during ethionine-induced carcinogenesis, hyperplastic nodules display decreased lipid peroxidation in comparison to normal liver, and this effect becomes more marked at the hepatoma stage. So, the extent of lipid peroxidation in tumour tissues may represent a measure of their anaplasia. From this point of view, therefore, the problem of lipid peroxidation as a regulatory mechanism for cell proliferation remains open. According to Burlakova (1967) lipid peroxidation might display its "regulatory" influence on mitosis mostly by acting on mitotic spindle formation. We know now that tubulin, the function protein of mitotic spindle microtubules, is affected both by aldehydes and by lipid peroxidation, as induced by CCl_4-treatment (Miglietta *et al.*, 1981). This point, apparently in favour of Burlakova's view, is, however, limited by the fact that tubulin inhibition *in vitro* requires rather high aldehyde concentrations. The most effective aldehyde, from this point of view is, at present, HNE, whose influence can occur within the micromolar range. An important point is whether such concentrations can really be reached within the cells in any physiological moment. Of course, the experiments we did *in vitro* are very artificial; this might increase the aldehyde concentrations needed to see an effect, especially due to a redistribution of endogenous thiols or of other antioxidants preventing the contact between the aldehyde and its target. This clearly results from the data published by Poli *et al.* (1981a) from my laboratory. These authors have found that SAMD-sensitivity to aldehydes increases with an increasing purification of the enzyme. The fact that in CCl_4-poisoning, where lipid purification is stimulated *in vivo*, there is definite damage both to tubulin and to SAMD, may favour this interpretation. In fact, aldehyde production in this intoxication *in vivo* certainly does not reach the concentrations needed for aldehyde action *in vitro*. Of course, we cannot exclude the possibility that tubulin or SAMD inhibitions seen *in vivo* after CCl_4 are related to mechanisms different from aldehyde production, so this argument is in no way conclusive. In principle, however, it is not necessary to think that a homogeneous distribution of aldehyde within the cell is required for action. In fact, the active concentration is needed only at the level of the target. As lipid peroxidation occurs mainly in SER, and possibly in mitochondria and in other membranes, one might think that intracellular structures and enzymes being more intimately connected with such sites represent more probable targets for aldehydes.

The present experiments introduce a possible new mechanism for lipid peroxidation control of cell proliferation, i.e. regulation of polyamine synthesis. The main fact to support this possibility is the demonstration that SAMD activity is inhibited by very low concentrations of aldehydes known to be produced during lipid peroxidation, as well as by other aldehydes, such as MG. Furthermore, Poli and Gravela (see their communication in this book) observed that in CCl_4-induced stimulation of lipid peroxidation in intact hepatocytes, an inactivation occurs of ornithine decarboxylase, which is the rate limiting enzyme of polyamine metabolism.

Another possible mechanism of aldehyde regulation of metabolic reactions might be at the level of plasmamembrane adenylate cyclase, which undergoes strong changes in the presence of extremely low concentrations of HNE. As adenylate cyclase is a key enzyme in cAMP regulation of a lot of biochemical reactions in living cells, this point increases the attention to be given to aldehydes as regulatory products.

Other mechanisms for lipid peroxidation control of cell proliferation might be represented by inhibition of protein or nucleic acid synthesis, and even by lysosomal damage. In the case of protein and DNA synthesis, the concentrations of aldehydes needed to produce damage *in vitro* are rather high, but HNE is much more effective than the other aldehydes. So, the same type of reasoning described above for tubulin may be applied to this parameter. As far as regards lysosomes, the present experiments show that MG-treated liver displays an increased level of autophagy, the RLA of acid phosphatase being significantly increased. The influence of lysosomal enzyme activation in cell multiplication is still controversial, and the observed increased autophagy might represent an aspect of aspecific damage. So, at the moment, we have no conclusion to provide on this point.

In any case, the results of the experiments on hepatoma cell cycle are suggestive for some effect *in vivo* of the aldehydes on cell multiplication. From this point of view, what seems very interesting is not only the fact that the aldehydes increase the length of the

S-phase, but especially that they decrease the growth-fraction; in consequence, the proliferating compartment becomes smaller. This indicates that a certain proportion of treated cells do not behave anymore as cancer cells from this point of view. A deeper interpretation, of course, needs more experiments, but the first results are encouraging enough to continue this work.

As far as regards the question why tumour cells are more sensitive to the actions of aldehydes than normal cells, I think that the present experiments on aldehyde dehydrogenases represent a good key for explanation. In fact, we saw that aldehyde dehydrogenase activity is much lower in tumour than in normal tissue; moreover, it has a different intracellular distribution, favouring the activity of injected aldehydes on definite intracellular targets, such as mitochondria and microsomes. In addition, tumour mitochondria have only the high affinity and low Km enzyme, sited in the matrix and in the inner membrane, and do not possess the low affinity and high Km enzyme sited in the outer membrane. So, low aldehyde concentrations can act on mitochondria without being destroyed by aldehyde dehydrogenases, as distinct from the case of normal liver. Of course, further mechanisms to explain why tumour cells are more sensitive to aldehydes than normal cells might be the higher functional level in tumour cells of systems involved in cell multiplication, such as microtubule functioning, protein and DNA synthesis, polyamine synthesis, membrane adenylate cyclase activity, that represent at the same time good targets for aldehyde action.

In conclusion, the problems remain completely open, but there are good reasons to continue on this line of work.

SUMMARY

We have studied the influence of several aldehydes, and especially of those originating during peroxidative degradation of unsaturated lipids, on several biochemical parameters of either normal or neoplastic liver cells. The mitochondrial acceptor control ratio is decreased by aldehydes, the most effective among those that have been used being HNE. Aldehyde dehydrogenase distribution among cell fractions is different in liver and in hepatoma cells. In fact, in normal liver almost 30% of the activity is present in each of the following subfractions: mitochondria, microsomes and cytosol; in the tumour, more than 80% of the activity is in the cytosol. Moreover, the enzyme activity present in the tumour is less than one third of that found in normal liver cells. At the level of the mitochondria, it is possible to show two aldehyde dehydrogenases occur in normal liver cells, the first one having low affinity and high Km, the second having high affinity and low Km. Tumour mitochondria display only the high affinity and low Km enzyme sited on the outer membrane. These facts may explain why tumour mitochondria, and tumour cells generally, are more sensitive to aldehydes than normal cells.

The studies done on the lysosome-vacuolar system are in favour of increased autophagy in aldehyde-treated normal rats.

Aldehydes produce a block of both protein and DNA synthesis, as well as of lipoprotein secretion from isolated hepatocytes. In all these experiments, HNE seemed the most active among the substances used. HNE was very inhibitory, at micromolar concentration, on plasma-membrane adenylate cyclase. Tubulin function was more affected by HNE than by other aldehydes. S-adenosylmethionine decarboxylase (putrescine-activated) was inhibited by aldehydes, the most effective being HPE. The degree of inhibition depended upon the degree of purity of the enzyme. MG and HPE have been shown to display a definite action on cell cycle of hepatoma cells growing in the ascite fluid of rats. The most important points are an increase in the length of the S-phase and a decrease of the proliferating compartment. These results are discussed with special reference to the problem of a possible regulatory action of lipid peroxidation on cell multiplication and to that of the higher susceptibility of hepatoma cells to aldehyde action.

REFERENCES

Albano, E., Gravela, E., Poli, G. and Chiarpotto, E. (1981a). *In* "Recent Advances in Lipid Peroxidation and Tissue Injury" (Eds. T.F. Slater and A. Garner), Brunel University Biochemistry Department, London.

Albano, E., Poli, G., Chiarpotto, E. and Gravela, E. (1981b). *Boll. Soc. Ital. Biol. Sper.* (in press).

Bartoli, G.M. and Galeotti, T. (1979). *Biochim. Biophys. Acta* 574, 537-541.

Benedetti, A., Comporti, M. and Esterbauer, H. (1980). *Biochim. Biophys. Acta* 620, 281-296.

Burlakova, E.B. and Palmina, N.P. (1967). *Biofisika* 12, 1032-1036.
Conroy, P.J. (1979). *In* "Submolecular Biology and Cancer" Ciba Foundation Series 67, pp.271-300. Excerpta Medica, Amsterdam.
De Duve, C., Pressman, B.C., Giannetto, R., Wattiaux, R. and Appelmans, F. (1955). *Biochem. J.* 60, 604-617.
Deter, R.L. and De Duve, C. (1967). *J. Cell Biol.* 33, 437-449.
Dianzani, M.U. (1979). *In* "Submolecular Biology and Cancer" Ciba Foundation Series 67, pp.245-270. Excerpta Medica, Amsterdam.
Dianzani, M.U., Gabriel, L., Gravela, E. and Paradisi, L. (1976). *In* "International Meeting on Recent Advances in Biochemical Pathology: Toxic Liver Injury" (Eds. M.U. Dianzani, G. Ugazio and L.M. Sena), pp.310-319. Minerva Medica, Torino.
Feo, F., Canuto, R.A. and Garcea, R. (1973). *Eur. J. Cancer* 9, 203-214.
Feo, F., Canuto, R.A., Garcea, R. and Gabriel, L. (1975). *Biochim. Biophys. Acta* 413, 116-134.
Fonnesu, A., Del Monte, U. and Olivotto, M. (1966). *Sperimentale* 116, 353-372.
Gabriel, L., Bonelli, G. and Dianzani, M.U. (1977). *Chem. Biol. Interact.* 19, 101-109.
Gerlach, U. and Hiby, W. (1974). *In* "Methods of Enzymatic Analysis" (Ed. H.U. Bergmeyer), pp.871-873. Springer Verlag, Berlin.
Gravela, E., Feo, F., Canuto, R.A., Garcea, R. and Gabriel, L. (1975). *Cancer Res.* 35, 3041-3047.
Gravela, E., Poli, G., Albano, E. and Dianzani, M.U. (1977). *Exp. Mol. Pathol.* 27, 339-352.
Keirns, J.J., Wheeler, M.A. and Bitensky, M.W. (1974). *Anal. Biochem.* 61, 336-348.
Kovacs, J. and Rez, G. (1979). *Acta Biol. Acd. Sci. Hung.* 30, 177-199.
Lash, E. (1966). *Arch. Biochem. Biophys.* 115, 332-336.
Lebsack, M.E., Petersen, D.R., Collins, A.C. and Anderson, A.D. (1977). *Biochem. Pharmacol.* 26, 1151-1154.
Lowry, O.H., Rosebrough, N.J., Farr, A.L. and Randall, R.J. (1951). *J. Biol. Chem.* 193, 265-275.
Mendelsohn, M.L. (1962). *J. Natl. Cancer Inst.* 28, 1015-1029.
Miglietta, A., Bonelli, G. and Gabriel, L. (1981). *IRCS Med. Sci.* 9, 77-78.
Paradisi, L., Panagini, C., Parola, M., Ribotta, P.B., Carasso, M.C. and Dianzani, M.U. (1981). submitted to *Chem. Biol. Interact.*
Pipeleers, D.G., Pipeleers-Marichal, M.A., Sherline, P. and Kipnis, D.M. (1977). *J. Cell Biol.* 74, 341-350.
Player, T.Y., Mills, T.Y. and Horton, A.A. (1977). *Biochem. Soc. Trans.* 5, 1506-1508.
Poli, G., Gravela, E., Albano, E. and Dianzani, M.U. (1979). *Exp. Mol. Pathol.* 30, 116-127.
Poli, G., Chiarpotto, E. and Gravela, E. (1981a). *Boll. Soc. Ital. Biol. Sper.* (in press).
Poli, G., Cheeseman, K., Slater, T.F. and Dianzani, M.U. (1981b). *Chem. Biol. Interact.* (in press).
Rez, G., Kiss, A., Bucsek, M.J. and Kovacs, J. (1976). *Chem. Biol. Interact.* 13, 77-78.
Rumpelt, H.J., Albring, M. and Thomes, W. (1974). *Virchows Arch. B* 16, 195-203.
Rumpelt, H.J. and Weisbach, T. (1978). *Am. J. Pathol.* 91, 49-55.

Ugazio, G., Burdino, E. and Gabriel, L. (1968). *Boll. Soc. Ital. Biol. Sper.* 44, 30-34.
Ugazio, G., Gabriel, L. and Burdino, E. (1969). *In* "Atti del Congresso della Soc. Ital. di Patologia, XI Congresso, Roma 29-31 Ottobre 1969.
Utsumi, K., Yamamoto, G. and Inaba, K. (1965). *Biochim. Biophys. Acta* 105, 368-371.
Zuretti, M.F., Bouma, J.W.M, Messina, M., Barrera, G. and Baccino, F.M. (1980). *Exp. Mol. Pathol.* 33, 316-322.

DISCUSSION

Slater: Thank you for the presentation of a huge amount of data in a characteristically modest and elegant fashion. Two things come immediately to my mind. The first point that I wish to raise is that you showed in one of your early slides that a hepatoma produces a more vigorous thiobarbituric acid reaction than the control. Now bearing in mind what we heard from Professor Esterbauer earlier, where generally speaking the thiobarbituric acid reaction represents mainly the production of malonaldehyde, that the hepatoma-lines shown at the bottom of that slide, where in fact there is very little TBA positive material, is it worth checking that these hepatoma-lines are in fact producing non-malonaldehyde-like products?

Dianzani: This point of course needs to be checked. We are in contact with Professor Esterbauer and he has started a collaboration with us to measure the pattern of aldehydes produced during peroxidation of various hepatoma cell lines. He already noticed a considerable difference in the aldehyde patterns compared to normal. The results I presented are very recent. In fact the results with the MH_1C_1 hepatoma peroxidation were the surprise of the last week for us.

Slater: For my second point I was very impressed with your studies relating to the effects of aldehydes at different stages of the cell cycle, and it makes me think of some studies with methyl glyoxyl on dividing *Escherichia coli*. The study I'm thinking of, using synchronised *E. coli* cells, was done by Fraval and McBrien (1980), and one of those authors is indeed our present editor. I wonder whether Dr McBrien would like to comment on this point.

Dianzani: Of course, synchronisation in the cell lines that I described was not very good, and in consequence the peaks shown on the graphs were not very sharp but it is not easy to obtain better synchronisation by the method that we used. The results I showed were obtained with 4-hydroxy-pentenal. As far as methyl glyoxal is concerned, I must say it produces the same type of decrease in the proliferation compartment but does not increase Ts. This may suggest a different mechanism of action for methyl glyoxal compared to 4-hydroxy-pentenal.

McBrien: In reply to the chairman's invitation to comment on those of our results relevant to those presented by Professor Dianzani (Fraval and McBrien, 1980), in cultures of *E. coli* we found, as expected, that the methyl glyoxal inhibited protein synthesis very strongly, but also DNA synthesis was inhibited. We used synchronised cultures to try to determine how the effect of methyl glyoxal on DNA synthesis occurred. What we observed in synchronised cultures was that methyl glyoxal inhibited the initiation of DNA synthesis; DNA synthesis that had already started continued. If methyl glyoxal was added within about 20 min of cell division then that division did not take place. This result ties in with other observations on the cell cycle in *E. coli* where particular proteins have to be synthesised within that time period prior to cell division and, therefore, we concluded that the effect of methyl glyoxal on DNA synthesis and on cell division arose as a result of the inhibition of protein synthesis.

Dianzani: Well, in reply to those interesting comments of Dr McBrien I forgot to mention that at the same time as we measured the incorporation of thymidine into DNA we also measured the incorporation of uridine into RNA and of leucine into protein. We got about 40% inhibition of DNA synthesis, about 30% of inhibition of RNA synthesis and about 20% inhibition in the synthesis of protein. But of course, your system, Dr McBrien, is very much less complicated than the one we were studying using hepatoma cells seeded into the peritoneal cavity.

McBrien: When Hadrian Fraval and I published the work I referred to we were aware of other work in this area using other types of cell but we used a somewhat different method for measuring the effects on protein, RNA and DNA synthesis. In our experiments we pulsed the samples for very short periods of time (around 4 min) so that we were measuring absolute rates of incorporation at specific times in the cell cycle, whereas most people who have done this type of work use much longer pulse times. If you do take a long time for incubation then you don't see such a strong effect on DNA synthesis.

Dianzani: Well, in any case you were measuring much shorter times than we did. The results with the hepatomas, for example, cover periods up to 18 h.

Esterbauer: Professor Dianzani, have you measured alcohol dehydrogenase activity in mitochondria in hepatomas for example? I ask that because aldehyde dehydrogenase may cooperate in a detoxification system for the aldehydes. I just mentioned this because with 4-hydroxy-nonenal, for instance, on incubation with liver homogenate and adding NADH or NADPH one can convert most of the aldehyde to the alcohol.

Dianzani: There is no alcohol dehydrogenase activity in normal liver mitochondria. In fact, this enzyme is mostly found in the cytosol. There is another enzyme attacking ethanol which occurs in microsomes, the so-called microsomal ethanol oxidising system. But in mitochondria there is really no such activity and the small amount that one finds in mitochondrial suspension probably results from contamination by microsomes and cell sap. But, in any case, one should add that it seems that acetaldehyde is the most important factor damaging mitochondria in ethanol induced liver injury.

Adams: It is always good to hear a rational explanation for a difference in response between normal and malignant tissue and I found your talk interesting in that respect. In cancer therapy the response of cells of the intestinal epithelium or of the haemopoietic system is often a limiting factor. What is the position in regard to the effects on such cells of the aldehydes that you have described?

Dianzani: Of course, I agree with you. I feel in any case that the ideas of Burlakova are rather theoretical ones in principle. However, there was something attractive theoretically in her ideas concerning the inverse relationship between cell division and the peroxidation rate.

Slater: I think what Professor Dianzani is referring to in his last remarks is that the ideas for studying any relationship between lipid peroxidation and cell division came in the beginning from studies of Burlakova (1975). Dr Burlakova's group showed that in a number of normal tissues with widely ranging rates of cell division and in various tumours there was indeed an inverse relationship between the rate of cell division and of peroxidised products. And she based a lot of her writings around that initial finding and there seems no doubt that lipid peroxidation goes on in the cells of the body under physiological conditions. And as Professor Dianzani has just said it is very hard to extrapolate from the studies of Burlakova which concerned essentially the anti-oxidant status of tissues with modern concepts of anti-cancer treatment and the rates of cancer cell division.

Dianzani: Yes, generally I think the exact correlations proposed from those early studies are rather approximate, but the overall idea is rather good. They did not of course suggest any exact mechanism for the inverse relationship between lipid peroxidation and the rate of cell division. Of course, basically what they said was that the rate of lipid peroxidation can regulate cell division but they never developed an explanation for that basic idea. They tried to link up their work with the well known studies of ionising radiation on cell division. That was, I think, a philosophical approach.

Stier: Was the reduction in cytochrome P_{450} content observed *in vivo* or *in vitro*?

Dianzani: It was observed *in vitro*. The aldehydes were added, in these experiments done by Dr Poli, directly to isolated hepatocyte suspensions.

Stier: So these results were obtained with isolated hepatocytes. You have no results with microsomes where you added the aldehydes under conditions involving mixed function oxygenation?

Dianzani: A few years ago in Turin we added methyl glyoxal to microsome suspensions *in vitro* to study effects on drug metabolism. With the concentrations we used we obtained only a small inhibitory effect. As far as experiments *in vivo* are concerned, Professor Gravela did some experiments some years ago where he injected aldehyes directly into the peritoneal cavity and observed some inhibition of protein synthesis in the liver, but we have no studies on cytochrome P_{450}.

Esterbauer: Taking up the point of Professor Stier, do you mean whether we have any results with aldehydes added directly to microsomes?

Stier: Yes.

Esterbauer: Well, we have done some studies in this direction and the concentration of aldehydes required to inhibit cytochrome P_{450} in isolated microsomes was about 200 μM.

Slater: Yes, I think going back to the *in vivo* situation that Professor Dianzani was referring to, the few experiments that have been done with aldehyde injected into rats have produced no significant changes in liver P_{450}. And as far as I know, no one has looked at the overall rate of drug metabolism *in vivo* following injection of the types of aldehyde discussed by Professors Esterbauer and Dianzani.

Stier: Then I can rephrase my question referring to the very specific effect of cytochrome P_{450} by allyl isopropyl acetamide. Perhaps one could expect a similar decrease in cytochrome P_{450} induced by some of the aldehydes described, especially those with the allylic function, since this type of group seems to lead to a rather specific destruction of this hemoprotein (De Matteis and Cantoni, 1979).

Slater: I think that is a very interesting question and it surely relates to work done, for example, by Dr De Matteis at Carshalton where I think he has now shown that there is a specific methylation involved in the destructive action of allyl isopropyl acetamide on cytochrome P_{450} in rat liver, and in the resultant accumulation of porphyrin precursors and the experimental prophyria that results from the administration of the toxic agent. I think that this treatment must cause a diversion of the normal bio-synthetic P_{450} pathway and loss of control of P_{450} levels. From that point of view I think it's a different aspect to the work described by Professor Dianzani where it is the products of lipid peroxidation that are interesting us in relation to the sequence of events giving toxic liver injury.

Magee: In relation to the endogenous peroxidation that you are speaking about with reference to the regulation of cell proliferation - to what extent does it vary from organ to organ in relation to the corresponding rates of cell division?

Dianzani: Professor Slater and Dr Benedetto studied the lipid peroxidation rate in a wide range of tissues from the rat and the highest activity was found in the liver. Some peroxidation activity was found in most other tissues with some doubt relating to the activity in the brain and in the lungs. But the problem was in fact the lack of cytochrome P_{450} in these tissues. By using very sensitive spectrophotometric measurements they were able to find cytochrome P_{450} even in those tissues. But I think perhaps Professor Slater is probably better able to answer this point himself.

Slater: Basically, the endogenous rate is low in most tissues except liver of course, but if you add a reducing substrate such as ascorbate or NADPH then you can accelerate the rate of lipid peroxidation in more or less all tissues under these conditions; for example, in brain you can get then a very rapid rate of lipid peroxidation in the presence of ascorbate. Although as we heard this morning, if you increase the concentration of ascorbate too far then it stops acting as a pro-oxidant and acts instead as an anti-oxidant and stops the peroxidation process. So in these senses then all tissues have some endogenous peroxidation, but in this study which was done largely by Chiara Benedetto, we measured only malonaldehyde and oxygen uptake and I think that really one should go back to those studies and look at other aldehydic products that are produced during peroxidative reactions. And also to look at the disappearance of the polyunsaturated fatty acid itself in the membrane fractions during endogenous peroxidation. But that would be a rather massive extension of the study where we measured I think 23 tissues, and even with measurement only of malonaldehyde and oxygen uptake P_{450} and the NADPH-flavoprotein it took us rather a large amount of effort. In summary, I suppose we can say that by and large liver is by far the most active tissue in relation to endogenous peroxidation as measured by malonaldehyde production.

Magee: So that the extent of lipid peroxidation does not correlate with the basic mitotic index of the tissue since the liver does not divide very much?

Slater: I agree; I think this is a very pertinent point. I think another relevant issue is that in some tissues such as lung, whilst we measure P_{450} in microsomal fractions prepared from lung homogenates as a measure of P_{450} dependent peroxidative reactions, we know that P_{450} occurs only in certain types of cell in that complex tissue so that really we should be measuring the malonaldehyde production or the oxygen uptake or the disappearance of polyunsaturated fatty acid in that particular type of cell that has the concentrated amount of P_{450} in it. We actually have that type of project in mind because Dr Nöhammer from Graz now has methods for allowing us to measure aldehyde production in single cells so as part of the overall Brunel-Graz-Turin collaboration we will be looking at aldehyde production in single cells to see whether in tissues that turn over fast or turn over slowly there are related changes in peroxidation in the relevant cell types.

Magee: You have obviously thought around this problem, i.e. in brain there are neuronal cells which apparently can't divide at all and glial cells that can divide very well, and in that sense you have contrasting cell populations with regard to cell division.

Dianzani: We studied peroxidation, some years ago, in testis where there is a high rate of cell division, and in muscle where of course there is a very slow rate of cell division. In both tissues, the rate of lipid peroxidation was low. The low lipid peroxidation in muscle tissue had been observed also by the Russian group, who explained it by the presence of a high concentration of endogenous anti-oxidant. The natural anti-oxidant suggested by them was imidazole.

Player: I have studied in my short time in this area, lipid peroxidation in brain microsomes where there is a low level of cytochrome P_{450} and low, but quite easily measurable, levels of NADPH-cytochrome c reductase so that there are some features of the peroxidising system in brain. In fact, the first project on lipid peroxidation that I was involved in concerned work on the sarcoplasmic reticulum of chicken breast muscle and the effects of lipid peroxidation on calcium and on ATPase. So that from my experience, peroxidation is certainly detectable even if rather low in different tissues.

Dianzani: We must remember first of all that there is not a homogeneous composition of cells in different tissues. If we consider lipofuschin production, for example, this is rather high in the cortical cells in old people. Lipofuschin production is generally considered to be a proof of the occurrence of lipid peroxidation. Other brain cells, however, show only a low rate of lipofuschin production.

Slater: But I think Professor Magee has put his finger on a very interesting point in relation to the general peroxidation hypothesis. Because on the basis of the inverse relationship proposed by the Burlakova group we would expect tissues which have a very low rate of cell division like brain to have a high peroxidation rate and tissues like liver to have a rather lower rate of peroxidation. But in fact what we find, of course, is that liver is by far the most active and brain is very low in lipid peroxidation rate unless supplemented in certain specific fashions.

Riley: If one is to pursue that kind of argument then I would think it possible to distinguish between tissues where growth is possible and, therefore, has to be related and tissues where growth is switched off completely and, therefore, no physiological regulation is required. So I think it is possible to exclude brain and muscle on that basis.

Player: Of course, most of our discussion so far has centred around peroxidation in isolated microsomes but when we consider the whole cell situation we have to bear in mind the organised anti-oxidant capabilities of an organised cell.

Slater: Of course, I'm sure that is right.

Riley: Going back to your study of the effects of aldehydes on synchronised cells I think the results you showed concerning the action of aldehydes on tubulin are not consistent with the conclusion you reached with respect to inhibition in the G_1 phase of the cell cycle because if the aldehydes are acting by interaction with tubulin then you would expect the inhibition to be at the G_2/M stage.

Dianzani: We must consider of course that about 30% of the cells enter into G_0. I agree with you that the evidence for the tubulin mechanism being the major one for the aldehyde effect is rather feeble.

REFERENCES to Discussion

Burlakova, E.B. (1975). *Russ. Chem. Rev.* 44, 871-880.

De Matteis, F. and Cantoni, L. (1979). *Biochem. J.* 183, 99-103.

Fraval, H.N.A. and McBrien, D.C.H. (1980). *J. Gen. Microbiol.* 117, 127-134.

Effects of Low Concentrations of Aldehydes on Tumour Cells and Tumour Growth

E. SCHAUENSTEIN

REVIEW

A new group of α,β-unsaturated aldehydes, the 4-hydroxyenals, have been detected in, and isolated from watery suspensions of linoleic acid in the course of autoxidation under air in pure distilled water at 40°C, in work which started in our laboratory in 1964 (Schauenstein *et al.*, 1964a).

A striking chemical feature of these substances is the fact that, at neutral pH, they react exclusively with SH-groups (of both proteins and nonproteins) in the cell. Moreover, they discriminate between different types of thiols. For example, when acting *in vitro* on Ehrlich ascites tumour cells in concentrations exceeding 3 mM, the entire sub-cellular content of nonprotein thiols (which mainly consists of glutathione) is consumed by reaction with the hydroxyalkenals, whereas only 50% of the soluble cell protein thiols react (Rindler and Schauenstein, 1970). Among the latter are functional thiols of cytoplasmic enzymes of both glycolysis and respiration, as well as of nuclear enzymes of nucleic acid biosynthesis and protein synthesis (Bickis *et al.*, 1969; Schauenstein *et al.*, 1970). As a consequence, respiration is strongly inhibited and glycolysis and protein and nucleic acid biosynthesis completely stopped (Bickis *et al.*, 1969). The cells show drastic morphologic damage (Fig. 1) and ultimately are killed as shown by the trypan blue reaction (Schauenstein *et al.*, 1964b; Schauenstein *et al.*, 1968).

If the concentration is reduced to 0.2 mM, it becomes apparent that hydroxyalkenals also discriminate between cytoplasmic and nuclear protein thiols. It is the latter that possess the highest sensitivity to hydroxyalkenals (Khoschsorur *et al.*, 1981).

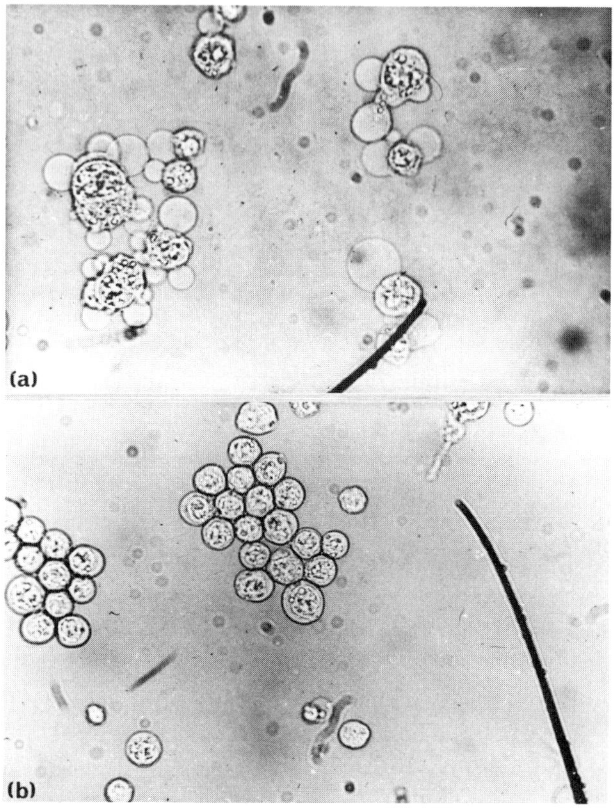

FIG. 1 Ehrlich ascites tumour cells incubated 30 min in (a) 3 mM HPE and in (b) 0.9% NaCl.

For these investigations the cells were homogenised, and cytoplasmic and nuclear fractions were separated according to Mamaril *et al.* (1970). The yield of pure intact nuclei was approximately 90%. From both fractions the soluble proteins were isolated by column chromatography according to Rindler and Schauenstein (1970) and the thiols quantitatively determined with DTNB. Table 1 shows the different effects of hydroxypentenal (HPE) on both cytoplasmic and nuclear protein thiols after 30 min *in vitro* incubation. The loss of the SH-content of the soluble proteins of the cytoplasm amounts to 10 nmoles/mg (7% decrease) compared with 26 nmoles/mg of the soluble nuclear proteins (21%). Table 2 demonstrates the effects with the 9-carbon-

TABLE 1 Sulphydryl content of the soluble proteins of Ehrlich ascites tumour cells after 30 min incubation *in vitro* in 0.2 mM HPE or 0.9% NaCl

	Sulphydryl composition of soluble protein	
	Cytoplasm (n moles/mg prot.)	Nucleus (n moles/mg prot.)
A. Controls (0.9% NaCl)	143.5	125.3
B. HPE 0.2 mM	133.3	98.9
Difference (A-B)	10.2 ± 1.2	26.4 ± 0.8
(A-B) as a %	7.1 ± 0.8	21.4 ± 0.8
n	4	4

n: number of single experiments.

TABLE 2 Sulphydryl content of the soluble proteins of Ehrlich ascites tumour cells after 30 min incubation *in vitro* in 0.2 mM HNE or 0.9% NaCl

	Sulphydryl composition of soluble protein	
	Cytoplasm (n moles/mg prot.)	Nucleus (n moles/mg prot.)
A. Controls (0.9% NaCl)	130.0	162.8
B. HNE 0.2 mM	127.7	118.0
(A-B)	2.3 ± 0.5	44.8 ± 1.0
(A-B) as a %	1.7 ± 0.3	27.4 ± 0.6
n	4	4

n: number of single experiments

homologue 4-hydroxynonenal (HNE). This aldehyde seems to be of special biological interest since its biogenic formation has recently been established by Benedetti *et al.* (1980) in liver cell microsomes. It can be seen that the cytoplasmic proteins lose only 2.3 nmoles SH/mg (1.7%), which is insignificant, whereas nuclear soluble proteins lose 45 nmoles SH/mg (27%). This difference is highly significant.

TABLE 3 The soluble protein and sulphydryl content of Ehrlich ascites tumour cells

	Cytoplasm	Nucleus	Complete cell
Soluble protein (mg/g wet weight)	30.6 ± 3.9	1.4 ± 0.7	26.5 ± 1.7
SH content (n moles/mg prot.)	136.5 ± 21.0	133.9 ± 21.8	126.0 ± 2.0

Of the total soluble proteins of the whole cell only 5% are soluble nuclear proteins whereas 95% are located in the cytoplasm. Both protein fractions have approximately the same SH-content as Table 3 shows. So approx. 1.5% of the total soluble protein thiols are attacked by hydroxynonenal and they are situated in the nucleus. The remainder being still unaffected are largely in the cytoplasm. In excellent accordance with these findings are the results obtained by Bickis *et al.* (1969) on the metabolic activities of the cells after incubation with 0.2 mM HPE *in vitro*. Respiration of the cell remains practically unaffected, and anaerobic glycolysis is inhibited only by some 15%. Both processes are controlled by SH enzymes. But DNA synthesis is inhibited up to 90% after 30 min incubation (cf. also Schauenstein and Esterbauer, 1979).

Still more impressive is the biological behaviour of tumour cells preincubated *in vitro* in 0.16 mM HNE which is shown in Fig. 3. The percentage of both stalagmotic and trypan blue-positive cells in the controls do not differ essentially from those observed with the HNE-treated cells, but when the latter were reimplanted into healthy mice, considerable inhibitions of tumour growth occurred. When cells which have been preincubated 120 min in 0.16 mM HNE were implanted, 90% of animals remained absolutely tumour-free after 10 days, and 10% of the animals showed considerable inhibition of tumour growth; no animal showed unchanged tumour growth.

It should be noted that after 30 min of incubation, when the biosynthesis of DNA has already been extensively inhibited, the reimplanted cells still do not show an inhibition of tumour growth, the full inhibition appearing only after 120 min incubation. A possible

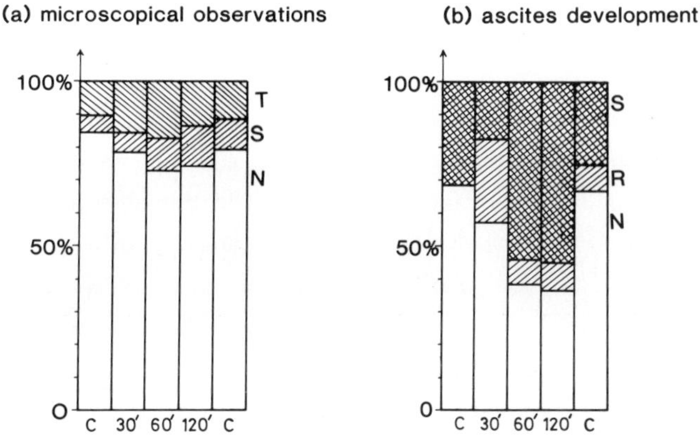

FIG. 2 Effects of 0.2 mM HPE after incubation *in vitro* for various times with Ehrlich ascites tumour cells. (a) T = % cells stainable with Trypan blue, S = % cells with "stalagmosis" (cf. Fig. 1a), N = normal cells. (b) Effects on development of ascites tumour 10 d after re-implantation; S = animals macroscopically free of ascites tumour, R = tumour development retarded, N = normal tumour development. C = controls.

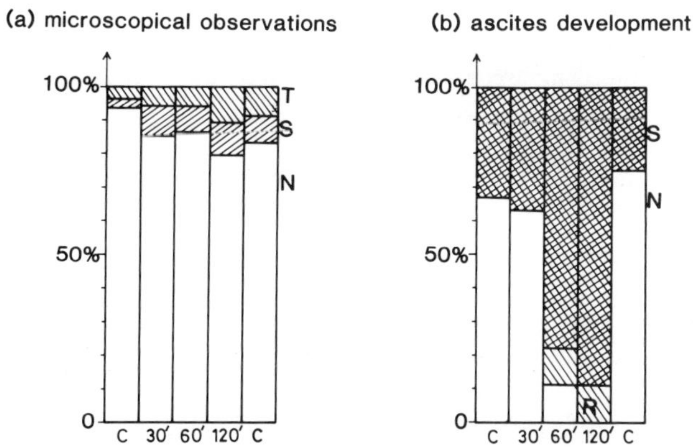

FIG. 3 Effects of 0.16 mM HNE after incubation *in vitro* for various times with Ehrlich ascites tumour cells. Symbols as in Fig. 2.

explanation could be that the amount of cells which have been arrested by HNE in the late S-phase increases with increasing incubation time.

Figure 2 shows that similar effects have also been observed with HPE which, in comparison with HNE, produces more extensive morphological damage to the cells but exerts a distinctly weaker cytostatic effect on the re-implanted tumour cells. Thus, as can be seen from

Tables 1 and 2, the influence of the lipophilic aliphatic chain on the biochemical properties of the hydroxyalkenals becomes evident again.

Returning again to the effects on HNE, the most plausible explanation of the results may be to assume that the substance penetrates the cells, a proportion of which reaches the nucleus and reacts there with some thiols of the soluble proteins causing an inhibition of DNA polymerase. This enzyme, as is well known (Chiu *et al.*, 1977) has functional thiol groups. Possibly biosynthesis of RNA and protein might also be involved. The absolute number of the nuclear soluble protein thiols attacked by HNE can be approximately calculated as 0.2 f moles/single cell.

Nöhammer (1981) determined quantitatively by means of cytospectrophotometry both the amount of protein SH-groups as well as the protein-bound carbonyls per single cell after incubation in 0.16 mM HNE. According to these measurements one single cell loses about 1.2 f moles SH, and approximately the same quantity of protein-bound carbonyl appears. That means that in addition to the sensitive SH-groups of the soluble nuclear proteins also thiols have been attacked by HNE belonging to structural proteins and this may also contribute to the inhibition of cell division.

An important question arises now: How does HNE reach the nucleus and what happens on its way through the cytoplasm? Following a valuable suggestion of T. Slater we examined the incubation medium during incubation for amounts of HNE still present in the medium (Esterbauer *et al.*, 1981). The results are shown in Fig. 4, which shows a drastic decrease of the HNE content of the incubation medium amounting to 50%. That indicates a considerable turnover of the substance: 0.5 μ moles of HNE disappeared from 6 ml of incubation medium. On the other hand the 30 million cells bind 0.07 to 0.08 μ moles of HNE in reaction with total protein- and nonprotein-SH. This indicates a metabolism of HNE in the cytoplasm probably by an aldehyde oxidoreductase. As this reaction apparently is the predominant one, the HNE-sensitive SH-groups of the cytoplasmic respiratory and glycolytic enzymes remain unchanged, the energy supplying pathways continue to run, and the cell is still alive. However, small amounts of HNE

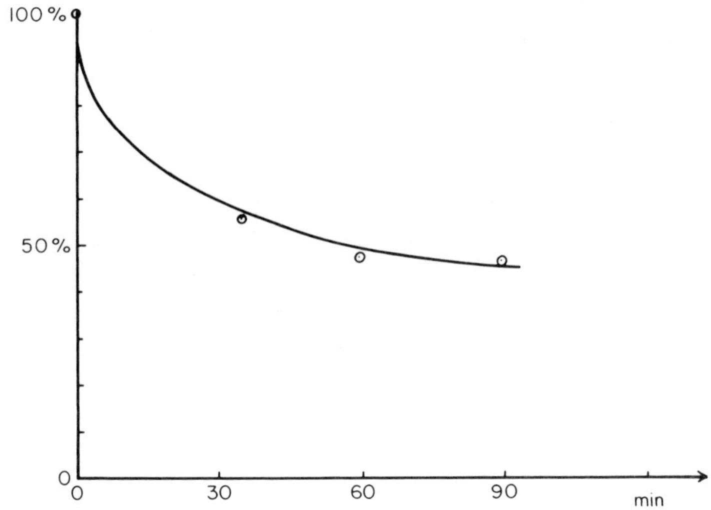

FIG. 4 % decrease of HNE (0.16 mM in isotonic saline) during incubation of Ehrlich ascites tumour cells *in vitro*.

actually reach the nucleus and attack there selectively the highly sensitive SH-groups of the systems which are responsible for cell division.

ACKNOWLEDGEMENTS

This paper is dedicated to Professor Dr Erich Ziegler on the occasion of his 70th birthday.

REFERENCES

Benedetti, A., Comporti, M. and Esterbauer, H. (1980). *Biochim. Biophys. Acta* 620, 281-296.

Bickis, J., Schauenstein, E. and Taufer, M. (1969). *Monatsch. Chem.* 100, 1077-1104.

Chiu, J.F., Hnilica, L.S., Belanger, L. and Morris, H.P. (1977). *Adv. Exp. Med. Biol.* 92, 181-203.

Esterbauer, H., Schauenstein, E. and Tillian, H.M. (1981). (prepared for publication).

Khoschsorur, G., Schaur, R.J., Tillian, H.M. and Reiter, M. (1981). *Z. Naturforsch. Teil C* 36 (in press).

Mamaril, F.P., Dobrjansky, A. and Green, S. (1970). *Cancer Res.* 30, 352-356.

Nöhammer, G. and Schauenstein, E. (1981). (Prepared for publication).

Rindler, R. and Schauenstein, E. (1970). *Z. Naturforsch. Teil B* 25, 739-744.

Schauenstein, E., Esterbauer, H., Jaag, G. and Taufer, M. (1964a). *Monatsch. Chem.* 95, 180-183.
Schauenstein, E., Zangger, J. and Ratzenhofer, M. (1964b). *Z. Naturforsch. Teil B* 19, 923-929.
Schauenstein, E., Wohl, W. and Kramer, I. (1968). *Z. Naturforsch. Teil B* 23, 530-537.
Schauenstein, E., Verdino, H. and Taufer, M. (1970). *Monatsch. Chem.* 101, 1189-1202.
Schauenstein, E. and Esterbauer, H. (1979). *In* "Submolecular Biology and Cancer", Ciba Foundation Series 67 (new series), pp.225-244. Excerpta Medica, Amsterdam.

DISCUSSION

Professor Schauenstein was unable to present his paper at the meeting and the following is a discussion of a related presentation by Professor Esterbauer.

Willson: I have two questions - one an *in vitro* question and the second an *in vivo* question. I will deal with the *in vivo* question first. It concerns the use of tumours of the type you have particularly used in your study. An old colleague, Dr Harold Hewitt used to call these "Joe Bloggs" tumours, in the sense that they have a name to them and that they are relatively old tumours. Dr Hewitt has written an article in which he pointed out that these tumours have been induced, often chemically, many years ago and they are no longer isogeneic with the recipient animals into which they are injected or implanted (Hewitt, 1978). Have you considered this? Do you think that a larger animal study should be done, using an inbred colony, with tumours that have arisen spontaneously in it. This will, of course, be very expensive.

Esterbauer: I completely agree, but for a preliminary screening we prefer to use the simple test system of EATC in mice. More intensive studies including transplanted solid tumours as well as spontaneous tumours are underway in Graz. But it takes a long time to establish the different tumour lines and the methodology. I completely agree that one has to go from the simple system of EATC tumours to solid tumours and finally to spontaneous tumours. The therapeutic effects of 4-hydroxypentenal have been tested on a number of different transplanted solid tumours of mice. Subcutaneous peritoneal application of this aldehyde (dose 1 x 0.2 mg to 3 x 0.2 mg per 10 g body weight) definitely inhibited the growth of Ehrlich solid tumour, sarcoma 180, Nemeth-Kellner lymphosarcoma and Harding-Passey melanoma (Schauenstein *et al.*, 1977).

Willson: Thank you, and can I now ask my *in vitro* question, I am very interested in the equilibrium that you have observed. You suggested that it was perhaps due to a polymerase which could be activated by dithiothreitol. Have you tried giving your aldehyde and then adding the dithiothreitol? If it's an equilibrium, you may be able to reverse the situation.

Esterbauer: Not in this case, not with DNA polymerase. But we have done it with some other isolated enzymes and in each case it was possible to activate the enzymes using the proper concentration of a reactivating agent. So one can, for example, reactivate glycerin-aldehyde-3-phosphate dehydrogenase very easily by adding glutathione or cysteine and removing the aldehyde again. So it is always a question of affecting the equilibrium Prot-SH + aldehyde $\rightleftharpoons$ Prot-S-aldehyde by a competitive aldehyde binding reaction Prot-S-aldehyde + RSH $\rightleftharpoons$ Prot-SH + RS-aldehyde.

Willson: Are you suggesting this system as a control system for cell growth or division?

Esterbauer: It could be, yes. But only in theory, since these are not very fast reactions. The reverse reactions (Prot-S-aldehyde + RSH $\rightleftharpoons$ Prot-SH + RS-aldehyde) requires at least, on average, one hour to go to completion.

Willson: Does that go against it being a control system, or can control systems act slowly?

Riley: Can I follow that up? Isn't it rather surprising then that if all these SH groups are in equilibrium with aldehydic reagents, that you actually end up with some specific process being affected in the way that you have demonstrated. It seems odd that the nuclear SH groups are so specifically selected in this way.

Esterbauer: The problem is much more complicated than I could show here. It is reasonable to assume that due to the reaction of the aldehydes with SH groups the complete SH/SS status of the cell is affected both in the cytoplasm and in the nucleus.

Riley: Are you saying that there is a reduction of glutathione levels before you get binding to the SH groups in the DNA polymerase or whatever the sensitive component is?

Esterbauer: There is a significant loss of glutathione at concentrations which give an inhibition of mitochondrial respiration or glycolysis. But there is probably only a much lower loss of glutathione, if any, at aldehyde concentrations which do inhibit DNA synthesis to 50% and more. Even if there is no measurable decrease of GSH, it is not possible to say whether GSH did not react at all or whether the consumed GSH was replaced (resupplied) from the glutathione pool of the proteins. To clear this question, radioactive aldehydes should be applied. Such studies are not in progress.

Garner: If these compounds, specifically HPE, can inhibit DNA synthesis at $^{1}/_{100}$th the concentration required to knock out for instance the average protein SH group, there must be a very specific reaction involved if the target in the nucleus is a protein SH group, and it would tend to indicate that this is not an equilibrium reaction.

Esterbauer: What I wanted to point out is the rather specific effect of HNE on the nuclear SH proteins and that the target in the nucleus is most probably DNA polymerase. The total decrease of protein SH in the nucleus is around 30% and so about 70% are not affected. In the cytoplasm, on the other hand, no measurable reaction with protein SH groups takes place.

The amount of the aldehyde reacting with the nucleus and producing inhibition is only a small fraction (less than 10%) of the total aldehyde taken up by the cell. Per single cell the upper limit (estimated by cytospectrometric measurements) is 1.2 femtomole/nucleus; the lowest possible amount is 0.2 femtomole/nucleus (measured as decrease of soluble nuclear protein SH groups).

Slater: We saw in an earlier slide of Professor Esterbauer's that when 4-hydroxy-alkenals react with something like glutathione the product is a furan type derivative, almost an analogue of deoxyribose; so whether by reacting a hydroxy-alkenal in a certain way with an SH group on DNA polymerase the enzyme becomes blocked in some very specific way at the nucleotide site, is an interesting speculation. Such an interaction may help to explain the powerful effects you mentioned at 1.2 femtomoles per nucleus.

Stier: That's quite a lot. There are 10^8 molecules per nucleus. How large are the levels of DNA polymerase in the nucleus? I guess it is not that large.

Esterbauer: You mean that we should consider how many of the protein molecules in the nucleus have been modified. According to Kornberg there are four different types of eukaryotic DNA polymerases and from each type the single cell certainly contains many thousands of molecules. It is certainly right that the absolute number of aldehyde molecules bound in the nucleus or the total number of modified protein molecules is still very high. In terms of percentage proportion the measurement showed that out of ten protein SH groups, three were modified by the aldehyde.

Magee: I was thinking about this - about half way through your talk you mentioned that a concentration of about 100 micromolar of the aldehyde will inhibit DNA synthesis in kidney cells. This was kidney cells *in vitro?*

Esterbauer: Yes, that is right.

Magee: Now would it be possible to achieve this concentration in the kidney of an intact animal, without actually killing it? Do you know what the toxicity, the LD_{50}, would be of the aldehyde?

Esterbauer: No, it is not possible to reach this concentration. The LD_{50}s are known (see Schauenstein *et al.*, 1977), they are around 1-1.5 mmole/kg body weight in mice. The highest concentration that could be reached just for toxicity reasons and rate of detoxification is certainly not above 10 micromolar. That is probably also the concentration that Professor Dianzani obtained in the animals, when he saw the various effects on mitosis in bone marrow.

Riley: Can I return to the DNA polymerase. It seems to me that if you are now speculating or estimating that there are, say, three out of 10 DNA polymerase molecules affected in this way, all that this would be expected to do is to extend the period of DNA synthesis. It would not completely prevent a cell from synthesising DNA and in that case it makes it very difficult to explain for example the results that were obtained by reimplantation with your tumour.

Esterbauer: Yes, that is true. But we do not mean that only 30% of the DNA polymerase molecules have been blocked by the aldehyde. On the contrary, we know that at least 90% of the DNA polymerase activity disappeared after incubation of EATC in 0.2 mM aldehyde, and therefore it was concluded that the loss of SH groups in the nucleus is almost due to the loss of SH in the DNA polymerase. If this inhibition is irreversible, it would explain without difficulty the results of reimplantation presented in this paper.

Nöhammer: I think that I have an answer because this problem is much more complex than one might think. We investigated the effects of 2.10^{-4} molar HNE on Ehrlich ascites tumour cells microspectrometrically and found not only a decrease of SH groups within the nucleus, but also an equal increase of protein-bound carbonyls. There is also a decrease of the glutathione - the protein-bound glutathione - within the cytoplasm. But, in addition, there is an increase of the protein-bound glutathione within the nucleus, and this I think is the effect we should consider, because as you know Mannervik (1980) reported this effect saying that this protein-bound glutathione can act as a switch-on switch-off mechanism of SH enzymes. I think, besides the possibility of the direct binding of HNE and HPE to SH groups of proteins, we should take much more notice in the future of this special effect of the alkenals, the effect of secondary blockade of SH enzymes by protein-bound glutathione. It is an additional effect to the direct, the primary blockage of SH enzymes by hydroxyalkenals. Professor Dianzani reported above about an increase of the nuclear proteins during the incubation: that means - in my opinion - that the cell cycle must be influenced, to be slower or stopped (for example, at G_2+M-phase), so that some of the cells had no chance to divide. The result must be an increase of nuclear proteins, calculated per single cell, just as we found with our microspectrometrical investigations. The treatment of living cells with hydroxyalkenals is seen to be a very complex problem.

Willson: Just a very quick one with reference to Dr Riley's comment and my first comment. Is there any information on whether these compounds stimulate the immune response - has anybody done this or looked at it?

Esterbauer: We have not done such experiments but perhaps Professor Dianzani has some more data?

Dianzani: I think you refer to the immune response? If so, I don't have many data to tell you on this. I remember that Professor Ugazio in Turin did some experiments in collaboration with Dr Forni of the Institute of Microbiology. They found some decrease of the immune response but I cannot remember their experimental details concerning dose, etc.

Slater: I think generally the aldehydes, given parenterally, are immuno-suppressant, that the aldehyde-ascorbate adducts, which have been tested, are immuno-stimulatory (Champion *et al.*, 1981).

REFERENCES to Discussion

Champion, J., Hudson, K. and Slater, T.F. (1981). *IRCS Med. Sci.* 9, 540-549.

Hewitt, H.B. (1978). *Adv. Cancer Res.* 27, 149-200.

Mannervik, B. and Axelsson, K. (1980). *Biochem. J.* 190, 125-130.

Schauenstein, E., Esterbauer, H. and Zollner, H. (1977). "Aldehydes in Biological Systems", pp.77-78, Pion, London.

Lipid Peroxidation in Rat Liver, Hepatomas and Regenerating Liver

T.J. PLAYER

INTRODUCTION

Lipid peroxidation is thought to be involved with a number of normal and abnormal physiological processes. Normal conditions include prostaglandin synthesis and aging while abnormal conditions include haemolytic anaemia and lung damage. Lipid peroxidation largely results from free radical reactions in biological membranes which are rich in polyunsaturated fatty acids. Not only will oxidation affect the structure of complex lipids, but there may also be an effect on proteins and nucleic acid via free radical-mediated interactions. This reflects a major difficulty in interpreting the biological significance of results which are largely studied *in vitro* and therefore which often are not subject to constraints which may exist in the intact cell.

The connection between lipid peroxidation and cellular aging is the accumulation of fluorescent pigments, including lipofuscin, formed from the products of oxidised unsaturated lipids polymerised with denatured proteins. *In vitro* liver microsomal lipid peroxidation has also been shown to decrease the activity of certain enzymes while not affecting others and this appears to correlate with the situation in aging cells (Koster and Slee, 1980).

Mitochondria exhibit a high content of polyunsaturated acids and oxidation catalysts which may lead them to be particularly suited to peroxidative damage (Hunter *et al.*, 1963) and these organelles are known to undergo age-dependent deteriorative changes with respect to the functioning of the inner membrane (Barrett and Horton, 1976). It was shown in our laboratory that an enzyme lipid peroxidation system

TABLE 1 Requirements for mitochondrial enzymic lipid peroxidation

Additions	Malonaldehyde production (nmol/mg protein)
ADP + Fe + NADPH	9.50
ADP + Fe	0.25
ADP + NADPH	2.65
Fe + NADPH	4.25
ADP + Fe + 0.5 mM NADH	0.92
ADP + Fe + 1.0 mM NADH	1.03
ADP + Fe + NADPH + Heat treated mitochondria	0.00

The reaction medium contained: 0.15 M Tris-HCl (pH 7.4), 1.0 mM KH_2PO_4 and 1 mg mitochondrial protein per ml in a final volume of 5 ml. Additions of 0.4 mN NADPH, 4 mM ADP, 0.05 mM $FeCl_3$ and 0.5 mM or 1.0 mM NADH were made as indicated. The reaction vessel was shaken at 25°C. Heat denaturation of the mitochondria was at 80°C for 5 min, employing a Potter Elvehjem homogeniser for resuspension. After 30 min incubation, 0.5 ml samples were taken for MDA determination. Mitochondria were isolated from 6 month old rats. From Player *et al.* (1977).

exists in rat liver mitochondria and has the requirements shown in Table 1. Assay of glucose-6-phosphatase activity indicated 4-5% microsomal contamination in these preparations. Due to the high level of NADPH-dependent lipid peroxidation exhibited by the microsomal fraction, mitochondria were prepared by sucrose density gradient centrifugation which led to a 2% level of microsomal contamination, but resulted in increased mitochondrial lipid peroxidation by 20%.

The NADPH-dependent peroxidation of endogenous lipids in the liver microsomal fraction has been well studied and documented from its initial discovery in 1963 (Hochstein and Ernster, 1963). The reaction is dependent on Fe^{+++}, ADP or ATP as well as NADPH. The enzyme NADPH cytochrome c reductase mediates the reaction which is part of the mixed function oxidase system (Hrycay and O'Brien, 1973).

The mechanism for the reaction in mitochondria is unproven, but is thought to utilise the non-energy dependent transhydrogenase (Pfeifer and McCay, 1972). This agrees with the observation of Takeshige *et al.* (1980) that NADPH dehydrogenase is essential for the reduction of the ADP-Fe^{+++} chelate in electron transport particles prepared from beef heart mitochondria.

RESULTS AND DISCUSSION

Mitochondria were isolated from the livers of rats varying in age; Fig. 1 shows that the extent of enzymic lipid peroxidation increases from foetal and neonatal isolates through young (6 months) to old (24 months) animals. NADPH-dependent lipid peroxidation in rat liver microsomal fractions also exhibited age-related differences (Fig. 2). The initial rates of NADPH-dependent lipid peroxidation show no significant difference between young and old animals up to 15 min. NADPH cytochrome c reductase activity is not significantly different between the two fractions (Table 2). A significant increase in docosahexanoic acid and a decrease in linoleic acid from microsomal and mitochondrial fractions from animals aged 24 months compared with animals aged

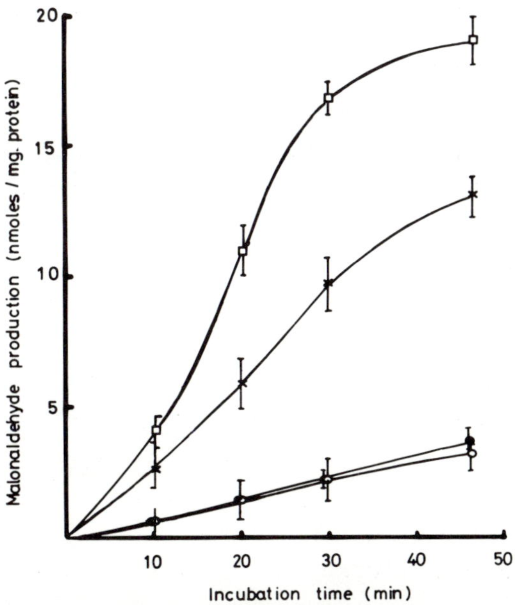

FIG. 1 Malonaldehyde production by mitochondria (1 mg/ml) from old (□), young (x), neonatal (●) and foetal (○) rat livers, suspended at 25°C with vigorous shaking in 0.15 M Tris-HCl (pH 7.4), 1 mM KH_2PO_4, 4 mM ADP, 0.4 mM NADPH and 0.05 mM $FeCl_3$. The values are the means ± SD of separate experiments with mitochondria isolated from three animals or three litters of each age group. From Player *et al.* (1977).

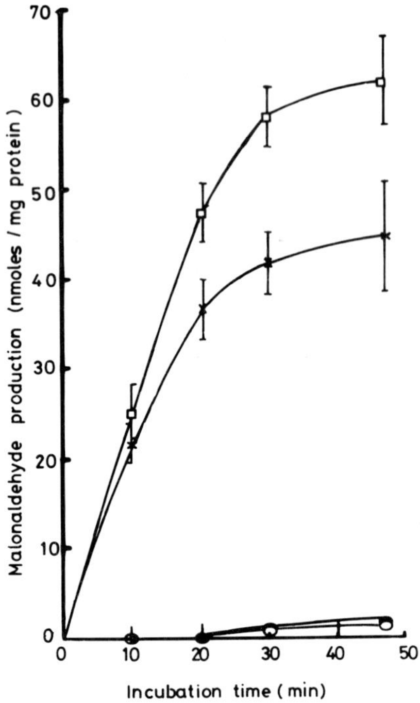

FIG. 2 Malonaldehyde production by microsomal fractions (1 mg/ml) from old (□), young (x), neonatal (●) and foetal (○) rat livers. Reaction medium and number of experiments as in Fig. 1. From Player *et al.* (1977).

TABLE 2 NADPH-cytochrome c reductase in microsomal fractions from rat liver.

Source	NADPH-cytochrome c reductase (nmol/min/mg protein)
Old	153.6 ± 9.4
Young	145.0 ± 6.6
Neonatal	31.4 ± 1.0
Foetal	28.2 ± 1.4

From Player *et al.* (1977).

6 months has been reported by Grinna (1977) and this may explain the results reported here. Lipid peroxidation in foetal and neonatal microsomal fractions was virtually absent. The level of arachidonic

acid (identified as the main substrate for the reaction by Niehaus and Samuelson, 1968) was 2-3% less than in fractions from 6 month animals and the level of NADPH-cytochrome c reductase activity was very low.

It has been reported that tissue homogenates from mature animals, which do not exhibit a rapid rate of mitosis, readily undergo lipid peroxidation (e.g. brain, liver, kidney) whereas those tissues which are not susceptible to lipid peroxidation (e.g. testis and intestinal epithelium) undergo rapid cell division (Barber and Wilbur, 1959). We therefore decided to investigate changes in enzymic lipid peroxidation in liver cells which were transformed into a rapidly dividing state as a result of partial hepatectomy.

Partial hepatectomy was performed according to Higgins and Anderson (1931). The median and left lateral lobes of the liver were removed which together accounted for 60-70% of the total liver weight. Control animals underwent surgery without removal of any liver tissue. After partial hepatectomy the remaining tissue goes into a phase of increased mitotic activity and growth to compensate. The precise time of maximum mitotic activity after partial hepatectomy varies not only with different cell types (Widmann and Fahimi, 1975) but also between different laboratories. Whereas O'Connor (1971) reported that the first peak of DNA synthesis occurs 20 h after partial hepatectomy, Goldenberg *et al.* (1975) stated the first mitotic wave is observed after 24-36 h and Wolfson *et al.* (1956) quote 48 h after surgery as the time of maximum mitotic activity.

Animals were sacrificed periodically over the following 7 d and microsomal fractions prepared. NADPH-dependent lipid peroxidation and NADPH cytochrome c reductase activities were then measured. Figure 3 shows that there is a significant decrease in both these activities which reaches a minimum at about 48 h after partial hepatectomy which corresponds approximately to the time of maximum mitosis. The fatty acid compositon from rat liver microsomes from regenerating liver showed little variation from that of controls (Table 3) suggesting that substrate is unlikely to be responsible for restricting lipid peroxidation in this case.

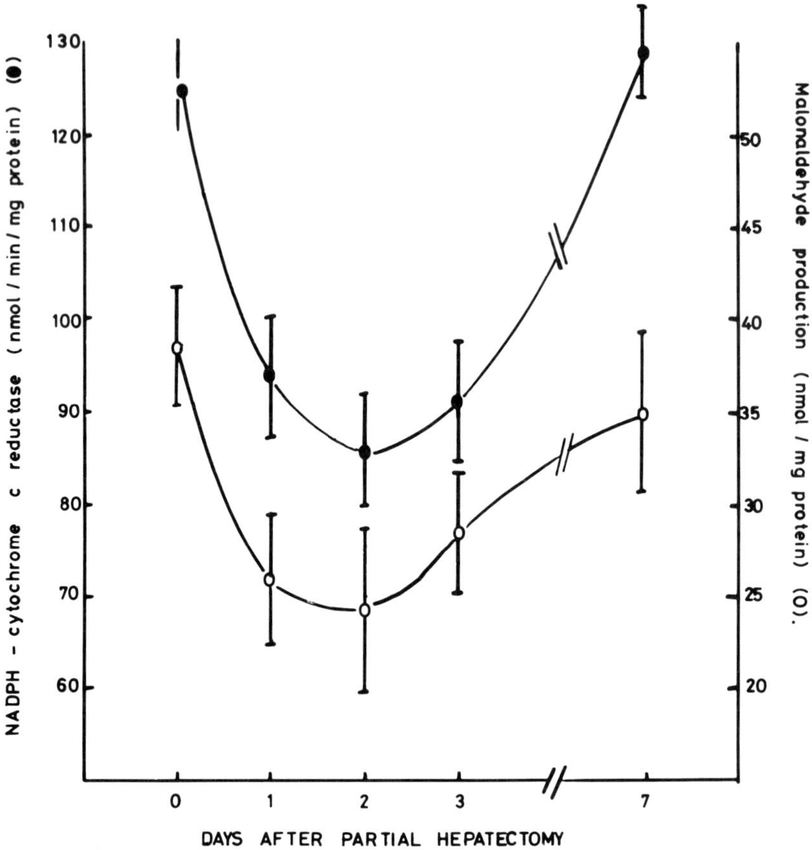

FIG. 3 Liver microsomal NADPH-cytochrome c reductase activity and NADPH-dependent lipid peroxidation (expressed in terms of MDA production) following partial hepatectomy. Samples were taken at regular intervals for MDA analysis throughout a 45 min incubation period. The data presented represent MDA production after 30 min incubation. Each point represents the mean ± SD of assays of separate microsomal fractions from three animals (control or partially hepatectomised) performed in triplicate. For regenerating livers 48 h after partial hepatectomy: (a) NADPH-dependent lipid peroxidation was significantly different from controls; P = 0.02 by Student's t test; (b) NADPH-cytochrome c reductase activity was significantly different from controls: P = 0.01 by Student's t test.

TABLE 3 Total fatty acid analysis of liver microsomes

Time between hepatectomy and killing	fatty acid*				
	16:0	18:0	18:1	18:2	20:4
Control	26.2 ± 1.0	26.1 ± 1.5	12.0 ± 2.0	15.3 ± 1.2	20.4 ± 2.1
24 h	25.8 ± 1.0	25.9 ± 1.1	10.3 ± 1.5	17.7 ± 1.0	21.1 ± 1.6
48 h	26.1 ± 0.8	24.1 ± 0.8	11.9 ± 0.9	16.9 ± 1.4	20.8 ± 0.7
72 h	25.8 ± 0.6	26.8 ± 2.0	12.0 ± 0.6	16.4 ± 0.5	19.0 ± 2.5
168 h	25.1 ± 1.2	27.1 ± 1.5	13.5 ± 1.2	14.8 ± 0.8	19.5 ± 1.9

*Data presented as peak area percentages. (Means ± SD for at least three animals at each time.)

Wolfson *et al.* (1956) had previously reported a decrease in ascorbic acid-induced lipid peroxidation in whole liver homogenates (1 g tissue/ 15 ml Na^{+}-K^{+} phosphate buffer, pH 7.4) 48 h after partial hepatectomy. This was not confirmed in our laboratory. Possible differences in the antioxidant capacity of regenerating and control rat liver were therefore investigated by measuring lipid peroxidation over a range of dilutions of liver homogenates. Lipid peroxidation was induced either by an ascorbic acid or NADPH system and no significant differences were found in MDA production between equivalent dilutions of regenerating liver homogenate and controls (Figs. 4 and 5). These figures do illustrate the diluting out of antioxidant control exerted by the soluble fraction. At higher levels of dilution the antioxidant systems are unable to limit lipid peroxidation which increases rapidly in both controls and regenerating liver. This effect was also demonstrated by dilution of the soluble fraction from control and regenerating livers, adding the microsomal fractions as substrate and incubating in the presence of ascorbic acid (Fig. 6).

Work done prior to this in our laboratory had indicated that the soluble fraction from rat liver of various ages, hepatomas and livers of animals bearing hepatomas do vary in terms of their influence on microsomal lipid peroxidation (Player and Horton, 1978). Soluble fractions of these tissues were prepared and various dilutions added to an incubation system including the microsomal fraction from mature (6 months) rat liver and the cofactors necessary for NADPH-dependent

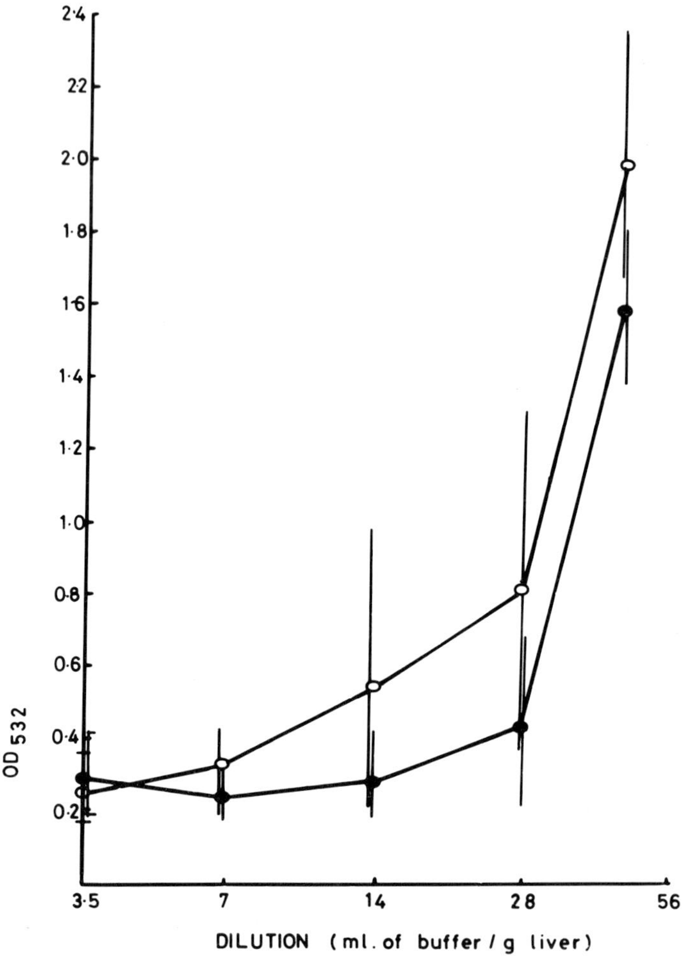

FIG. 4 Production of MDA (expressed as OD_{532}) in whole liver homogenates from control animals (O) and animals 48 h after partial hepatectomy (●) incubated in the presence of sodium ascorbate. Livers were homogenised in 0.15 M Tris-HCl (pH 7.4) (1 g liver: 3.5 ml buffer). The homogenates were serially diluted as indicated. Samples (2 ml) of each dilution were incubated in the presence of 0.2 mg sodium ascorbate/ml at 37°C for 1 h in a shaking water bath. The results of the assay of MDA in separate homogenates of livers from three control and three partially hepatectomised animals at the dilutions indicated and performed in triplicate are expressed as the means ± S.D.

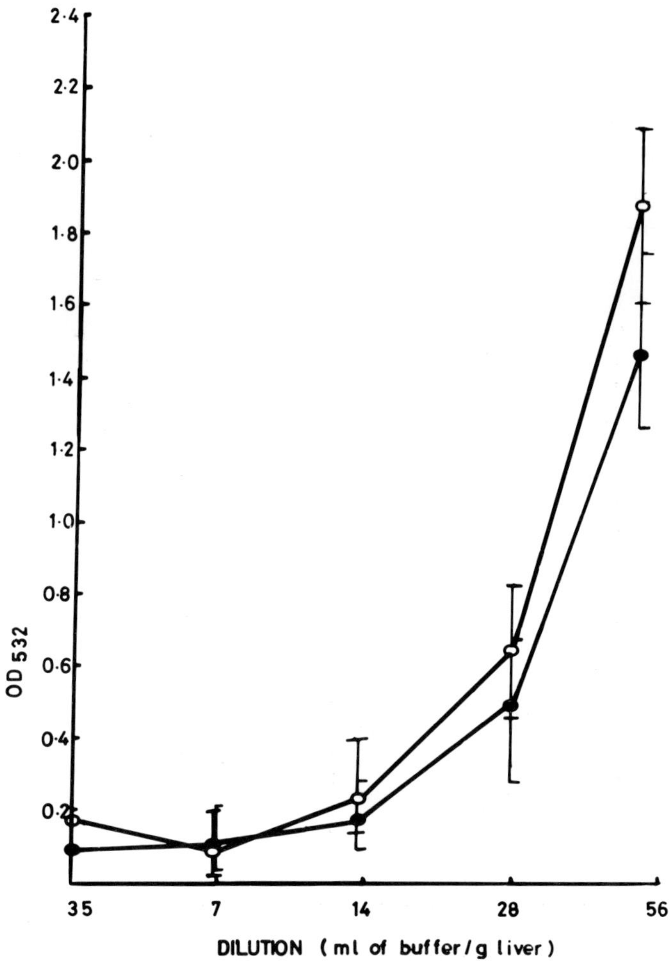

FIG. 5 Production of MDA (expressed as OD_{532}) in whole liver homogenates from control animals (O) and animals 48 h after partial hepatectomy (●) incubated in the presence of an NADPH-generating system. Livers were homogenised in 0.15 M Tris-HCl (pH 7.4) (1 g liver:1.75 ml buffer) and serial dilutions made as indicated. Samples (1 ml) of each dilution were incubated with an NADPH-generating system (1 ml), the final concentrations being 0.15 M Tris-HCl (pH 7.4), 4 mM ADP, 1 mM KH_2PO_4, 0.05 mM $FeCl_3$, 0.8 mM $NADP^+$, 10 mM glucose-6-phosphate and glucose-6-phosphate dehydrogenase (3 units/ml). Incubation was at 25°C for 1 h in a shaking water bath. The results of the assay of MDA in separate homogenates of livers from three control and three partially hepatectomised animals at the dilutions indicated and performed in triplicate are expressed as the means ± S.D.

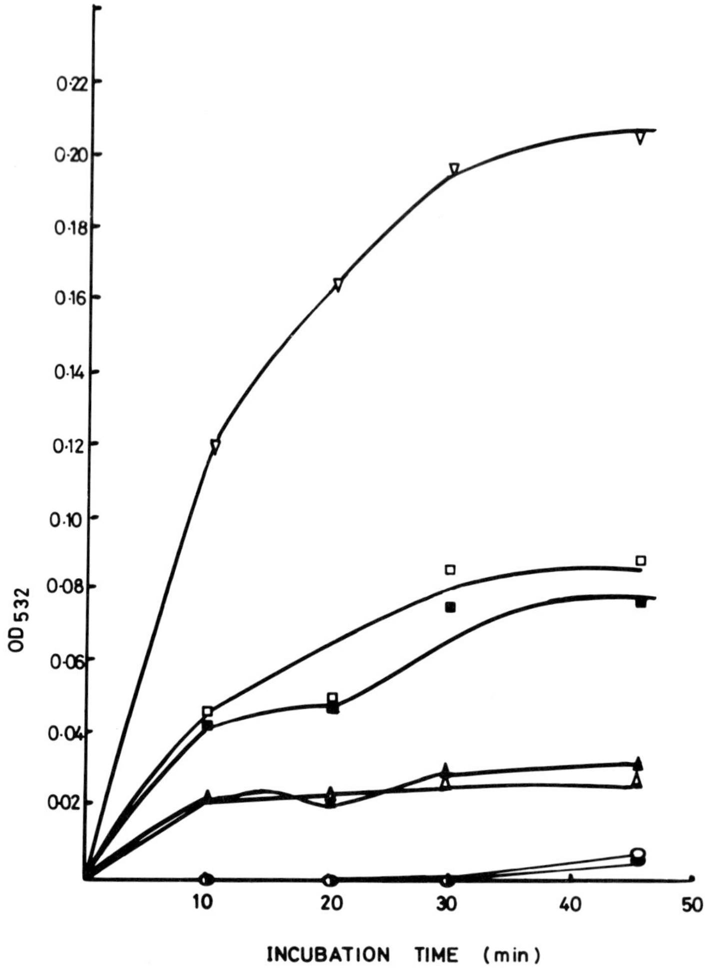

FIG. 6 Effect of the soluble fraction of liver from control animals (closed symbols) and animals 48 h after partial hepatectomy (open symbols) on ascorbic acid-incuded lipid peroxidation. Soluble fractions were prepared by centrifugation of the liver homogenates 0.15 M Tris-HCl (pH 7.4) at 105,000 × g av. for 60 min in an MSE Superspeed 50 centrifuge. Soluble fraction (3 ml), microsomal fraction (0.25 mg/ml) (previously prepared and stored at -20°C) and ascorbic acid (0.2 mg/ml) were incubated in a shaking water bath at 37°C. Samples were taken at regular intervals for assay of MDA. Dilutions of the soluble fractions were 1 g liver:1.5 ml 0.15 M Tris-HCl (pH 7.4) (O), 1 g: 3.0 ml (△), 1 g:4.5 ml (□) and 0.15 M Tris-HCl (pH 7.4) alone (▽). Results are the means of experiments with separate soluble fractions from two control and three partially hepatectomised animals, performed in triplicate.

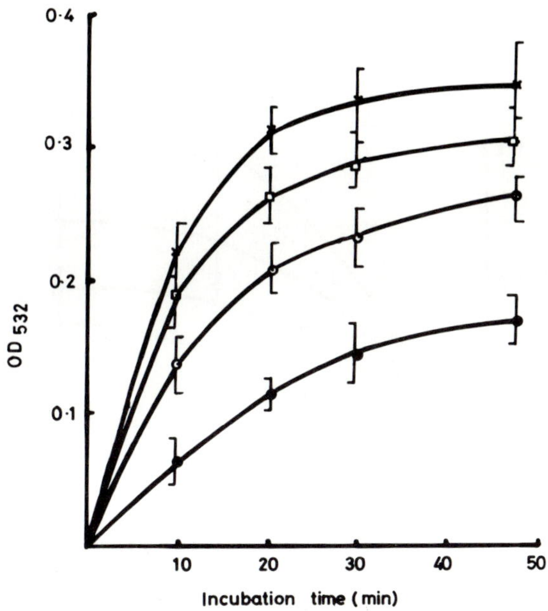

FIG. 7 Effect of the soluble fraction from mature rat liver on microsomal lipid peroxidation. The incubation systems contained 0.25 mg microsomal protein/ml and soluble protein concentrations of 0 (●), 2.7 (x), 5.5 (□) and 8.2 (O) mg/ml. The results are the mean ± SD of three experiments. From Player *et al.* (1978).

lipid peroxidation. Figure 7 shows that the presence of the soluble fraction from mature animals at a relatively high dilution resulted in stimulation of microsomal lipid peroxidation but, with increasing concentration of the soluble fraction, increasing inhibition of lipid peroxidation resulted. Figure 8 demonstrates that when the soluble fraction from neonatal rat liver was used, lipid peroxidation was stimulated and increased stimulation resulted from increased concentration.

These results may reflect the differences between the two systems in balance of antioxidant and pro-oxidant factors. An increase in superoxide dismutase (SOD) activity of liver cytosol from birth (10.8 units/mg protein) to maturity (22.6 units/mg protein) has been measured in this laboratory. Sharma (1977) has demonstrated a decrease in iron content of rat liver from birth (25.2 mg/100 g tissue) to 8 months (9.9 mg/100 g tissue). While iron acts as a catalyst for enzymic

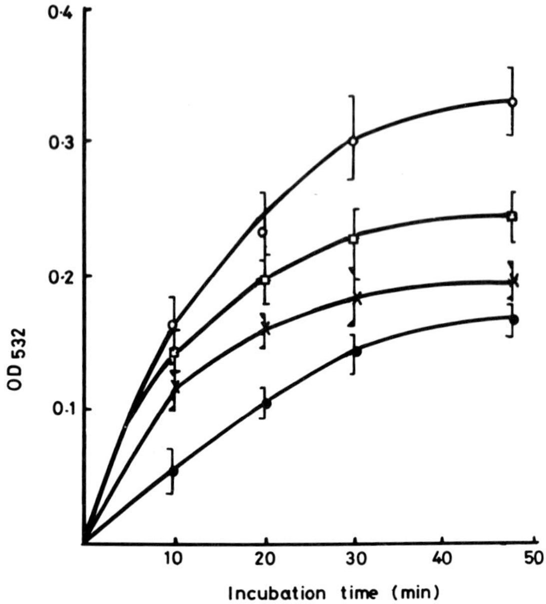

FIG. 8 Effect of the soluble fraction from neonatal rat liver on microsomal lipid peroxidation. The incubation systems contained 0.25 mg microsomal protein/ml and soluble protein concentrations of 0 (●), 6 (x), 9 (□), and 18 (O) mg/ml. The results are the mean ± SD of three experiments. From Player *et al.* (1978).

lipid peroxidation, it is doubtful whether this increase in the neonatal soluble fraction could influence the reaction here, where adequate levels of Fe^{+++} ions are included in the incubation medium. The possible protection afforded to the system by SOD has been suggested by Utsumi *et al.* (1977) where an increase in SOD activity concomitant with a decrease in liver peroxidation of rat liver homogenates incubated in buffer alone has been shown to occur with increase in age from birth.

The lipid peroxidation potential of subcellular fractions and antioxidant potential of the soluble fraction of transformed liver cells has also been examined. Primary hepatomas examined were induced by feeding 4-dimethyl-aminoazobenzene (DAB) and antigenically typed hepatomas D23, D30 and D192A were maintained by subcutaneous passage and harvested 2-3 weeks after implantation.

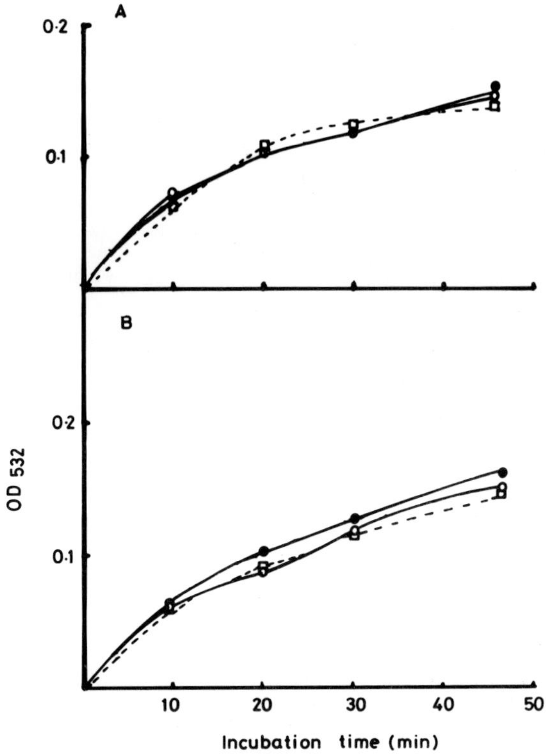

FIG. 9 Effect of the soluble fraction from (A) hepatoma D192A and (B) hepatoma D30 on microsomal lipid peroxidation. Each system contained 0.25 mg microsomal protein/ml and soluble protein concentrations of 0 (●), 4.2 (O) and 8.3 (□) mg/ml. The average values for two experiments in each case are shown. From Player *et al.* (1978).

None of the soluble fractions from any of the hepatomas had any effect on liver microsomal NADPH-dependent lipid peroxidation (Fig. 9). However, when the soluble fraction from liver bearing a primary hepatoma was prepared, after carefully removing and discarding hepatoma tissue, and added to a liver microsomal lipid peroxidation system, a lag in the initial rate of lipid peroxidation was observed (Fig. 10). A lag effect was also observed when supernatants were prepared from livers of rats 3-4 weeks after subcutaneous implantation of hepatomas D30 and D192A (Fig. 11). Thsi inhibitory effect was shown to be sensitive to heat treatment ($100^{o}C/5$ min). Increases in inhibition of lipid peroxidation have been reported to occur when animals have

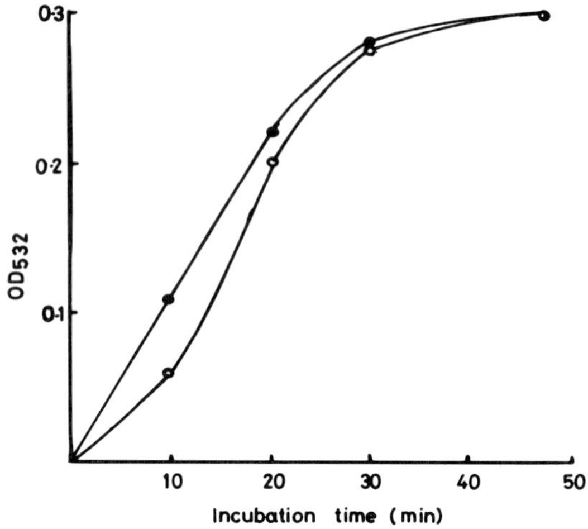

FIG. 10 Effect of the soluble fraction of rat liver from animals with primary hepatomas on microsomal lipid peroxidation. The incubation systems contained 0.20 mg microsomal protein/ml and soluble protein concentrations of 2.5 mg/ml. Hepatoma-bearing rats (O), control rats (●). The results show the mean values of two experiments performed in duplicate. From Player *et al.* (1978).

received a fat-free, high carbohydrate diet (Talcott *et al.*, 1976) or dosage with carbon tetrachloride (Kamataki *et al.*, 1977). In the former case, the inhibitor responsible is thought to be incorporated into the microsomal membrane. This is clearly not the case with the hepatoma-induced inhibitor.

With regard to enzymic microsomal lipid peroxidation exhibited by primary and passaged hepatomas activity was shown to be extremely low or absent altogether (Table 4). Lipid peroxidation was also found to be virtually absent when these fractions were incubated in the presence of ascorbic acid. The activity of NADPH-cytochrome c reductase was also measured (Table 5) and found to be present at low levels in each of the hepatomas investigated. However, it is unlikely that these reduced enzyme levels are entirely responsible for the lack of NADPH-dependent lipid peroxidation, due to the absence of peroxidation in the presence of ascorbic acid.

Fatty acid analysis of the hepatoma microsomal fractions demonstrated substantial levels of arachidonic acid in the phospholipid component (Table 6). While it may be seen that a different ratio of

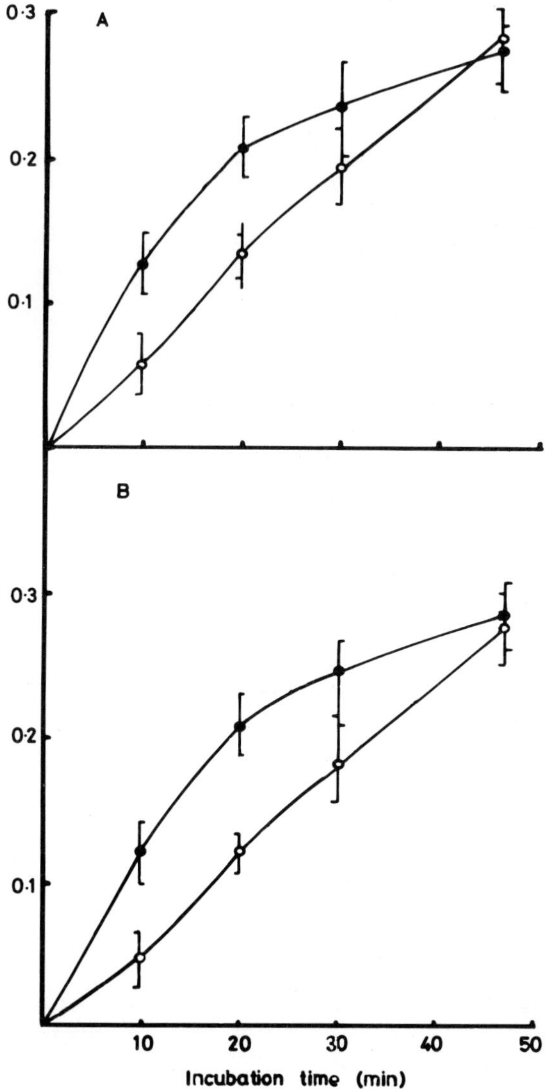

FIG. 11 Effect of the soluble fraction of rat livers from animals bearing (A) hepatoma D192A and (B) hepatoma D30 on microsomal lipid peroxidation. The incubation systems contained 0.25 mg microsomal protein/ml and soluble protein concentrations of 7.5 mg/ml. Hepatoma-bearing animals (O), control animals (●). The results are the mean ± SD of three experiments. From Player *et al.* (1978).

TABLE 4 Microsomal lipid peroxidation induced by the NADPH system or the ascorbic acid system

Tissue	MDA production (nmol/mg protein)[a]	
	NADPH	Ascorbic acid
Liver	33.0	35.8
D23	0.21	0.42
D30	0.58	1.04
D192A	0.00	0.42
D30 (heat treated)[b]		1.04
Liver from DAB treated rats	38.7	40.8
Primary DAB-induced hepatoma	3.3	5.4

[a]After incubation for 45 min. Means of two separate experiments each using a microsomal fraction from a different animal and performed in duplicate. [b]Microsomal fraction was heated at 80°C for 5 min in a water bath. See Fig. 1 for incubation conditions. From Player *et al.* (1979).

TABLE 5 Activity of NADPH-cytochrome c reductase in microsomal fractions from liver and hepatoma[a]

Tissue	NADPH-cytochrome c reductase activity (nmol/mg protein/min)
Liver	122.3 ± 10.9
D23	16.9 ± 5.8
D30	14.1 ± 6.4
D192A	9.0 ± 4.3

[a]Values are expressed as means ± SD for three separate experiments each using one animal.

phospholipid (PL) to neutral lipid (NL) was found in the hepatoma fractions in comparison with liver, it may be assumed that adequate substrate for detectable peroxidation is present. In fact, when hepatoma lipid was extracted from hepatoma microsomes it was shown to be capable of supporting ascorbic acid-induced lipid peroxidation (Table 7). Similarly when the phospholipid fractions were incubated in the same fashion there was no significant difference between malonaldehyde production/mg phospholipid from liver or hepatoma microsomal fractions.

TABLE 6 Analysis of microsomal lipid from liver and hepatomas[a]

	Fatty acid					PL[b] Content (%)
	16:0	18:0	18:1	18:2	20:4	
Liver						
NL[b]	36.1[c]	27.1	14.7	22.1	-[d]	90
PL[b]	29.2	26.7	16.2	10.2	17.7	
D23						
NL	26.6	36.4	27.4	9.6		79
PL	24.5	27.2	25.4	8.9	14.3	
D30						
NL	30.3	35.7	19.5	12.2	2.3	75
PL	22.9	32.9	19.0	6.9	18.3	
D192A						
NL	31.6	26.8	24.1	17.5	-	60
PL	22.5	22.3	20.4	10.4	24.7	

[a]Averages of two experiments each using one animal and performed in duplicate. [b]NL neutral lipid, PL phospholipid. [c]Peak area percentages. [d]1% of total fatty acids.

TABLE 7 Ascorbic acid-induced malonaldehyde production in extracted microsomal lipids from liver and hepatomas[a]

(i) Total extracted lipid	MDA production (OD_{532})
Liver (6)	0.473 ± 0.120
D30 (4)	0.481 ± 0.105
D192A (3)	0.460 ± 0.100

(ii) Phospholipid and neutral lipid	MDA production (OD_{532})	
	PL	NL
Liver (4)	0.545 ± 0.150	0.075 ± 0.025
D30 (4)	0.420 ± 0.100	0.055 ± 0.020
D192A (3)	0.380 ± 0.126	0.065 ± 0.030

[a]Results are expressed as mean ± SD and the numbers of samples from separate animals are shown in parentheses.

TABLE 8 Reconstituted NADPH-dependent lipid peroxidation system from NADPH cytochrome c reductase and liver microsomal lipid - effect of enzyme concentration

NADPH cytochrome c reductase[a] (mg protein)	Lipid peroxidation activity (nmol MDA/min/ml)
0	0.15
0.1	1.05
0.2	1.35
0.3	1.32
0.4	1.38
0.5	1.42

Incubation conditions were: 0.25 M Tris/HCl (pH 6.8), 0.25 M NaCl, 0.5 μmol lipid P liposomes, 2 mM ADP, 0.4 mM NADPH, 0.22 mM $Fe(No_3)_3$, 0.1 mM EDTA, NADPH cytochrome c reductase preparation. Incubate at 37°C for 15 min. [a]Activity of enzyme preparation was 3.5 μmol/min/mg.

TABLE 9 Effect of liver and hepatoma microsomal lipid fractions in the reconstituted NADPH-dependent lipid peroxidation system[a]

Substrate	Lipid peroxidation activity (nmol MDA/min/ml)
Liver total lipid	1.12
Liver phospholipid	0.05
Hepatoma total lipid	0.01
Hepatoma phospholipid	0.05
Liver total + liver phospholipid	2.30
Liver total + hepatoma phospholipid	2.35
Liver total + liver neutral lipid (2 mg)	1.12
Liver total + hepatoma neutral lipid (2 mg)	0.06

[a]Incubation conditions were as described in Table 8.

We have attempted to reconstitute the NADPH-dependent lipid peroxidation system using a partially purified NADPH-cytochrome c reductase with total, PL and NL fractions from hepatoma and liver microsomal fractions. The enzyme was prepared by trypsin digestion and Sephadex G100 chromatography according to the method of Omura and Takesue (1970) to give activities between 3 and 4 μmoles/min/mg protein. Lipids were sonicated in 0.25 M Tris/HCl (pH 6.8), 0.25 M NaCl and equilibrated at 37°C prior to enzyme addition to start the reaction. Table 8 describes the conditions employed for the incubation, where the effect of enzyme concentration was examined in combination with total liver microsomal lipid. Table 9 shows the rate of lipid peroxidation in the presence of various lipid fractions from liver and hepatoma microsomes.

The results demonstrate firstly the necessity for the total lipid component rather than just the PL fraction for maximum lipid peroxidation under the conditions imposed. This may indicate the requirement for the NL for either binding the enzyme or in binding the cofactors necessary for activity. Also shown is that purified hepatoma PL will act as a substrate equal in efficiency to liver PL, but that the total hepatoma microsomal lipid fraction results in very little lipid peroxidation activity. When liver or hepatoma PL was added to the total liver lipid and sonicated together prior to the addition of the enzyme, both resulted in increased activity, acting as additional substrate for the reaction and still permitting interaction of the enzyme or cofactors with the lipid. When NL prepared from the liver microsomal lipid was added back to the total liver lipid prior to sonication, there was no effect on the rate of peroxidation whereas the addition of NL prepared from hepatoma microsomal lipid caused a 50% reduction in rate, clearly demonstrating an inhibitory function of this fraction.

SUMMARY

In summary, this paper describes the variation in lipid peroxidation activity and antioxidant potential in subcellular fractions from rat liver over the lifespan of the animal as well as mature liver cells which have been induced to a state of increased mitotic activity and from transformed liver cells. Microsomal NADPH-dependent lipid peroxidation activity has been shown to increase with aging of the animal and is reduced in cells exhibiting increased mitotic activity and growth, and some possible explanations have been discussed. The antioxidant/pro-oxidant capacity of the soluble fraction appears to change from birth to maturity but appears to have no significant effect in the case of the hepatoma soluble fractions. However, an inhibitory factor appears to be produced in the liver soluble fraction as a result of the animal bearing either a primary or passaged hepatoma.

REFERENCES

Barber, A.A. and Wilbur, K.M. (1959). *Radiat. Res.* 10, 167-175.
Barrett, M.C. and Horton, A.A. (1976). *Biochem. Soc. Trans.* 4, 64-66.
Goldenberg, H., Huttinger, M., Bock, P. and Kramar, R. (1975). *Histochemistry* 44, 47-56.
Grinna, L.S. (1977). *Mech. Ageing Dev.* 6, 197-205.
Higgins, G.M. and Anderson, R.M. (1931). *Arch. Pathol.* 12, 186-202.
Hochstein, P. and Ernster, L. (1963). *Biochem. Biophys. Res. Commun.* 12, 388-394.
Hrycay, E.G. and O'Brien, P.J. (1973). *Arch. Biochem. Biophys.* 157, 7-22.
Hunter, F.E., Gebicki, J.M., Hoffsten, P.E., Weinstein, J. and Scott, A. (1963). *J. Biol. Chem.* 238, 828-835.
Kamataki, T., Sugita, O., Kitada, M., Naminohara, S. and Kitagawa, H. (1977). *Res. Comm. Chem. Pathol. Pharmacol.* 17, 205-273.
Koster, J.F. and Slee, R.G. (1980). *Biochim. Biophys. Acta* 620, 489-499.
Niehaus, W.G. and Samuelson, B. (1968). *Eur. J. Biochem.* 6, 126-130.
O'Connor, P.J. (1971). *Biochim. Biophys. Acta* 238, 186-189.
Omura, T. and Takesue, S. (1970). *J. Biochem. (Tokyo)* 67, 249-257.
Pfeifer, P.M. and McCay, P.B. (1972). *J. Biol. Chem.* 247, 6763-6769.
Player, T.J. and Horton, A.A. (1978). *FEBS Lett.* 89, 103-106.
Player, T.J., Mills, D.J. and Horton, A.A. (1977). *Biochem. Biophys. Res. Commun.* 78, 1397-1402.
Player, T.J., Mills, D.J. and Horton, A.A. (1978). *FEBS Lett.* 89, 103-106.
Player, T.J., Mills, D.J. and Horton, A.A. (1979). *Br. J. Cancer* 39, 773-778.
Sharma, O.P. (1977). *Biochem. Biophys. Res. Commun.* 78, 469-475.
Takeshige, K., Takajanagi, R. and Minakami, S. (1980). *Biochem. J.* 192, 861-866.
Talcott, R.E., Denk, H., Eckerstorfer, R. and Schenkman, J.B. (1976). *Chem. Biol. Interact.* 12, 355-361.
Utsumi, K., Yoshioka, T., Yamanaka, N. and Nakuzawa, T. (1977). *FEBS Lett.* 79, 1-3.
Widmann, J. and Fahimi, H.D. (1975). *Am. J. Pathol.* 80, 349-366.
Wolfson, N., Wilbur, K.M. and Bernheim, F. (1956). *Exp. Cell Res.* 10, 556-558.

DISCUSSION

Slater: Perhaps I could start with just a general comment. We have been working along similar lines to those that you initiated some years ago, and we are also now very interested in neutral lipid fractions as shown in your last slide. We have just started a collaboration with Dr Keith Ingold in Ottawa, basically to look in particular for α-tocopherol and its related products in the neutral lipid fraction of tumour fractions obtained from animals and human samples. Have you specifically looked at such materials in your studies?

Player: We haven't done much in actually investigating the various anti-oxidant substances involved, or pro-oxidant substances involved in the soluble fractions due to the resources we had available. It would require a considerable amount of time, but these are observations with very few explanations at the moment.

Dianzani: Several years ago in Torino, Professor Ugazio saw that the supernatant from Yoshida hepatoma was strongly inhibitory on lipid peroxidation in normal liver. We thought at that time that anti-oxidant substances, or some other type of inhibitor, were present in the supernatant fractions of these tumours. When repeating the experiments last year we were surprised to see that if we used different amounts of supernatant from normal liver we got different amounts of malonaldehyde production according to the different amount of added protein. Dilution increased the amount of TBA-reacting substance produced. Just the same happened if we used fresh serum or commercial beef albumin. At this point we tried to add the protein at the end of the incubation time and we were surprised to see that the simple addition of the proteins at the end of the incubation time decreased strongly the production of colour. So we concluded that the added protein can trap some malonaldehyde so falsifying the thiobarbituric test. Of course, by comparing the results obtained with the supernatant of tumours with those obtained from normal liver we are still convinced that some inhibitor is present in the supernatant of tumours, but I wonder if you have tried to add more protein at the end of the incubation time to see if your dilution experiments can be explained in this way.

Player: But, don't you think that in the mature liver when you increase the protein you in fact increase the anti-oxidant potential, whereas in the neonatal one when you increase the protein content it goes the other way, and you can vary the protein concentration of the tumour and you get no effect? Unless it is one specific protein, of course.

Dianzani: Yes, but did you try to add the protein at the end of the incubation?

Player: No.

Poli: With regard to the ADP/iron stimulated lipid peroxidation in mitochondria from animals of different age, did you check also the aldehyde dehydrogenase activity in mitochondria from the different aged animals?

Player: I believe this work has been done by Dr A. Horton at the University of Birmingham.

Ts'o: In your study of the relationship between anti-oxidant states or potentials and aging, what is the relationship between enzyme systems in defence of oxygen radicals, like superoxide dismutase and aging? Do you know any of that?

Player: Yes, we have measured a difference in superoxide dismutase in the newborn animal where it is about 10 units per milligram of protein up to mature levels where it reaches about 22 units per milligram.

Ts'o: Yes, but what about aging, really old animals?

Player: Really old? No.

Magee: I think there is a theory of aging, isn't there, that relates increased lipid peroxidation to age or aging? Do you want to comment on that?

Player: In terms of lipofuscion accumulation are you talking about? That is the whole correlation between lipid peroxidation and aging, that oxidising lipids react with denatured proteins to produce insoluble compounds, one of which is lipofuscion. They accumulate in various organs in the body such as the hair and the skin, the latter probably being the most noticeable. That is the original connection between lipid peroxidation and aging.

Magee: Yes, but what is the standing of that view now? Is it thought to be supportable? Is it a good idea?

Player: I think it's not disproved.

Slater: There is the possibility of peroxidation products cross-linking proteins; we know from Herman Esterbauer's work that this certainly occurs.

Stier: Just a quick question about the arachidonic content which didn't change during regeneration. I remember that Comporti and Benedetti (Benedetti *et al.*, 1976) found that the lipid peroxidation takes place first in the phosphatidylethanolamine fraction. Do you know whether during regeneration the arachidonic acid is primarily bound to the phosphatidylcholines or phosphatidylethanolamines?

Player: No, I haven't done that. I haven't done a TLC analysis of the phosphatides, just looking at the fatty acids from the phospholipid fraction. But that is a very good point.

Mason: This question has a possible one word answer. Are you willing to speculate on the initiating species in microsomal lipid peroxidation?

Player: There are so many theories that we should discuss that at length afterwards; so the answer is no!

REFERENCE to Discussion

Benedetti, A., Canini, A., Ferrali, M. and Comporti, M. (1976). *Panminerv. Med.* 18, 433.

Effects of Scavengers and Inhibitors on Lipid Peroxidation in Rat Liver Microsomes

K.H. CHEESEMAN

INTRODUCTION

This study is part of a continuing investigation into carbon tetrachloride (CCl_4)-induced lipid peroxidation and liver injury begun by Slater and co-workers approximately 15 years ago (for reviews see Slater, 1972, 1978, and this Symposium). During that time many others have contributed greatly to the study of this topic, which is an important model system of chemical carcinogenesis and tissue injury (for reviews see Plaa and Witschi, 1976; Recknagel and Glende, 1973; Reynolds and Moslen, 1980; Slater, 1972, 1978).

Lipid peroxidation is considered to be an important feature in the cellular injury brought about by chemical agents such CCl_4, paraquat and ozone, and by such physical phenomena as ionising radiation (see Slater, 1979a; Plaa and Witschi, 1976). In these instances lipid peroxidation is thought to be a consequence of the production of highly reactive free radicals that act as initiators of the peroxidative chain reaction. The targets of this attack are the polyunsaturated fatty acids of cell membranes such as the plasma membrane and endoplasmic reticulum.

The main features of lipid peroxidation are presented below where the initiating radical ($R^\bullet$) abstracts a hydrogen from a polyunsaturated fatty acid (PUFAH) to form the fatty acid radical ($PUFA^\bullet$). Reaction with oxygen yields the corresponding peroxy radical ($PUFAOO^\bullet$) and chain propagation ensues, leading ultimately to degradation of the lipid to a wide range of products including aldehydes and gases such as ethane and pentane.

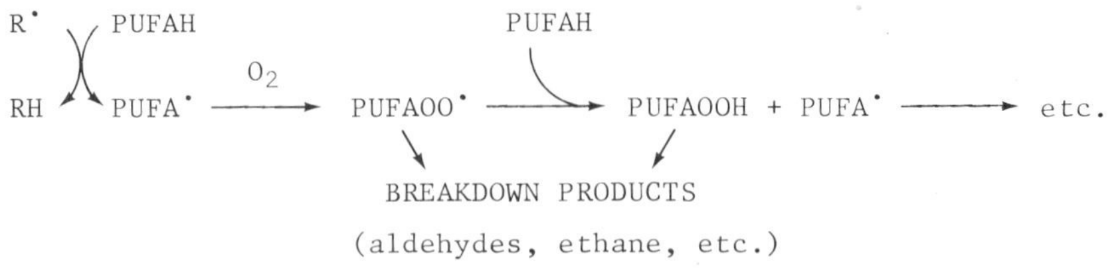

The amount of one of the aldehydic products, malonaldehyde (MAA), is estimated by the thiobarbituric acid (TBA) test which is probably the most commonly used assay method for *in vitro* lipid peroxidation. This method, and the process of lipid peroxidation in general, have been extensively reviewed (for example see Slater, 1972; Dianzani and Ugazio, 1978).

In biological membranes the presence of enzymes and of heme and non-heme iron increases the complexicity of the peroxidation process. In this field of study the most widely investigated biological membrane is the endoplasmic reticulum, fragments of which (microsomes) are isolated for experiments *in vitro*. Liver microsomes contain the drug metabolising system, an electron transport chain consisting of a flavoprotein (P_{450} reductase, also known as NADPH-cytochrome c reductase) that transports electrons from NADPH to cytochrome P_{450}. Xenobiotics are detoxified by this system (see Parke, 1968). A non-heme iron protein may also be present (Salerno and Ingledew, 1975). This system, as a whole and as individual components, is implicated in many types of lipid peroxidation.

The flavoprotein (P_{450} reductase) may be responsible for producing reactive oxygen species such as the hydroxyl radical, OH• (Lai *et al.*, 1979) and the superoxide radical, $O_2^{\bullet -}$ (Aust *et al.*, 1972). In the much-studied peroxidation system dependent on NADPH and ADP/iron (Hochstein and Ernster, 1963) the reductase plays a key role in keeping the catalytic ADP-Fe^{2+} complex in the reduced state. The actual initiator in this system has been suggested to be the OH• radical (Fong *et al.*, 1973) but other workers consider the initiator to be the ADP-perferryl ion (ADP-Fe^{++}-O_2) with singlet oxygen ($^1O_2$) important in the propagation stages (Svingen *et al.*, 1978).

Cytochrome P_{450} may be important in catalysing the breakdown of lipid peroxides (Hrycay and O'Brien, 1971) to a variety of reactive products which may contribute to chain propagation. Among these may be peroxy and alkoxy radicals (Svingen *et al.*, 1979), $OH^{\cdot}$ radicals (O'Brien and Hawco, 1978) and singlet oxygen (Hawco *et al.*, 1977; Svingen *et al.*, 1979). This property of cytochrome P_{450} is utilised in the peroxidation of microsomes induced by cumene hydroperoxide, CU-OOH (O'Brien and Rahimtula, 1975), a system used in this study with slight modification. The precise mechanism involved is unclear. Theoretical considerations have ruled out the participation of $^{1}O_2$ (Hawco *et al.*, 1977) and cumene hydroperoxide apparently produces only a very low concentration of $OH^{\cdot}$ radicals (O'Brien and Hawco, 1978). Spin trap studies have suggested the production of alkoxy and methyl radicals (Griffin and Ting, 1978). Presumably, peroxy radicals would also be produced, by the reaction:

$$\text{CU-OOH} + P_{450}(Fe^{3+}) \longrightarrow \text{CU-OO}^{\cdot} + H^{+} + P_{450}(Fe^{2+}).$$

The P_{450} system as a whole can produce damaging free radicals as a result of misguided metabolism, such that a foreign compound, rather than being detoxified, is converted to a reactive intermediate (see Slater, 1979a). An example of a compound activated in this way is CCl_4 and it is the study of microsomal CCl_4 metabolism and the consequent lipid peroxidation which forms the core of this investigation.

When CCl_4 is added to an NADPH-fortified microsomal suspension it is metabolised to the trichloromethyl radical ($CCl_3^{\cdot}$) as a result of dissociative electron capture:

$$CCl_4 + e^{-} \longrightarrow (CCl_4^{\cdot -}) \longrightarrow CCl_3^{\cdot} + Cl^{-}$$

This radical reacts with lipid and protein components of the microsomal membrane and binds irreversibly (covalently). Lipid peroxidation may be initiated by this radical (by hydrogen abstraction) or more probably, by the more reactive species $CCl_3OO^{\cdot}$ which forms extremely rapidly in aerobic solutions (Slater, 1981). The many years of research have not provided convincing evidence of the precise locus and mechanism of CCl_4 activation; both the flavoprotein and cytochrome P_{450} are possible sites of $CCl_3^{\cdot}$ production (Glende, 1972; Slater and Sawyer, 1971b).

When CCl_4 is added to a suspension of liver microsomes a type I difference spectrum is obtained (McLean, 1967) indicative of a substrate-type interaction with cytochrome P_{450}. This, together with the fundamental dogma of xenobiotic metabolism, suggests cytochrome P_{450} as the site of activation. However, certain results with specific inhibitors of the microsomal electron transport chain apparently conflict with this hypothesis (Slater and Sawyer, 1971b). This has led to the suggestion that more than one site of activation of CCl_4 exists along the electron transport chain (see Slater *et al.*, 1980; and Slater, in this Symposium). This work with inhibitors and radical scavengers has been extended and a selection of the results obtained are presented here. The earlier studies used lipid peroxidation as the index of CCl_4 metabolism; here, this parameter is again measured but it is supplemented by the measurement of the covalent binding of radio-labelled metabolites of CCl_4 to microsomal protein. This technique utilises[^{14}C]CCl_4 and enables covalent binding and lipid peroxidation to be measured simultaneously. The binding of [^{14}C]CCl_4 to microsomal components is probably a better index of $CCl_3^{\bullet}$ production than is lipid peroxidation (as measured by malonaldehyde production) and there are some interesting differences between the results obtained using the two methods. For comparison, the effects of these various scavengers and inhibitors on the metabolism of aminopyrene, a classical type I substrate of cytochrome P_{450}, were also measured. Moreover, cumene hydroperoxide-mediated lipid peroxidation system, which is P_{450} dependent, provided further information. The comparison of these four processes (CCl_4-lipid peroxidation; CCl_4-covalent binding; aminopyrene demethylase; cumene hydroperoxide-lipid peroxidation) is of interest with regard to the elucidation of the locus of CCl_4 activation. It also sheds light upon the effects of "specific" inhibitors and scavengers on microsomal lipid peroxidation and on the enzymes of the drug metabolising system.

METHODS

Preparation of Microsomes

The rats used were albino females (Charles River CD strain) of 200-300 g body weight. They were fasted overnight before preparation of microsomes. Liver microsomes were prepared as described by Slater and Sawyer (1971a). Pellets were stored at -20°C for up to 10 d before use when they were resuspended in 0.15 M KCl such that 1 ml was equivalent to 1 g wet weight of original liver.

Metabolism of Carbon Tetrachloride

Microsomes were incubated aerobically with an NADPH-generating stock solution (Slater and Sawyer, 1971a) at 37°C in 10 ml stoppered glass tubes, with shaking, in the dark. Stock solutions (2.2 ml) were mixed with 0.3 ml microsome suspension (equivalent to about 6 mg protein) and 0.5 ml of an aqueous solution of the agent under study. Carbon tetrachloride was added to appropriate tubes as 10 μl of a CCl :DMSO mixture (1:4, v/v). Controls without CCl_4 were also incubated. Where covalent binding was to be measured $[^{14}C]CCl_4$ was used such that each tube received approximately 0.24 μCi. After incubation for 15 min the reaction was stopped by the addition of 6.0 ml trichloracetic acid (10%, w/v) and malonaldehyde determined in the protein-free supernatant by the thiobarbituric acid (TBA) reaction (Slater and Sawyer, 1971a). CCl_4-induced peroxidation was estimated by subtracting control values. The precipitate was extracted to remove lipid, RNA and unbound $[^{14}C]CCl_4$ by the method of Rao and Recknagel (1969). The dry protein was weighed and dissolved in Soluene (Packard Instrument Ltd.) and Dimilume scintillation fluid (Packard Instrument Ltd.) was added. Radio-activity was measured in a Packard 2425 scintillation counter. Efficiency correction was made using sample channels ratio.

Metabolism of Aminopyrene

Aminopyrene demethylase activity was estimated using a modification of the method of Orrenius (1965) as described by Slater and Sawyer (1971b). Incubations were for 10 min at 37°C, with shaking, in the dark.

Cumene Hydroperoxide-Mediated Lipid Peroxidation

Microsomes (approx. 2 mg protein) were incubated with 150 nmoles cumene hydroperoxide, 24 μmoles tris buffer (pH 7.4) and 73 μmoles KCl in a total volume of 1.5 ml; incubations were for 15 min at 37°C with shaking. At the end of the incubation 3 ml trichloracetic acid (10% w/v) was added and malonaldehyde estimated as above; control values were subtracted.

RESULTS AND DISCUSSION

Lipid-soluble thiol-blocking reagents can block drug metabolism by penetrating into the membrane of the endoplasmic reticulum and impeding electron flow from the flavoprotein (P_{450} reductase) to cytochrome P_{450} (Orrenius, 1965; Franklin and Estabrook, 1971). Thus, the requirement for electron flow to P_{450} in any of the four systems under study can be assessed by the use of p-chloromercuribenzoate (p-CMB). This reagent was studied at low concentrations (up to 200 μM) so as to maintain this site-specific effect and not to convert cytochrome P_{450} to its denatured form, P_{420}. The results obtained with p-CMB are shown in Fig. 1. As expected aminopyrene demethylase

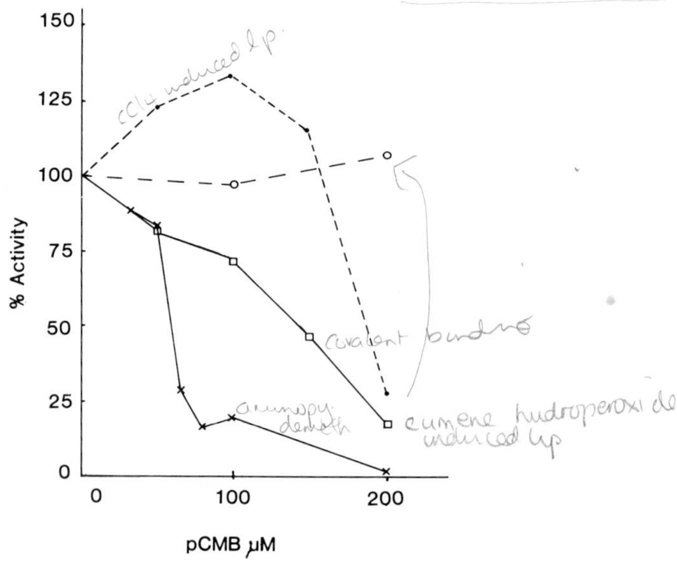

FIG. 1 The effect of p-CMB on CCl_4-induced lipid peroxidation (•------•), cumene hydroperoxide-induced lipid peroxidation (○----○), covalent binding of $[^{14}C]CCl_4$ to protein (□——□) and aminopyrene demethylation (×——×).

is strongly inhibited whereas CU-OOH-induced lipid peroxidation, which requires no NADPH, is unaffected. The covalent binding of [^{14}C]CCl_4 is strongly inhibited, but the CCl_4-dependent lipid peroxidation shows a completely different pattern of response. With concentrations of p-CMB up to 100 μM malonaldehyde production is actually increased but at higher concentrations a crossover-effect occurs and the peroxidation is strongly inhibited. The results in the CCl_4 systems are thus very interesting in that [^{14}C]CCl_4 binding (presumed to be the better indication of CCl_4 activation) qualitatively parallels aminopyrene metabolism whereas CCl_4-dependent lipid peroxidation does not. This difference in response between the two CCl_4 systems is also striking when the effects of SKF 525A (Table 1) are considered, although in this instance [^{14}C]CCl_4 binding does not parallel aminopyrene demethylation. SKF 525A inhibits microsomal drug metabolism by blocking cytochrome P_{450} (for a review, see Anders, 1973) and so aminopyrene demethylase is very strongly inhibited. CU-OOH-induced microsomal peroxidation is also P_{450}-dependent and thus SKF 525A

TABLE 1 The effects of inhibitors of P_{450} function upon microsomal functions

		Function as % change from control			
Agent	Conc. (mM)	CCl_4 lipid peroxidation	[^{14}C]CCl_4 covalent binding	Aminopyrene demethylase	CU-OOH lipid peroxidation
SKF 525A	0.02	-	-	-54	-
	0.05	-17	+ 5	-	-
	0.10	-16	+20	-	-50
	0.20	-26	+47	-	-
	0.25	-	-	-70	-76
	0.50	-62	+95	-	-
Metyrapone	0.5	+ 9	-53	-71	-28
	1.0	+ 5	-67	-72	-
Imidazole	1.0	+ 5	+21	-41	- 8
Pyrazole	5.0	- 5	+ 3	-65	+ 6
Nicotinamide	20.0	+73	-66	-24	+ 3

inhibits malonaldehyde production (Table 1) and also oxygen uptake (O'Brien and Rahimtula, 1975) from that reaction. However, CCl_4-induced lipid peroxidation is only weakly inhibited and the covalent binding of $[^{14}C]CCl_4$ is actually stimulated; neither index of CCl_4 activation, therefore, parallels P_{450}-dependent drug metabolism. It should be noted that Sipes *et al.* (1977), in a similar system, found no effect of SKF 525A on the covalent binding of $[^{14}C]CCl_4$; they did report, however, a stimulation of the covalent binding of $[^{14}C]CBrCl_3$, a related compound. The conflicting results may be due to the differences in the strain of rat used and the use of phenobarbital induction by Sipes *et al.* (1977). Moreover, when using relatively high concentrations of SKF 525A the possibility that it is acting through mechanisms other than that for which it was used, must be considered. This compound does possess surface-active properties (Lee *et al.*, 1968) and in the lipid peroxidation systems the weak antioxidant property of SKF 525A (Miles *et al.*, 1980) may also be a pertinent factor.

SKF 525A is a type I inhibitor of cytochrome P_{450} reactions; several type II inhibitors were also tested. These were metyrapone, imidazole, pyrazole and nicotinamide (Table 1). As expected, all of these inhibited aminopyrene demethylase, to varying degrees. Surprisingly, CU-OOH-induced peroxidation was relatively insensitive to these compounds. Metyrapone and imidazole were less inhibitory to CU-OOH-induced lipid peroxidation than they have been reported as being to CU-OOH-induced oxygen uptake (O'Brien and Rahimtula, 1975). With the exception of the stimulation produced by a high concentration of nicotinamide, CCl_4-induced lipid peroxidation was also rather insensitive to these compounds. CCl_4-induced peroxidation and covalent binding were again noticeably different in their response to these agents. Only metyrapone was capable of strongly inhibiting the covalent binding of $[^{14}C]CCl_4$. Therefore, with regard to inhibitors of P_{450} reactions, CCl_4 activation and aminopyrene metabolism do not correlate well.

An interaction with P_{450} may well be involved in the effects of the metal-chelating agents 1,10-phenanthroline and 2,2'-bipyridine on CCl_4 metabolism (Table 2). Both phenanthroline and bipyridine

TABLE 2 The effects of metal chelating agents upon microsomal functions

Agent	Conc. (mM)	Function as % change from control: CCl_4 lipid peroxidation	Function as % change from control: $[^{14}C]CCl_4$ covalent binding
1,10-phenanthroline	2.2	+107	+303
	1.0	+ 89	+224
	0.1	+ 25	+ 76
2,2'-bipyridine	5.0	+ 5	+ 72
	1.0	- 23	+ 18
	0.5	- 27	+ 11

enhanced the covalent binding of $[^{14}C]CCl_4$ and phenanthroline also stimulated CCl_4-dependent malonaldehyde production. The quantitative relationship between covalent binding and lipid peroxidation suggests that the perceived effect on lipid peroxidation may represent a balance between increased production of initiating radical and decreased propagation of peroxidation due to iron chelation. These two structurally related compounds were originally tested because of their iron-chelating ability but in microsomal systems they also have other significant properties. Both compounds are known to enhance the metabolism of type II drugs by cytochrome P_{450} (Anders, 1973; Powis *et al.*, 1977). However, the metabolism of type I compounds is normally inhibited by these compounds and so the apparent enhancement of metabolism of CCl_4, itself a type I compound, is especially surprising.

Differences in the CCl_4 systems and the demethylase and CU-OOH systems are again apparent when their responses to menadione are considered (Table 3).

Menadione (menapthone, vitamin K_3) can uncouple the microsomal electron transport chain, probably by withdrawing electrons from the flavoprotein. It inhibits drug metabolism and lipid peroxidation induced by NADPH and by ascorbate (Wills, 1972). Wills concluded that, especially in view of its inhibitory properties in the ascorbate-dependent system, menadione had an antioxidant property which was independent of its ability to stimulate NADPH oxidation. Wills studied the inhibitory properties of menadione on aminopyrene

TABLE 3 The effects of menadione upon microsomal functions

Conc. (μM)	% inhibition of function			
	CCl_4 lipid peroxidation	$[^{14}C]CCl_4$ covalent binding	Aminopyrene demethylase	CU-OOH lipid peroxidation
0.2	42	0	–	0
0.5	77	–	–	–
1.0	85	13	–	0
4.0	94	19	0	–
10.0	100	–	–	–
50.0	100	–	–	18
100.0	100	86	85	18

demethylation over a range of 10-100 μM, reporting 50% inhibition at around 20 μM; our results are consistent with this. However, at much lower concentrations, menadione has a profound effect on CCl_4-induced lipid peroxidation; 50% inhibition is achieved with less than 0.5 μM menadione. At these sub-micromolar levels, the covalent binding of $[^{14}C]CCl_4$ indicative of CCl_4 activation, is completely unimpaired. Covalent binding, like aminopyrene demethylation, is only inhibited when menadione concentrations are increased to levels which, presumably, completely inhibit electron flow to cytochrome P_{450}. Moreover, lipid peroxidation induced by CU-OOH is practically immune to the antioxidant properties of menadione. Considered together, these data suggest that menadione inhibits CCl_4-dependent lipid peroxidation by scavenging a radical species not involved in covalent binding of $[^{14}C]CCl_4$ or in CU-OOH-dependent lipid peroxidation; the trichloromethylperoxy radical, $CCl_3OO^{\bullet}$, therefore seems a candidate. However, to scavenge $CCl_3OO^{\bullet}$, menadione needs to be reduced. Since the reduced form of menadione reacts rapidly with oxygen (to form $O_2^{\bullet -}$) (Talcott *et al.*, 1979), this hypothesis requires menadione to be reduced by the flavoprotein and to react with $CCl_3OO^{\bullet}$ more rapidly than with O_2. No convincing explanation for the effects of menadione in the CCl_4 activation systems can be made at this time.

Lipid peroxidation can be inhibited by scavengers which react with initiating and propagating radicals and yield harmless products (see Slater, 1972, 1978). Because of their rates of reaction many scavengers are generally considered as relatively "specific" for certain radicals. Consequently, many workers have utilised "selective" scavengers in lipid peroxidation systems in order to identify the radical species involved. The interpretation of results obtained with "selective" scavengers is, however, fraught with difficulties, especially in biological systems. These difficulties are illustrated in this study where scavengers putatively specific for the $OH^{\bullet}$ radical were tested. The three $OH^{\bullet}$ scavengers tested were mannitol, *t*-butanol and thiourea; all have very high rate constants for reaction with the $OH^{\bullet}$ radical. Urea was also included; it has a relatively low rate constant for reaction with $OH^{\bullet}$ and serves as a control for thiourea. Mannitol and *t*-butanol, at concentrations up to 50 mM had no significant effects in any of the four systems studied. The CU-OOH dependent lipid peroxidation system is inhibited by high concentrations of thiourea (high concentrations are required to compete with bio-molecules for $OH^{\bullet}$ radicals). However, since urea was only slightly less inhibitory and as the breakdown of CU-OOH is postulated not to produce $OH^{\bullet}$ radicals (O'Brien and Hawco, 1978), thiourea may be acting in a non-selective manner. Thiourea was strongly inhibitory in the CCl_4-dependent peroxidation system and less so in the covalent binding system. It may, therefore, scavenge peroxy radicals of lipids and/or CCl_4. Incidentally, the use of high concentrations of urea illustrated again the difference between the CCl_4 systems of peroxidation and covalent binding. The mechanism of action of urea in inhibiting CCl_4-dependent peroxidation is unclear. Urea is an unlikely radical scavenger and the concentrations used here are not expected to affect cytochrome P_{450} significantly (Franklin, 1972).

Three radical scavengers which strongly inhibit the CCl_4-dependent peroxidation of microsomes are promethazine, propyl gallate and catechin (Slater, 1968, 1979b; Slater and Sawyer, 1971c). These compounds, which are not generally considered to be "selective", are potent inhibitors at micromolar concentrations (Table 4) and also inhibit CCl_4-induced peroxidation of isolated rat hepatocytes (Poli *et al.*, 1978). They are, though, much less effective in inhibiting the covalent binding of $[^{14}C]CCl_4$, suggesting that they do not scavenge $CCl_3^{\bullet}$ (Table 4; also see Cheeseman, 1981). In the case of

TABLE 4 The effects of free radical scavengers upon microsomal function

Agent	Conc. (mM)	% inhibition of function		
		CU-OOH lipid peroxidation	CCl_4 lipid peroxidation	$[^{14}C]CCl_4$ covalent binding
Thiourea	8	–	75	26
	10	20	–	–
	20	39	–	–
Urea	20	27	–	–
	50	49	34	4
	100	51	63	11
Catechin	0.02	27	51	6
	0.05	41	70	6
Promethazine	0.001	0	62	17
	0.01	15	87	16
	0.1	76	97	34
Propyl gallate	0.01	20	83	13
	0.02	41	87	12
	0.05	70	90	26

promethazine, pulse radiolysis studies have verified that this scavenger reacts much less rapidly with $CCl_3^{\cdot}$ than with $CCl_3OO^{\cdot}$ (Packer *et al.*, 1978). In the CU-OOH-mediated peroxidation system the three scavengers are inhibitory, but less so than in the CCl_4-mediated peroxidation system. At the higher concentrations used an inhibition of the electron transport chain may occur, as evidenced by inhibition of aminopyrene demethylase (see Slater, 1981). In summary, the strong inhibition of CCl_4-induced lipid peroxidation seen with these three radical scavengers at low micromolar concentrations is probably due to a scavenging of the $CCl_3OO^{\cdot}$ radical as well as certain propagating radicals common to the CCl_4 and CU-OOH systems.

CONCLUSION

From the results above, it can be seen that, by the use of certain inhibitors and free radical scavengers, the processes of CCl_4-induced lipid peroxidation and the covalent binding of radical products of $[^{14}C]CCl_4$ can be dissociated. These data, together with fundamental data from pulse radiolysis studies, have led to the conclusion that whilst the $CCl_3^{\cdot}$ radical is the species which preferentially produces covalent binding, it is the $CCl_3OO^{\cdot}$ radical which preferentially initiates lipid peroxidation (see Slater, 1981). Of course, $CCl_3^{\cdot}$ is only "unreactive" in comparison to $CCl_3OO^{\cdot}$ and is certainly capable of initiating lipid peroxidation itself. Moreover, $CCl_3OO^{\cdot}$ may have a small role in covalent binding, not directly (as it would yield unstable products) but via the formation of phosgene. This unstable compound would break down and bind, as it does to cysteine (to form oxothiazolidine carboxylic acid) in the method used for its entrapment (Shah *et al.*, 1979).

The results above also stress the apparent differences between on the one hand both models of CCl_4 metabolism (peroxidation and covalent binding) and on the other hand classical, P_{450}-dependent drug metabolism as exemplified by aminopyrene demethylation. A better correlation exists between aminopyrene metabolism and $[^{14}C]CCl_4$ binding than with aminopyrene metabolism and CCl_4-induced peroxidation. If covalent binding is assumed to be the better model of CCl_4 activation, then CCl_4 metabolism may be said not to be totally dissimilar to classical drug metabolism. However, the differences apparent between these processes require explanation. Possibly the reductive nature of CCl_4 metabolism is part of the explanation (aminopyrene metabolism is oxidative in nature) but it is clear that these data are not inconsistent with a mechanism of CCl_4 activation involving more than one site.

REFERENCES

Anders, M.W. (1973). *Fortschr. Arzneimittelforsch.* 17, 11-32.

Aust, S.D., Roerig, D.L. and Pederson, T.C. (1972). *Biochem. Biophys. Res. Commun.* 47, 1133-1137.

Cheeseman, K.H. (1981). *In* "Recent Advances in Lipid Peroxidation and Tissue Injury" (Eds. T.F. Slater and A. Garner) Brunel Biochemistry Department, London.

Dianzani, M.U. and Ugazio, G. (1978). *In* "Biochemical Mechanisms of Liver Injury" (Ed. T.F. Slater), pp.669-708, Academic Press, London.

Fong, K.L., McCay, P.B., Poyer, J.L., Keele, B.B. and Misra, H. (1973). *J. Biol. Chem.* 248, 7792-7797.

Franklin, M.R. (1972). *Mol. Pharmacol.* 8, 711-721

Franklin, M.R. and Estabrook, R.W. (1971). *Arch. Biochem. Biophys.* 143, 318-329.

Glende, E.A. (1972). *Biochem. Pharmacol.* 21, 1697-1702.
Griffin, B.W. and Ting, P.L. (1978). *FEBS Lett.* 89, 196-200.
Hawco, F.J., O'Brien, C.J. and O'Brien, P.J. (1977). *Biochem. Biophys. Res. Commun.* 76, 354-361.
Hochstein, P. and Ernster, L. (1963). *Biochem. Biophys. Res. Commun.* 12, 388-394.
Hrycay, E.-G. and O'Brien, P.J. (1971). *Arch. Biochem. Biophys.* 147, 14-27.
Lai, C.-S., Grover, T.A. and Piette, L.H. (1979). *Arch. Biochem. Biophys.* 193, 373-378.
Lee, I.P., Yamamura, H.I. and Dixon, R.L. (1968). *Biochem. Pharmacol.* 17, 1671-1681.
McLean, A.E.M. (1967). *Biochem. Pharmacol.* 16, 2030-2033.
Miles, P.R., Wright, J.R., Bowman, L. and Colby, H.D. (1980). *Biochem. Pharmacol.* 29, 565-570.
O'Brien, P.J. and Hawco, F.J. (1978). *Biochem. Soc. Trans.* 6, 1169-1171.
O'Brien, P.J. and Rahimtula, A. (1975). *J. Agric. Food Chem.* 23, 154-158.
Orrenius, S. (1965). *J. Cell Biol.* 26, 713-723.
Packer, J.E., Slater, T.F. and Willson, R.L. (1978). *Life Sci.* 23, 2617-2620.
Parke, D.V. (1968). "The Biochemistry of Foreign Compounds" Pergamon, London.
Plaa, G.L. and Witschi, H. (1976). *Ann. Rev. Pharmacol. Toxicol.* 16, 125-141.
Poli, G., Chiono, M.P., Slater, T.F., Dianzani, M.U. and Gravela, E. (1978). *Biochem. Soc. Trans.* 6, 589-591.
Powis, G., Lyon, L. and McKillop, D. (1977). *Biochem. Pharmacol.* 26, 137-141.
Rao, K.S. and Recknagel, R.O. (1969). *Exp. Mol. Pathol.* 10, 219-228.
Recknagel, R.O. and Glende, E.A. (1973). *Crit. Rev. Toxicol.* 2, 263-297.
Reynolds, E.S. and Moslen, M.T. (1980). *In* "Free Radicals in Biology" (Ed. W.A. Pryor) Vol. 4, pp.49-94. Academic Press, New York.
Salerno, J.C. and Ingledew, W.J. (1975). *Biochem. Biophys. Res. Commun.* 65, 618-624.
Shah, H., Hartmann, S.P. and Weinhouse, S. (1979). *Cancer Res.* 39, 3942-3947.
Sipes, I.G., Krishna, G. and Gillette, J.R. (1977). *Life Sci.* 20, 1541-1548.
Slater, T.F. (1968). *Biochem. J.* 106, 155-160.
Slater, T.F. (1972). "Free Radical Mechanisms in Tissue Injury" Pion Ltd., London.
Slater, T.F. (1978). *In* "Biochemical Mechanisms of Liver Injury" (Ed. T.F. Slater) pp.745-801. Academic Press, London.
Slater, T.F. (1979a). *In* "Drug Toxicity" (Ed. J.W. Garrod) pp.123-132. Taylor and Francis, London.
Slater, T.F. (1979b). *In* "Oxygen Free Radicals and Tissue Damage" pp.143-163. Ciba Foundation Series 65. Excerpta Medica, Amsterdam.
Slater, T.F. (1981). *In* "2nd International Symposium on Biological Reactive Intermediates" (Ed. F. Snyder). Plenum, New York.
Slater, T.F. and Sawyer, B.C. (1971a). *Biochem. J.* 123, 805-814.
Slater, T.F. and Sawyer, B.C. (1971b). *Biochem. J.* 123, 815-821.

Slater, T.F. and Sawyer, B.C. (1971c). *Biochem. J.* 123, 823-828.
Slater, T.F., Ahmed, M., Benedetto, C., Cheeseman, K., Packer, J.E., Willson, R.L. and Dianzani, M.U. (1980). *Int. J. Quantum Chem.* 7, 347-356.
Svingen, B.A., Buege, J.A., O'Neal, F.O. and Aust, S.D. (1979). *J. Biol. Chem.* 254, 5892-5899.
Svingen, B.A., O'Neal, F.O. and Aust, S.D. (1978). *Photochem. Photobiol.* 28, 803-809.
Talcott, R.E., Shu, H. and Wei, E.T. (1979). *Biochem. Pharmacol.* 28, 665-671.
Wills, E.D. (1972). *Biochem. Pharmacol.* 21, 1879-1883.

DISCUSSION

Marsh: Copper-phenanthroline is used as a cross-linking reagent (Murphy, 1976). Is it possible that any reaction of this type is taking place?

Cheeseman: I did look at some papers on the cross-linking of cytochrome P_{450} molecules (McIntosh *et al.*, 1980; McIntosh and Freedman, 1980) but they did not seem to have a great deal of relevance to the enhancing effect. It seemed to be a rather different system in that they use, as you say, copper-phenanthroline complexes rather than phenanthroline (or bipyridine) *per se*. I think that this enhancement, or apparent enhancement, of carbon tetrachloride metabolism is more likely to be related to the enhancement of type II metabolism that has already been seen and is well documented. But, as I indicated, carbon tetrachloride is a type I compound and so if it is being metabolised by cytochrome P_{450}, it seems to be acting, in this instance, as a type II compound, which is rather strange.

Slater: There is some evidence now in the literature that carbon tetrachloride reacts specifically with a particular type of P_{450}, whereas, of course, when we started these studies many years ago we referred to P_{450} as if it was one substance. Do you think that the conflicting results that you showed might represent differential effects on particular types of P_{450}?

Cheeseman: That is certainly a possibility. The literature reports on specific forms of P_{450} being inactivated by CCl_4 are, as far as I know, only in the abstract stage at the moment (Head *et al.*, 1980; McCay *et al.*, 1980, 1981) which is rather frustrating, so it is difficult to make any conclusions about these.

Certainly, one of the main problems concerning the comparison of our results to other results in the literature is that there is, we now know, a multiplicity of cytochrome P_{450}s (Lu and West, 1980). These may be different in different strains of rat and they are certainly different when induction methods are used. I used no induction here, which makes it rather hard to compare with the results of people who use phenobarbitone to induce P_{450}, for instance, which is also considered to induce specific forms of P_{450}.

Asmus: I have a figure that might be of interest. You were talking about the reaction of the $CCl_3^\bullet$ radical with O_2. We have just been able to measure the absolute rate constant for this reaction in our studies of the oxidation of phenothiazines by the $CCl_3O_2^\bullet$ radical. The rate constant is $3.3 \times 10^9\ M^{-1}\ s^{-1}$ (Bahnemann, 1981). This is a figure which you would certainly expect, it is a practically diffusion controlled rate. It might be quite useful to have that handy. In connection with this, you can now predict what kinds of reactions the $CCl_3^\bullet$ radical would undergo if you know the exact O_2 concentration in the environment where you produce the $CCl_3^\bullet$ radical. How well do you know and how well can you control the O_2 concentration? That is my question.

Cheeseman: That's a very good question. We do not really know what the O_2 concentrations are in the local site where $CCl_3^\bullet$ may be produced and that is obviously going to be important in these radical reactions. Kieczka *et al.* (1981) have shown a strong dependence on O_2 concentration of the covalent binding of CCl_4 to either lipids or protein. For instance, at the O_2 concentrations I presume to have in my experiments, using their results, it would appear that I'm probably getting no covalent binding to lipids, whereas at lower concentrations of O_2 the covalent binding is *mainly* to lipids and less to proteins. So it is certainly a rather important effect.

Slater: Perhaps we can come back to that one.

Mason: I was involved in some work that demonstrated that there was an effect of oxygen on the ultimate metabolism of CCl_4 other than the reaction between $CCl_3^\bullet$ and O_2. We were looking at the disappearance of CCl_4 in microsomal incubations, not knowing what the products are, just its disappearance; and its disappearance is inhibited 99% by air

(Wolf *et al.*, 1980). So even though the $CCl_3^{\cdot}$ radical will react with O_2 to form $CCl_3O_2^{\cdot}$ there is much less *formation* of the $CCl_3^{\cdot}$ radical under aerobic conditions than there is under anaerobic conditions.

Slater: Yes, I think almost all, if not all, workers in the field would agree with that in the sense that anaerobic conditions in microsomal suspensions increase the production of $CHCl_3$ or covalent binding. I think there is no dispute. I think that the significance of Professor Asmus's remark is that if you can form $CCl_3^{\cdot}$ in the presence of dioxygen, the reaction rate is essentially diffusion controlled and what we know (and I will give you some figures, so will Dr Willson, later on) is that once we form even a small amount of $CCl_3O_2^{\cdot}$ radical it is so much more reactive than $CCl_3^{\cdot}$ in kinetic terms. But I think that we'll have to take that in the general discussion; I am going to give some data and so is Dr Willson on these points.

Connors: Can I go back to that result on the metal chelators. It is quite a remarkable result, the stimulation and the inhibition - the difference between the two. Have you tried a simple sort of pharmacological experiment where you take combinations of the two chelators and you titrate them to see if they are acting by independent pathways or if they are really antagonistic to one another?

Cheeseman: I am not sure that it is quite as simple as you make it sound. We know that metal chelators normally inhibit lipid peroxidation and my feeling here is that the *perceived* effects on the lipid peroxidation represent a balance between the increased production of the initiating radical and a decreased propagation of the peroxidation steps. But that is only a guess.

REFERENCES to Discussion

Bahnemann, D. (1981). Ph.D. Thesis. Technical University of Berlin.

Head, B., Moody, D.E., Woo, C.H. and Smuckler, E.A. (1980). *Fed. Proc.* 39, 1015.

Kieczka, H., Remmer, H. and Kappus, H. (1981). *Biochem. Pharmacol.* 30, 319-324.

McCay, P.B., Noguchi, T., Fong, K.-L., Olson, L., Lai, E.K., Alexander, S.S. and Poyer, J.L. (1980). *Fed. Proc.* 40, 1638.

McCay, P.B., Noguchi, T., Lai, E.K. and Fong, K.-L. (1980). *Fed. Proc.* 39, 612.

McIntosh, P.R. and Freeman, R.B. (1980). *Biochem. J.* 187, 227-237.

McIntosh, P.R., Kawato, S., Freedman, R.B. and Cherry, R.J. (1980). *FEBS Lett.* 122, 54-58.
Murphy, A.J. (1976). *Biochem. Biophys. Res. Commun.* 70, 160-166.
Wolf, C.R., Harrelson, W.G., Nastainczyk, W.M., Philpot, R.M., Kalyanaraman, B. and Mason, R.P. (1980). *Mol. Pharmacol.* 18, 553-558.

Lipid Peroxidation in Isolated Hepatocytes

G. POLI and E. GRAVELA

INTRODUCTION

The peroxidative breakdown of membrane polyunsaturated fatty acids, a consequence of the production and the propagation of free radicals, is involved in the pathogenesis of the liver injury induced by several chemicals. In order to check the influence of lipid peroxidation on different metabolic functions of the liver, a number of studies on the whole animal *in vivo* , and on the isolated perfused liver or on isolated organelles *in vitro* have been performed by several authors (for reviews see Slater, 1972; Dianzani and Ugazio, 1978).

More recently, suspensions of isolated rat hepatocytes have been employed for such studies (Hogberg *et al.*, 1975a; Sies and Summer, 1975; Weddle *et al.*, 1976; Poli *et al.*, 1978; Poli *et al.*, 1979a; Gravela *et al.*, 1979). Isolated liver cells provide certain advantages over the studies on the intact animal or on the isolated perfused liver, e.g. the possibility to avoid complications due to other organs, to study only parenchymal cells, to know exactly the concentration of the added substances reaching the cells under study. Furthermore, the use of intact hepatocytes represents a useful integration of experimental systems employing cell-free preparations or isolated organelles, since it allows the preservation of permeability barriers, of intracellular organisation and of controlling mechanisms for lipid peroxide formation. Because of improvements in the isolation procedure, it is possible now to obtain liver cells with reasonable amounts of NADPH, and physiological levels of GSH, both being very important in the regulation of lipid peroxidation.

We report here on studies to reproduce in the intact isolated hepatocyte model the pro-oxidant effect of several drugs. Deeper investigations have been performed with carbon tetrachloride (CCl_4), $FeCl_3$ and cumene hydroperoxide. Exposure of hepatocytes to these substances, in the presence or absence of promethazine, a free radical scavenger with strong antioxidant effect (Slater, 1972), has been carried out in order to check the effective role of lipid peroxidation in the pathogenesis of cell changes, such as intracellular enzyme inactivation, derangement of protein synthesis and of protein and lipoprotein secretion.

MATERIALS AND METHODS

Animals

Male rats of the Wistar strain (Nossan, Correzzana, Milano, Italy), weighing 200-250 g, were used. They were fed a semi-synthetic diet, devoid of any antioxidant (Piccioni, Brescia, Italy), with water *ad lib*. Operations were always performed between 10.00 and 12.00 a.m.

Reagents

All chemicals were of reagent grade and were obtained from the following sources: collagenase type I, amino acids, ethyleneglycol-bis-(β-amino-ethyl-ether) N,N'-tetraacetic acid (EGTA), N-2-hydroxyethyl-piperazine-N'-2-ethane-sulfonic acid (HEPES), pyridoxal phosphate, dithiothreitol, phenylmethylsulfonylfluoride, ascorbic acid, paraquat, from SIGMA Chemical Company, St. Louis, Missouri, USA; promethazine-HCl from May and Baker, Dagenham, UK; cumene hydroperoxide from Fluka AG, Buchs, Switzerland; malonaldehyde bis-dimethylacetal from Ralph N. Emanuel, Wembley, UK; other chemicals from Merck, Darmstadt, West Germany, and BDH Chemicals Ltd., Poole, UK. Radiochemicals were from the Radiochemical Centre, Amersham, UK; Pico-Fluor 30 was from Packard Instruments S.P.A., Milano, Italy.

Preparation of Isolated Liver Cells

Hepatocytes were prepared with the collagenase perfusion method described in preceding papers (Gravela *et al.*, 1977; Poli *et al.*, 1979a).

At the suggestion of other authors (Viña *et al.*, 1978), to prevent loss in cell glutathione content during cell isolation, 0.2 mM EGTA was included in the saline buffer used to wash the blood out of the liver before collagenase digestion; furthermore, in the cell incubation medium the amino acid mixture was replaced by 1 mM methionine during the first 10 min incubation step.

Only hepatocyte preparations with viable cells ranging from 85 to 95% were used. In fact, a range of 5-15% damaged cells does not interfere with lipid peroxidation detection in terms of malonaldehyde (Chiarpotto *et al.*, 1981).

Incubation of Liver Cells with Different Chemicals

The hepatocyte suspensions were diluted to 8 x 10^6 cells in a defined medium (Poli *et al.*, 1979a) where not indicated otherwise.

For cell treatment with CCl_4 or $CBrCl_3$, 2 ml aliquots of the suspensions were placed into the main compartment of 50 ml flasks, fitted with a centre well and closed with a screw cap. The halogenoalkanes were added in the centre well and allowed to diffuse in the closed system. The experiments which indicated the most convenient amount of CCl_4 per flask (7.5 μl, about 129 μM final concentration) have been reported elsewhere (Poli *et al.*, 1979a). As far as the experiments with $CBrCl_3$ are concerned, the cells were treated with the highest concentration of the drug not inducing severe damage to the cells, as measured by the Trypan blue exclusion test (Gravela *et al.*, 1977). As regards the other chemicals used to initiate lipid peroxide formation, they were added directly to the cell suspension. The concentration of the chemicals was chosen in such a way as not to induce overt damage to the cell plasma membrane, the integrity of which was monitored by measuring the cell release of lactate dehydrogenase and the cell stainability with Trypan blue (Gravela *et al.*, 1977).

The flasks containing hepatocyte suspensions, treated with the above mentioned drugs, with or without promethazine, were incubated at 37°C in a shaking water bath, for 30 or 60 min.

Determination of Malonaldehyde

Malonaldehyde production was taken as a measure of lipid peroxidation; it was determined according to Bernheim *et al.* (1948), with minor modifications previously reported (Poli *et al.*, 1979a). A calibration curve was constructed by using malonaldehyde-bis-dimethylacetal.

Determination of Microsomal Enzyme Activities

Cytochrome P_{450} content was measured on intact cells according to Kupfer and Orrenius (1970), using the millimolar extinction coefficient given by Omura and Sato (1964). Aminopyrene demethylation was measured, with the method of Slater and Sawyer (1971a), in the cell homogenate, obtained by ultrasonic disintegration (amplitude of vibrations 20 microns, for 5 sec). Also glucose-6-phosphatase activity was determined in the cell homogenate prepared as before, by using the method described by Poli *et al.* (1981b).

Evaluation of Valine Incorporation and Ornithine Decarboxylase (ODC) Activity

Hepatocytes were suspended in the previously mentioned medium (Poli *et al.*, 1979a) and diluted to 5 x 10^6 cells/ml. Aliquots of 2 ml of suspensions were placed into the above described 50 ml flasks; for each experimental condition three flasks were prepared. CCl_4 treatment was performed as above mentioned; promethazine or cycloheximide were added directly to the cell suspension. Flasks were incubated for 30 min at 37°C. Then two 0.1 ml aliquots of hepatocytes for each flask were taken to study the [^{14}C]valine incorporating activity by 30 min incubation at 37°C in the presence of 0.02 μCi/tube (0.02 mM) L-[U-^{14}C]valine. Incubation was stopped by adding 5 ml of 5% trichloroacetic acid (TCA). The determination of protein-bound radioactivity was carried out by collecting TCA precipitates on Whatman GF/C glass fibre filters. Protein material was rinsed three times with 5% TCA, three times with 2% TCA and finally with water; then the filters were air-dried and put into scintillation vials. Protein material on the filters was dissolved with 1 ml of 0.3 M NaOH, and after at least 3 h, 5 ml of Pico-Fluor 30 were added for radioactivity determination.

Hepatocytes remaining in the incubation flasks were harvested by centrifugation, rinsed with 5 ml of "homogenisation medium" (Olson and Russell, 1980), containing: 50 mM sodium-potassium phosphate buffer (pH 7.2), 0.04 mM pyridoxal phosphate, 1 mM dithiothreitol and 0.1 mM phenylmethylsulfonylfluoride, and suspended in the same homogenisation medium. Hepatocytes were homogenised by ultrasonic disintegration (as for cytochrome P_{450} determination) and centrifuged for 10 min at 48,000 x g (Olson and Russell, 1980). Aliquots of 90 µl of the supernatant fraction (3 aliquots for each sample) were assayed for ODC activity in a final volume of 100 µl, by using 8 ml tubes fitted with rubber plugs. ODC activity was determined by measuring the release of $^{14}CO_2$ from L-[1-^{14}C] ornithine. The latter (0.1 µCi/tube, final concentration 0.25 mM) was rapidly added and tubes were immediately closed with the rubber plug. Incubation was carried out at 37°C for 30 min, then 0.25 ml of 10% TCA were injected through the plug, and the released CO_2 was transferred to pre-evacuated 25 ml bottles, sealed with rubber plugs, containing 0.8 ml of 0.4 M KOH. This transfer was achieved with a plastic "U-tube" with a needle at each end. Then 5 ml of Pico-Fluor 30 were injected through the plug into the bottles and finally the mixture was transferred into scintillation vials. Preliminary studies, performed with a similar system by mixing known amounts of [^{14}C]sodium bicarbonate solution and TCA, showed that the $^{14}CO_2$ recovery was complete in the presence of CO_2 levels up to 5 nmol/tube.

Protein and Triglyceride Secretion from Pre-labelled Liver Cells

Hepatocytes suspended in the previously mentioned medium were centrifuged at 200 x g for 4 min. The pellets were resuspended in Ham's F-12 Medium (Ham, 1965), containing 10% horse serum, to give a concentration of 10^7 cells/ml. Cell protein, or triglyceride were labelled with [^{14}C]valine, or [^{14}C]sodium palmitate, as previously described (Gravela *et al.*, 1977; Poli *et al.*, 1979a). Suspensions of labelled hepatocytes were centrifuged at 400 x g for 4 min, then hepatocytes were suspended in the formerly used medium and diluted to 5 x 10^6 cells/ml. Aliquots of 2 ml of this suspension were incubated, in the above described 50 ml flasks, with or without CCl_4, or $FeCl_3$, or cumene hydroperoxide, in the presence or absence of promethazine. After 30 min incubation at 37°C cell suspensions were immediately centrifuged. Protein and lipoprotein triglyceride in supernatants were purified and processed for radioactivity determination as described elsewhere (Gravela *et al.*, 1977).

In all studies here above described radioactivity was measured by employing a Packard PRIAS liquid scintillation counter.

RESULTS AND DISCUSSION

Monitoring of Lipid Peroxidation in Intact Liver Cells

Lipid peroxidation may be divided into two sequential parts, i.e. initiation and propagation (Tam and McCay, 1970; Svingen *et al.*, 1978). Initiation is the generation of lipid hydroperoxides through an interaction of a reactive free radical with an unsaturated fatty acid, and it is characterised by low levels of malonaldehyde. Propagation is the breakdown of lipid hydroperoxides into reactive intermediates which prolongs the free radical reactions of lipid peroxidation; a rapid production of malonaldehyde corresponds to this step.

As regards the estimation of initiation reactions of lipid peroxidation in whole cells, the diene conjugation band is hardly detected (Hogberg *et al.*, 1975a; Stacey and Priestly, 1978) and lipid peroxides do not accumulate within the cell. The latter finding was obtained by our group in CCl_4-treated hepatocytes using two different methods of lipid peroxide determination, i.e. the iodimetric procedure described by Wills (1971) and a modification of the enzymatic method described by Heath and Tappel (1976) (P.H. Beswick, T.F. Slater, K. Cheeseman and G. Poli, unpublished experiments). Conversely, in the intact cell experimental model, the propagation of lipid peroxidation (the step during which peroxides, via radical reactions, give breakdown products) is better monitored and quantified than initiation.

Among the end products of lipid peroxidation, malonaldehyde is the compound, the production of which is routinely assessed in cell preparations treated with pro-oxidant drugs. The main advantages of this indirect method of lipid peroxidation measurement are represented by its sensitivity, reliability and reproducibility (Plaa and Witschi, 1976; Buege and Aust, 1978). Furthermore, for studies *in vitro* at least, on isolated microsomes, the malonaldehyde method gives more consistent results than other methods commonly employed, like determination of lipid peroxides, diene conjugation, or measurement of oxygen consumption (Beswick *et al.*, unpublished results; Buege and Aust, 1978).

Recently, analyses of the intracellular range of polar and unpolar aldehydes have been started in order to have a more complete monitoring of the extent of lipoperoxidative processes (Esterbauer *et al.*, 1981). Such measurements consist in the derivatisation of aldehydes with 2,4-dinitrophenylhydrazine then in the separation of the corresponding hydrazones by high pressure liquid chromatography (Benedetti *et al.*, 1981). Preliminary results have shown that both in isolated microsomes and in intact cells treated with the ADP-Fe^{3+} complex, several aldehydes are present, namely *n*-alkanals and 4-hydroxy-alkenals, having different toxicological implications (Esterbauer *et al.*, 1981). This finding moreover confirms the usefulness of integrating malonaldehyde detection with an analysis of the aldehydic patterns in the investigation of lipid peroxidation processes.

Hepatocyte Treatment with Different Pro-oxidant Chemicals

Experiments to reproduce lipid peroxidation processes in whole liver cells have been carried out by several authors over the last few years. In order to investigate the role of glutathione as intracellular defensive mechanism, Högberg *et al.* (1975a) induced lipid peroxide formation in rat hepatocytes by treating the cells with ADP-Fe^{3+} or with cumene hydroperoxide and followed the relationship between malonaldehyde production and glutathione content decrease. The pro-oxidant effect of cumene hydroperoxide was also investigated by Sies and Summer (1975), on isolated liver organelles and whole hepatocytes. More difficulties have been found in setting up the procedure of CCl_4 poisoning of intact liver cells than with the *in vitro* reproduction, in microsomal suspensions, of several effects exerted by the drug *in vivo*.

The direct addition of the halogenoalkane to hepatocyte suspensions gave controversial results. On one hand, Weddle *et al.* (1976) showed stimulation of malonaldehyde production by treating the cells with about 100 mM CCl_4. On the other hand, Lindstrom *et al.* (1978) with a concentration of CCl_4 20-40 times lower did not detect significant formation of malonaldehyde in cells isolated from untreated rats, but only in cells from phenobarbital pretreated rats. Furthermore, in both studies, cell integrity was not well preserved probably because of solvent effect due to the drug. A similar problem was found in direct treatment of cells with $CBrCl_3$ (Koster-Albrecht *et al.*, 1978). These disadvantages have been overcome by keeping cells and toxic agent in two different compartments of a closed system, and allowing CCl_4 to diffuse in it. In such a way, very low concentrations of the drug can be also achieved (Poli *et al.*, 1978; Stacey and Priestly, 1978; Poli *et al.*, 1979a). In Table 1 the lipoperoxidative effect of mentioned and other chemicals is reported, as measured in terms of malonaldehyde production.

TABLE 1 Pro-oxidant effect of different drugs on hepatocytes in single cell suspension

Treatment	Concentration of the drug	Malonaldehyde production	
		nmol/10^7 cells	$\frac{\text{exp.sample}}{\text{control}}$ ratio
Carbon tetrachloride	7.5 μl/flask	3.2	5.4
Bromotrichloromethane	0.5 μl/flask	19.4	32.9
Paraquat	1 mM	1.4	3.3
Cumene hydroperoxide	100 μM	2.8	5.7
Ascorbate	500 μM	0.5	0.9
$FeSO_4$	20 μM	35.0	66.0
$FeCl_3$	20 μM	1.9	3.6
Ascorbate + $FeSO_4$	500 μM + 20 μM	62.1	117.2
Ascorbate + $FeCl_3$	500 μM + 20 μM	3.2	6.0
$FeCl_3$	100 μM	11.2	21.0
ADP-$FeCl_3$	2.5 mM - 100 μM	17.2	32.5

Cell suspensions (2 ml, 1 x 10^7 cells) were incubated for 60 min at 37°C. For further details see Materials and Methods. For each group of substances a different control was carried out.

As regards the experiments with halogenoalkanes, a very low concentration of CCl_4 (about 129 μM, as determined by using [^{14}C]carbon tetrachloride) was able to induce significant stimulation of malonaldehyde production with preservation of cell integrity (Poli *et al.*, 1979a).

Much lower concentrations of $CBrCl_3$ gave a malonaldehyde stimulation 6-7 times higher than that obtained with CCl_4. The result fits well with the findings that homolysis of $CBrCl_3$ proceeds more rapidly than that of CCl_4 (Slater, 1972).

Evidence for lipid peroxidation induced by paraquat, a widely used herbicide, was also obtained, but only by testing liver cells with rather high concentrations of the toxic agent (1 mM).

With regard to the studies of initiation of lipid peroxidation with ascorbic acid and/or iron, an ascorbate concentration (500 μM) similar to that usually employed in experiments on liver microsomes (Hochstein and Ernster, 1963; see also Slater, 1972) did not show a pro-oxidant effect *per se*. On the contrary, the addition of small amounts of $FeCl_3$ and especially of $FeSO_4$ (20 μM) induced stimulation of malonaldehyde production by liver cells.

The ratio between the pro-oxidant effects of Fe^{2+} and Fe^{3+} was significantly higher than that commonly observed on liver microsomes treated with the same concentration of the two valency states of the metal (Kornbrust and Mavis, 1980). This evidence supports the hypothesis that mechanisms of competition with the reduction of ferric iron by the microsomal reductase are present within the cells. The effect of iron addition to the cells was doubled by the simultaneous treatment with ascorbate, confirming previous findings obtained with liver microsomes (Slater, 1972).

The effect of 100 μM $FeCl_3$, complexed or not with ADP, and of 100 μM cumene hydroperoxide on malonaldehyde production by isolated hepatocytes was also tested with the aim of comparing its pro-oxidant effect with that due to CCl_4, the concentration of which being similar. As reported in Table 1, while the halogenoalkane and the hydroperoxide showed similar peroxidative effect, the malonaldehyde production induced by $FeCl_3$ and ADP-$FeCl_3$ in cells was respectively 3-4 and 5-6 times higher.

Studies on the Role of Lipid Peroxidation in Microsomal Enzymatic Changes Induced by CCl_4, $FeCl_3$ or Cumene Hydroperoxide

It is widely accepted that CCl_4 may induce toxic liver injury through two main mechanisms, i.e. covalent binding of its metabolites to cell structure and lipid peroxidation. As regards the latter mechanism, it may produce cell damage either directly by membrane derangement, or indirectly by production of reactive intermediates such as lipid free radicals and peroxides, and of final products namely aldehydes

(Dianzani *et al.*, 1976; Benedetti *et al.*, 1979b). Moreover, the relative influence of lipid peroxidation and covalent binding in the pathogenesis of the different cell changes is not yet completely clear

In order to check the effective role of lipid peroxidation in the derangement of cell functions, we studied three experimental conditions in isolated hepatocytes in which a stimulation of lipid peroxidation occurs, i.e. treatment with similar concentrations of CCl_4, $FeCl_3$ and cumene hydroperoxide. Furthermore, the effect of promethazine addition to the three systems has been evaluated.

Promethazine has been shown to inhibit the stimulation of lipid peroxidation produced by CCl_4 *in vivo* (Jose and Slater, 1972) and *in vitro* on liver microsomes (Slater and Sawyer, 1971b) or on liver cells (Poli *et al.*, 1978). On the contrary, however, this substance has little effect on the covalent binding of the trichloromethyl radical ($CCl_3^{\bullet}$) to cell protein (Cheeseman, 1981). The explanation of this latter result has probably to be found in the slow reaction between $CCl_3^{\bullet}$ and the scavenger, as demonstrated using pulse radiolysis techniques (Packer *et al.*, 1978).

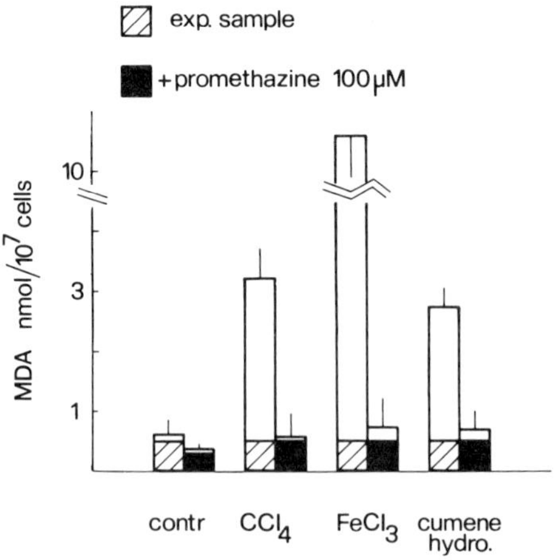

FIG. 1 Malonaldehyde production in the control and treated cells in the presence and absence of promethazine. Hepatocytes were incubated at 37°C for 60 min with 129 µM CCl_4, 100 µM $FeCl_3$, 100 µM cumene hydroperoxide or water. When used, promethazine was added at the concentration of 100 µM. For further experimental details see Materials and Methods section. Vertical bars denote the SD.

Figure 1 shows that 100 μM promethazine completely inhibits malonaldehyde stimulation due to 129 μM CCl_4, 100 μM $FeCl_3$ and 100 μM cumene hydroperoxide.

As far as the investigated microsomal enzyme activities are concerned, the liver cytochrome P_{450} was decreased by all of the three drugs (see Table 2). Carbon tetrachloride (129 μM) and cumene hydroperoxide (100 μM) gave similar percentages of inhibition(about 35%). A significantly larger decrease in the hemeprotein content was induced by iron treatment (about 50%). These results are in agreement with those obtained by several authors in the case of CCl_4 (for a review see Slater, 1978), by Högberg *et al.* (1975b) in the case of ADP-Fe^{3+} and of the peroxide, and by Bonkowsky *et al.* (1979) for ferric iron.

TABLE 2 Effect of carbon tetrachloride, $FeCl_3$ and cumene hydroperoxide in the presence and absence of promethazine on cytochrome P_{450} content of isolated rat hepatocytes

Treatment	Cytochrome P_{450} (nmol/10^7 cells)	
	without promethazine	with promethazine
None	0.17 ± 0.02 (10)	0.16 ± 0.01 (4)
Carbon tetrachloride	0.11 ± 0.01 (6)	0.10 ± 0.02 (4)
$FeCl_3$	0.08 ± 0.03 (10)	0.07 ± 0.03 (4)
Cumene hydroperoxide	0.11 ± 0.03 (8)	0.12 ± 0.04 (4)

Cell suspensions (2 ml, 1.6 x 10^7 cells) were incubated for 60 min at 37°C; where required, carbon tetrachloride (7.5 μl/2 ml) or $FeCl_3$ (100 μM) or cumene hydroperoxide (100 μM) were added at the start of the incubation. Promethazine was included to give 100 μM. The number of data is shown in parentheses. Values are means ± S.D.

The incubation in the presence of 100 μM promethazine did not protect the cells against the above mentioned changes induced by the three substances. With regard to the decrease of cytochrome P_{450} produced by CCl_4, a similar lack of protection by the free radical scavenger has been reported in studies *in vivo* (Slater and Sawyer, 1969) and, more recently, *in vitro*, on microsomes and intact hepatocytes (Poli *et al.*, 1978; Poli *et al.*, 1981b). Against a prominent role of lipid peroxidation in the CCl_4-mediated decrease of cytochrome P_{450} are also the results obtained by other authors using different

TABLE 3 Effect of carbon tetrachloride, $FeCl_3$ and cumene hydroperoxide in the presence and absence of promethazine on aminopyrene metabolism of isolated hepatocytes

Treatment	Aminopyrene metabolism (nmol of formaldehyde formed/min per 10^7 cells)	
	without promethazine	with promethazine
None	7.84 ± 1.54 (8)	8.41 ± 0.17 (4)
Carbon tetrachloride	1.44 ± 0.45 (6)	2.04 ± 0.58 (4)
$FeCl_3$	6.89 ± 1.83 (6)	7.74 ± 0.77 (4)
Cumene hydroperoxide	10.12 ± 0.28 (6)	8.16 ± 0.67 (4)

See Table 2 for experimental conditions.

experimental approaches (de Toranzo *et al.*, 1975; Guzelian and Swisher, 1979; de Groot and Haas, 1980).

As shown in Table 3, consistent with the decrease in cytochrome P_{450} content is the strong reduction (about 82%) of aminopyrene metabolism produced by CCl_4 in liver cells. Also in this case promethazine does not prevent at all the enzyme inactivation and the result confirms our earlier similar data obtained with isolated hepatocytes (Poli *et al.*, 1978). Conversely, cell treatment with $FeCl_3$ does not seem to significantly affect aminopyrene metabolism in spite of the considerably large decrease in cytochrome P_{450} content induced by the metal. The latter result needs to be confirmed since experiments not reported here, employing identical concentrations of ADP-Fe^{3+} complex instead of $FeCl_3$, showed a similar decrease of cytochrome P_{450} and also a significant reduction of aminopyrene demethylase activity (Chiarpotto, Pavia and Poli, unpublished data).

Data reported in Table 3 also show that cumene hydroperoxide stimulates aminopyrene metabolism. This result fits well with a number of reports describing hydroperoxide-supported oxidation activities of liver microsomes involving cytochrome P_{450} (Kadlubar *et al.*, 1973; Rahimtula and O'Brien, 1974; Hrycay *et al.*, 1975). The lack of stimulating effect by cumene hydroperoxide on aminopyrene metabolism in the presence of promethazine is consistent with recent evidence for the involvement of radical species in the oxidation of aminopyrene by this hydroperoxide (Griffin and Ting, 1978; Griffin, 1980).

TABLE 4 Effect of carbon tetrachloride, $FeCl_3$ and cumene hydroperoxide in the presence and absence of promethazine on glucose-6-phosphatase activity of isolated rat hepatocytes

Treatment	Glucose-6-phosphatase (nmol P/min per 10^7 cells)	
	without promethazine	with promethazine
None	517 ± 48 (4)	489 ± 30 (4)
Carbon tetrachloride	364 ± 60 (4)	536 ± 45 (4)
$FeCl_3$	456 ± 39 (4)	521 ± 17 (4)
Cumene hydroperoxide	418 ± 31 (4)	510 ± 21 (4)

See Table 2 for experimental conditions.

Contrary to the above mentioned data obtained with the analyses of cytochrome P_{450} content and aminopyrene metabolism are the conclusions arising from the investigation of glucose-6-phosphatase inactivation due to the treatment of cells with CCl_4, $FeCl_3$ and cumene hydroperoxide (Table 4). In the case of this enzyme a relationship is evident between degree of lipid peroxidation and degree of enzyme inactivation. In fact, promethazine completely prevents the decrease in glucose-6-phosphatase activity due to CCl_4 and cumene hydroperoxide. Table 4 shows that $FeCl_3$ gives little, if any, enzyme inactivation. It has been shown elsewhere that larger amounts of the metal produce significant decrease of glucose-6-phosphatase activity, especially when iron is complexed with ADP (Poli *et al.*, 1979b; Poli *et al.*, 1981a). These results give further evidence for a major role of lipid peroxidation in glucose-6-phosphatase inactivation occurring in experimental conditions characterised by enhanced peroxidative breakdown of biological membranes (see also Glende *et al.*, 1976; Benedetti *et al.*, 1977).

Studies on the Effect of Lipid Peroxidation on Protein Synthesis and Ornithine Decarboxylase Activity in Isolated Hepatocytes

Protein synthesis, as evaluated by [^{14}C]valine incorporation into protein, is strongly reduced in hepatocytes poisoned with CCl_4 (Poli *et al.*, 1979a). A relationship between inhibition of protein synthesis and lipid peroxidation is not evident. In fact, it has been observed (Gravela and Poli, unpublished data) that this change is not prevented by promethazine and that cumene hydroperoxide is only slightly inhibitory, and $FeCl_3$ is not inhibitory at all, to protein synthesis.

In the liver of rats poisoned with CCl_4 we have recently observed a decreased activity of ornithine decarboxylase (ODC), the initial rate-limiting enzyme in the polyamine biosynthetic pathway. This interference with polyamine metabolism represents a further mechanism in the hepatotoxic action of CCl_4. ODC has a peculiarly very fast rate of turnover, its decay seemingly mainly dependent on (or initiated by) SH-group oxidation (Williams-Ashman and Canellakis, 1979). No data have been reported about effects of CCl_4, or other pro-oxidant substances, on this very labile enzyme. In Fig. 2 it is shown that

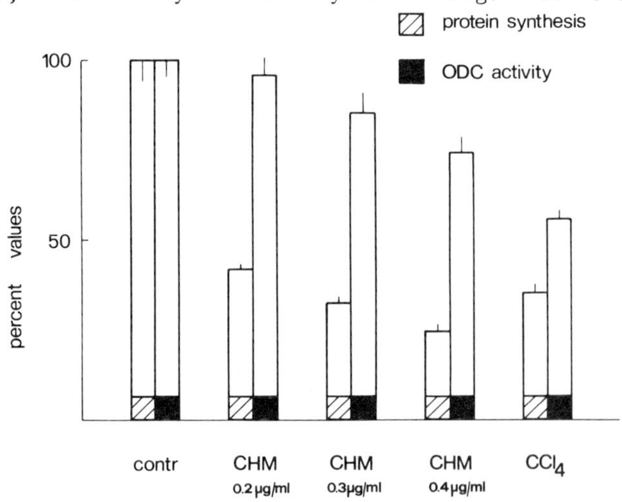

FIG 2 [^{14}C]valine incorporating activity, and ODC activity, of isolated liver cells poisoned with CCl_4, or cycloheximide. Hepatocytes were incubated at 37°C for 30 min with different concentrations of cycloheximide, or with 129 μM CCl_4. Then they were rinsed and tested for ODC activity. Experimental details are reported in the Materials and Methods section. Vertical bars denote the SD.

ODC activity is strongly reduced in isolated hepatocytes 30 min after CCl_4 poisoning. The short half-life of ODC and the inhibitory action of CCl_4 on protein synthesis suggest that the lower ODC activity in CCl_4-treated hepatocytes can be accounted for by the block in protein synthesis. In experiments reported in Fig. 2 the effect of CCl_4 has been compared to that of cycloheximide, a well known inhibitor of

TABLE 5 Effect of carbon tetrachloride, $FeCl_3$ and cumene hydroperoxide, in the presence and absence of promethazine, on ornithine decarboxylase activity of isolated rat hepatocytes

Treatment	Ornithine decarboxylase activity (pmol/mg protein/30 min)	
	without promethazine	with promethazine
None	61.1 ± 3.5 (12)	56.2 ± 3.6 (6)
Carbon tetrachloride	34.9 ± 1.9 (9)	33.7 ± 2.2 (6)
$FeCl_3$	59.9 ± 4.1 (6)	58.5 ± 5.0 (4)
Cumene hydroperoxide	211.1 ± 19.1 (5)	199.0 ± 22.7 (5)

Cells suspensions (2 ml, 10^7 cells) were incubated for 30 min at 37°C; where required, carbon tetrachloride (7.5 µl/2 ml), or $FeCl_3$ (100 µM), or cumene hydroperoxide (100 µM) were added at the start of the incubation, in the presence, or in the absence of 100 µM promethazine. Then hepatocytes were rinsed and processed for ornithine decarboxylase assay. Values are means ± SD; the number of data is shown in parentheses.

protein synthesis in eukaryotic cells. It is evident that cycloheximide concentrations (0.2-0.3 µg/ml) that reduce protein synthesis in hepatocytes by about 60-70%, as does CCl_4, do not cause great inhibition of ODC activity. This result indicates that CCl_4 acts through enzyme inactivation, rather than through inhibition of its synthesis. Experiments reported in Table 5 show that promethazine does not protect against the CCl_4-induced decrease of ODC activity. This effect of CCl_4, however, is not dependent on lipid peroxidation. Moreover, ODC activity is not affected by $FeCl_3$, in spite of the strong stimulation of lipid peroxidation exerted by this substance (see Table 1).

As far as regards the other lipid peroxidation initiator used in these studies, cumene hydroperoxide, it induces a strong increase of ODC activity, in the presence and in the absence of promethazine. No explanation can be given on this point. It is noteworthy, however, that three experimental conditions, all leading to increased lipid peroxidation, exert completely different effects (inhibition, no effect, stimulation) on ODC activity. A relationship between degree of lipid peroxidation and ODC activity is thus far from evident.

Effect of Lipid Peroxidation on Protein and Lipoprotein Secretion by Isolated Hepatocytes

Fatty liver produced by CCl_4 poisoning *in vivo* represents the most extensively studied model of fatty liver. Several sets of data (for a review see Dianzani and Ugazio, 1978) point out the block in lipoprotein secretion is a major cause of fatty accumulation. In isolated liver cells CCl_4 induces an impairment in protein and lipoprotein secretion (Poli *et al.*, 1979a); these changes do not appear to be mediated through the peroxidative stimulus produced by CCl_4 (Gravela *et al.*, 1979). Experiments reported in Fig. 3 strengthen the dichotomy

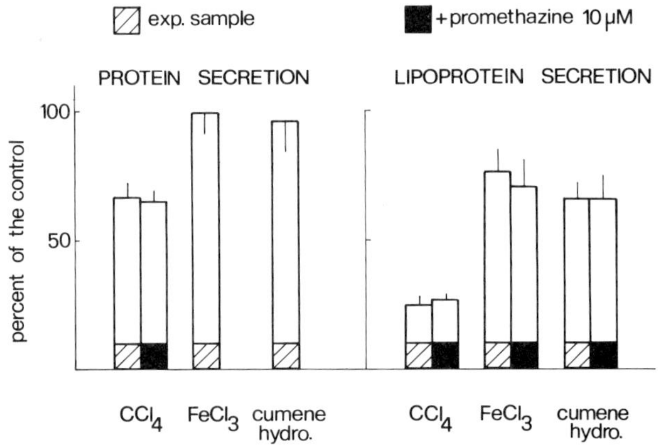

FIG. 3 Protein and lipoprotein triglyceride secretion in liver cells treated with CCl_4, $FeCl_3$ or cumene hydroperoxide. Effect of cell pretreatment with promethazine. Hepatocytes, of which protein or triglyceride were prelabelled *in vitro*, were incubated at 37°C for 30 min with 129 μM CCl_4, 100 μM $FeCl_3$, 100 μM cumene hydroperoxide, and the release of labelled molecules was measured (see also Materials and Methods). When used, promethazine was added at the start of the incubation to give a final concentration of 10 μM. Vertical bars denote the SD.

between the extent of lipid peroxidation and the degree of inhibition of secretion. Promethazine does not protect against the changes in secretion induced by CCl_4. Ferric chloride and cumene hydroperoxide do not affect protein secretion, whereas they slightly impair lipoprotein secretion. CCl_4 reduces the latter by about 75%; the concentration of $FeCl_3$ used (100 μM) stimulates malonaldehyde production much more than CCl_4 does (see Table 1), whereas it inhibits lipoprotein secretion by only 25%. Cumene hydroperoxide is a little more active than $FeCl_3$ in reducing lipoprotein secretion. Changes in secretion produced by $FeCl_3$, cumene hydroperoxide or CCl_4 are not prevented by promethazine.

CONCLUSIONS

The use of intact hepatocytes in single cell suspension has proved to be an important experimental model for studies *in vitro* on the effects of lipid peroxidation on metabolic cell functions. Some of the breakdown products of lipid peroxides are believed to cause loss of membrane structure, essential for the function of enzymes like glucose-6-phosphatase (Wills, 1971; Dianzani *et al.*, 1976; Benedetti *et al.*, 1979a,b). This point is well documented also by the results here and elsewhere reported (Poli *et al.*, 1981a,b) obtained with isolated hepatocytes.

Moreover, with regard to the pro-oxidant conditions examined in this paper, the experiments with intact cells suggest that the peroxidation is selective in causing loss of enzymatic activities. In fact, while a direct relationship between lipid peroxidation and change in glucose-6-phosphatase activity has been confirmed, the decrease in cytochrome P_{450} content due to CCl_4, $FeCl_3$ and cumene hydroperoxide and the inactivation of aminopyrene demethylase and of ornithine decarboxylase due to CCl_4 do not seem related to a pro-oxidant mechanism of injury.

Also the effects of CCl_4, $FeCl_3$ and cumene hydroperoxide on the investigated secretory pathways seem to be dependent on a mechanism involving free radical attack, not related to lipid peroxidation.

The discrepancy between the peroxidative effects of similar concentrations of the three substances used and the associated biological disturbances could be due to chemical and/or topographical differences in the initiation and the propagation mechanisms of lipid peroxidation. With regard to CCl_4 poisoning, in any case, there is increasing evidence for a prominent role of covalent binding of its reactive metabolites in early changes induced in liver cells.

SUMMARY

The peroxidative breakdown of membrane polyunsaturated fatty acids, a consequence of the production and the propagation of free radicals, represents one of the most investigated mechanisms of toxic liver injury. The use of intact hepatocytes in single cell suspension for studies "*in vitro*" on lipid peroxidation has provided the possibility to study both the intracellular controlling systems for a lipid peroxide formation and some consequences of lipoperoxidative phenomena in a more exact and reproducible way. A number of substances exert pro-oxidant effects in the intact isolated hepatocyte model; deeper investigations have been performed mainly with carbon tetrachloride, $FeCl_3$ and cumene hydroperoxide, powerful lipoperoxidation-stimulating agents. Hepatocyte exposure to these substances in the presence or in the absence of promethazine, a free radical scavenger with strong antioxidant effect, has been carried out in order to check the effective role of lipid peroxidation in the pathogenesis of cell changes like enzyme inactivation, or derangement of protein synthesis, and protein and lipoprotein secretion. In carbon tetrachloride-poisoned hepatocytes the following changes are not prevented by promethazine: decrease in cytochrome P_{450} content, decreases in aminopyrene demethylase and ornithine decarboxylase activities, protein synthesis and protein and lipoprotein secretion. Inhibition of glucose-6-phosphatase activity, on the contrary, is counteracted by promethazine. $FeCl_3$ and cumene hydroperoxide display evident effects only on cytochrome P_{450} and on lipoprotein secretion; these effects are not prevented by promethazine.

These results, together with other data, lead to the conclusion that the observed changes, with the exception of glucose-6-phosphatase inactivation, seem to be dependent on a mechanism involving free radical attack, not related to lipid peroxidation.

ACKNOWLEDGEMENTS

The authors wish to thank the National Foundation for Cancer Research, Turin Workshop, and the Consiglio Nazionale delle Ricerche, Rome, for supporting this research.

REFERENCES

Benedetti, A., Casini, A.F., Ferrali, M. and Comporti, M. (1977). *Exp. Mol. Pathol.* 27, 309-323.

Benedetti, A., Casini, A.F., Ferrali, M. and Comporti, M. (1979a). *Biochem. J.* 180, 303-312.

Benedetti, A., Casini, A.F., Ferrali, M. and Comporti, M. (1979b). *Biochem. Pharmacol.* 28, 2909-2918.

Benedetti, A., Comporti, M. and Esterbauer, H. (1980). *Biochim. Biophys. Acta* 620, 281-296.

Bernheim, F., Bernheim, M.L.C. and Wilbur, K.M. (1948). *J. Biol. Chem.* 174, 257-264.

Bonkowsky, H.L., Carpenter, S.J. and Healey, J.F. (1979). *Arch. Pathol. Lab. Med.* 103, 21-29.

Buege, J.A. and Aust, S.D. (1978). *In* "Methods in Enzymology" (Eds. S. Fleischer and L. Packer) Vol.52, pp.302-310. Academic Press, New York.

Cheeseman, K. (1981). *In* "Recent Advances in Lipid Peroxidation and Tissue Injury" (Eds. T.F. Slater and A. Garner). Brunel University Biochemistry Department, London.

Chiarpotto, E., Olivero, J., Albano, E., Poli, G., Gravela, E. and Dianzani, M.U. (1981). *Experientia* 37, 396-397.

De Groot, H. and Haas, W. (1980). *FEBS Lett.* 115, 253-256.

De Toranzo, E.G.D., Diaz Gomez, M.I. and Castro, J.A. (1975). *Biochem. Biophys. Res. Commun.* 64, 823-828.

Dianzani, M.U., Gabriel, L., Gravela, E. and Paradisi, L. (1976). *In* "International Meeting on Recent Advances in Biochemical Pathology. Toxic Liver Injury" (Eds. M.U. Dianzani, G. Ugazio and L.M. Sena) pp.29-38. Minerva Medica, Torino.

Dianzani, M.U. and Ugazio, G. (1978). *In* "Biochemical Mechanisms of Liver Injury" (Ed. T.F. Slater) pp.669-707. Academic Press, London.

Esterbauer, H., Cheeseman, K., Dianzani, M.U., Poli, G. and Slater, T.F. (1981). (in press).

Glende, E.A., Hruszkewycz, A.M. and Recknagel, R.O. (1976). *Biochem. Pharmacol.* 25, 2163-2170.

Gravela, E., Poli, G., Albano, E. and Dianzani, M.U. (1977). *Exp. Mol. Pathol.* 27, 339-352.

Gravela, E., Albano, E., Dianzani, M.U., Poli, G. and Slater, T.F. (1979). *Biochem. J.* 178, 509-512.

Griffin, B.W. (1980). *In* "Microsomes, Drug Oxidations, and Chemical Carcinogenesis" (Eds. M.J. Coon, A.H. Conney, R.W. Estabrook, H.V. Gelboin, J.R. Gillette and P.J. O'Brien) Vol.1, pp.319-322. Academic Press, New York.

Griffin, B.W. and Ting, P.L. (1978). *FEBS Lett.* 89, 196-200.

Guzelian, P.S. and Swisher, R.W. (1979). *Biochem. J.* 184, 481-489.

Ham, R.G. (1965). *Proc. Natl. Acad. Sci. USA* 53, 288-291.

Heath, R.L. and Tappel, A.L. (1976). *Anal. Biochem.* 76, 184-191.

Hochstein, P. and Ernster, L. (1963). *Biochem. Biophys. Res. Commun.* 12, 388-394.

Högberg, J., Orrenius, S. and Larson, R.E. (1975a). *Eur. J. Biochem.* 50, 595-602.

Högberg, J., Moldeus, P., Arborgh, B., O'Brien, P.J. and Orrenius, S. (1975b). *Eur. J. Biochem.* 59, 457-462.

Hrycay, E.G., Gustafsson, J., Ingelman-Sundberg, M. and Ernster, L. (1975). *Biochem. Biophys. Res. Commun.* 66, 209-216.

Jose, P.J. and Slater, T.F. (1972). *Biochem. J.* 128, 141P.

Kadlubar, F.F., Morton, K.C. and Ziegler, D.M. (1973). *Biochem. Biophys. Res. Commun.* 54, 1255-1261.

Kornbrust, D.J. and Mavis, R.D. (1980). *Mol. Pharmacol.* 17, 400-407.

Koster-Albrecht, D., Kappus, H. and Remmer, H. (1978). *Toxicol. Appl. Pharmacol.* 46, 499-505.
Kupfer, D. and Orrenius, S. (1970). *Mol. Pharmacol.* 6, 221-230.
Lindstrom, T.D., Anders, M.W. and Remmer, H. (1978). *Exp. Mol. Pathol.* 28, 48-57.
Olson, J.W. and Russell, D.H. (1980). *Cancer Res.* 40, 4373-4380.
Omura, T. and Sato, R. (1964). *J. Biol. Chem.* 239, 2379-2385.
Packer, J.E., Slater, T.F. and Willson, R.L. (1978). *Life Sci.* 23, 2617-2620.
Plaa, G.L. and Witschi, H. (1976). *Ann. Rev. Pharmacol. Toxicol.* 16, 125-141.
Poli, G., Poli Chiono, M., Slater, T.F., Dianzani, M.U. and Gravela, E. (1978). *Biochem. Soc. Trans.* 6, 589-591.
Poli, G., Gravela, E., Albano, E. and Dianzani, M.U. (1979a). *Exp. Mol. Pathol.* 30, 113-127.
Poli, G., Gravela, E., Chiarpotto, E., Albano, E. and Dianzani, M.U. (1979b). *IRCS Med. Sci.* 7, 558.
Poli, G., Gravela, E., Albano, E., Chiarpotto, E., Miglietta, A. and Dianzani, M.U. (1981a). *In* "Recent Advances in Lipid Peroxidation and Tissue Injury" (Eds. T.F. Slater and A. Garner), Brunel University Biochemistry Department, London.
Poli, G., Cheeseman, K., Slater, T.F. and Dianzani, M.U. (1981b). *Chem. Biol. Interact.* 37, 13-24.
Rahimtula, A.D. and O'Brien, P.J. (1974). *Biochem. Biophys. Res. Commun.* 60, 440-447.
Sies, H. and Summer, K.H. (1975). *Eur. J. Biochem.* 57, 503-512.
Slater, T.F. (1972). "Free Radical Mechanisms in Tissue Injury" Pion Ltd., London.
Slater, T.F. (1978). *In* "Biochemical Mechanisms of Liver Injury (Ed. T.F. Slater), pp.746-801. Academic Press, London.
Slater, T.F. and Sawyer, B.C. (1969). *Biochem. J.* 111, 317-324.
Slater, T.F. and Sawyer, B.C. (1971a). *Biochem. J.* 123, 815-821.
Slater, T.F. and Sawyer, B.C. (1971b). *Biochem. J.* 123, 823-828.
Stacey, N. and Priestly, B.G. (1978). *Toxicol. Appl. Pharmacol.* 45, 41-48.
Svingen, B.A., O'Neal, F.O. and Aust, S.D. (1978). *Photochem. Photo-Biol.* 28, 803-809.
Tam, B.K. and McCay, P.B. (1970). *J. Biol. Chem.* 245, 2295-2300.
Viña, J., Hems, R. and Krebs, H.A. (1978). *Biochem. J.* 170, 627-630.
Weddle, C.C., Hornbrook, K.R. and McCay, P.B. (1976). *J. Biol. Chem.* 251, 4973-4978.
Williams-Ashman, H.G. and Canellakis, Z.N. (1979). *Perspect. Biol. Med.* 22, 421-453.
Wills, E.D. (1971). *Biochem. J.* 123, 983-991.

DISCUSSION

Lohmann: In one of your slides you showed the effect of ferrous sulphate and ferric chloride; ferric chloride did not give any effect at all, while ferrous sulphate gave some effect. Do you think this might depend on the oxidation state of the iron or does it depend on the anion used? The second question is concerned with the effect you observed when you added ascorbate. How can you explain the stimulatory effect of ascorbate in the case of $FeSO_4$ but not in the case of $FeCl_3$?

Poli: First of all, the effect of ferric chloride at these concentrations is very small, perhaps not significant, but it is possible to see a stimulation of lipid peroxidation if I increase the concentration of ferric chloride. I don't know how, clearly, to explain the difference in the stimulation between ferric and ferrous iron. The ratio between the stimulation of lipid peroxidation between ferrous iron and ferric iron is higher in the cell system than that obtained with microsomes, suggesting perhaps some mechanism inhibiting the reduction of iron chloride by microsomal reductase.

Lohmann: Ferrous sulphate gave a better effect than ferric chloride. Why did you use then in your other investigations ferric chloride and not ferrous sulphate?

Poli: I started with ferric chloride because of reports in the literature and so as to be able to compare my results with them. At the beginning actually I started with ADP/ferric iron to compare my data with the data of Hogberg, Orrenius and various other groups working on lipid peroxidation induced by ADP/ferric iron. Afterwards, I changed my system slighly since ADP alone, by a mechanism I cannot so far explain, gave a non-specific effect on my protein/lipoprotein system - the main system I'm interested in.

Magee: The same question I was going to ask Mr Cheeseman I'll ask Dr Poli. I wonder if you've ever done any comparative studies with chloroform as well as carbon tetrachloride, because several groups, including Dr Sidney Weinhouse in our institute, have demonstrated the formation of phosgene from chloroform, and I wonder if this could be an intermediary in carbon tetrachloride metabolism and whether it might have any significance?

Poli: We haven't done any experiments on chloroform. It's a good suggestion, but we haven't done that.

Slater: Shall I reply for Mr Cheeseman? In relation to microsomes, of course we looked at chloroform - you'll see a slide on it in my lecture. The short answer is that $CHCl_3$ stimulates lipid peroxidation much more slowly compared with carbon tetrachloride. I will also refer to phosgene in my talk so perhaps we could come back to that. One feature, perhaps, that I think is of importance, and which comes out of Pippo Poli's paper, is that when you stimulate lipid peroxidation in microsomes or isolated liver cells in different ways, there appears to be different patterns of aldehydes, qualitatively, although we can't at the moment comment quantitatively on the significance of these differences. But the fact is, there does appear to be qualitative differences and yet peroxidation is routinely measured by the thiobarbituric acid reaction which, as Professor Esterbauer yesterday told us, is largely malonaldehyde. And so it raises, I think, the general point that the biological effects of peroxidation may reflect these different patterns of aldehydes. We heard from Professor Dianzani yesterday some of the aldehydes have specific effects at micromolar concentrations and yet in terms of our routine methods of analysis we measure malonaldehyde. In consequence, we may actually be seeing the same amount of malonaldehyde production but widely differing varieties of other aldehydes which will affect the cell or microsomes in different ways.

Swartz: This is a question, I think, primarily of my ignorance. When one makes that kind of analysis can confusion arise from the fact that the cell, or even the microsomes, may metabolise some of the aldehydes? If so, that which one sees in such an analysis is not necessarily what has been produced, but what has been produced minus what has been converted. If one observes different patterns of production of aldehydes is it possible to interpret these results?

Slater: I think you've put your finger with your usual unerring accuracy on a very difficult question. In the case of washed unsupplemented microsomes there appears to be a very small amount of aldehyde metabolism at least in the examples that we've tested. With homogenates, whole cells, or whole organs, of course metabolism is vastly increased and what is more there appears to be different routes of metabolism. In addition, there is the non-enzymic utilisation of aldehydes as discussed by Professor Esterbauer yesterday. So I'm sure you are absolutely right that what is measured at least in organised systems like isolated hepatocytes, is always the sum of production versus utilisation.

Asmus: I have one question in connection with some of your data. You showed the effect of promethazine which inhibited several of the processes which you were talking about. Would you think that this effect is due to the reaction of the $CCl_3O_2^{\cdot}$ radical with promethazine in the case of the carbon tetrachloride?

Poli: I think promethazine probably reacts with the peroxy radical, $CCl_3O_2^{\cdot}$ in the case of its protection on glucose-6-phosphatase derangement. My opinion is that the trichloromethyl radical is more important in covalent binding of carbon tetrachloride, rather than lipid peroxidation which is mediated by the trichloromethyl peroxy radical, and in the derangement of protein/lipoprotein secretion and perhaps in other cell functions.

Asmus: Well, if it was this reaction it is a process which occurs with a rate constant of $5.5 \times 10^8\ M^{-1}s^{-1}$ for the reaction of $CCl_3O_2^{\cdot}$ with promethazine. If you take metiazinic acid the reaction is even faster ($k = 1.3 \times 10^9\ M^{-1}s^{-1}$) (Bahnemann, 1981; Bahnemann, D., Asmus, K.-D. and Willson, R.L., to be published). So if the reaction of the $CCl_3O_2^{\cdot}$ radical with promethazine is responsible for the observed effect, you might try metiazinic acid which is much more easily oxidised, and you should see an enhanced effect.

Poli: I see, thank you.

Slater: Can we ask Mr Searle if he has tried metiazinic acid in microsomal lipid peroxidation systems?

Searle: Yes, I tried the effects of different phenothiazines on ferrous sulphate/cysteine stimulated lipid peroxidation. I think the order of effectiveness is promethazine, chlorpromazine, then metiazinic acid; so it would seem to be the other way round and not related to the rate constant in these circumstances.

Asmus: This could be because radical cations with oxidising properties are produced when you oxidise the phenothiazines, and in this case the promethazine radical cation is the best oxidant. It has an oxidation potential of 1.021 (Bahnemann, 1981; Bahnemann, D., Asmus, K.-D. and Willson, R.L., to be published). The radical cations from the other compounds are less effective, so you might think in terms of a consecutive reaction of the oxidised form, i.e. of the radical cation of the phenothiazines.

Willson: I think there's another point also. I'm not sure of the partition coefficients of these compounds. Some of them are charged and the accessibility of these compounds to a particularly vulnerable site in the cell is going to be most important. Their protective action will be partially dependent on the redox potential and kinetic parameters but on the other hand, also with the actual concentration of the particular compound at the vulnerable site. Little information is available about this.

Slater: Going back to Professor Asmus' point we were rather worried a year or two ago as to whether the failure of promethazine to protect against some of the changes seen by Pippo Poli who was working here at the time, perhaps reflected a biologically damaging action of the promethazine radical cation. In other words, scavenging the first entity, the trichloromethyl peroxy radical and in the process forming the promethazine radical, that was itself damaging. So what we did was to prepare this in two or three different ways and add it to microsomes and look at various changes in enzymes and it appears to be relatively inactive.

Willson: There are reports in the literature of the chlorpromazine radical cation inactivating enzymes (Levy and Burbridge, 1967; Akera and Brody, 1968, 1969, 1970, 1972).

Asmus: Well, these radical cations may readily react with vitamin E, vitamin C and cysteine, for example. If I say "react readily" that means with rate constants which are at least close to the diffusion limit, i.e. above 10^7. So chemically these radical cations are quite reactive (Bahnemann, 1981; Bahnemann, D., Asmus, K.D. and Willson, R. L., to be published).

Slater: I think what we looked at was just the decrease of cytochrome P_{450} and glucose-6-phosphatase; I cannot remember the concentrations of the radical cations that we added but they certainly weren't up in the millimolar range which we felt was too high to be realistic. Since we have a little time in hand, perhaps we could broaden the discussion to general aspects of lipid peroxidation.

Symons: Can I raise a point on the carbon tetrachloride story we heard earlier: it seems to me that the most difficult step to understand, and at the same time the key-step, is the actual initial attack on the carbon tetrachloride. You have shown conclusively that you get trichloromethyl radicals; I don't think anyone would argue about that and it's clear from several people's work that if you've got trichloromethyl radicals you must get some trichloromethylperoxy radicals. It is also clear that, in your system, the latter step is not particularly efficient because other things compete with the oxygen despite the fact that it reacts very rapidly. The difficult step is the generation of the trichloromethyl radical in the first place. Now, I take your point that it looks like an electron donation to make the radical - that's the most likely method of forming it. I certainly appreciate that solvated electrons will generate trichloromethyl radicals, but the question is will transition metal complexes react with carbon tetrachloride to give trichloromethyl radicals? Are there references in the straight chemical literature where strongly electron donating complexes react with carbon tetrachloride to give trichloromethyl radicals?

Willson: I agree with you that it is very difficult to see how carbon tetrachloride interacts with a simple iron complex but there is an indirect method how this can be achieved. The production of hydroxyl radicals can occur by an iron-catalysed reaction as you know. You can take an iron-complex as your electron donor and generate the hydroxyl radical which can then react with an alcohol or some other compound which yields an α-hydroxy radical. This radical can be oxidised by carbon tetrachloride to give the trichloromethyl radical and this can react with oxygen to give trichloromethyl peroxy radical. This can inactivate enzymes. So it's an indirect source but there must be a host of organic compounds in the cell like alcohols, sugars, for instance, that could enter into this type of reaction with carbon tetrachloride.

Symons: Well yes, but then are we really at that stage talking about electron transfer? I mean you can write the reaction: $R^{\bullet} + CCl_4 \rightarrow RCl + CCl_3^{\bullet}$, which is then homolytic displacement of trichloromethyl radical from carbon tetrachloride - is that perhaps not what is happening?

Willson: I would suggest that it *is* an electron transfer reaction. If it's an α-hydroxyl radical transferring electrons to carbon tetrachloride, a cation of some sort is left, but then this breaks down to give, in the case of the isopropanol radical, acetone. We can write the equation as an electron transfer reaction:

$$CH_3C(OH)CH_3^{\bullet} + CCl_4 \rightarrow CH_3C(OH)CH_3^{+} + CCl_4^{\bullet -}$$

Symons: But the alternative would be to chlorinate your alcohol radical to give you a chloro-alcohol radical and not, initially, the chloride ion. That can also break down to give you HCl.

Asmus: That would go slower because you have the reaction of the isopropanol radical, for example, with carbon tetrachloride. The kinetics of the chloride ion formation as measured by pulse radiolysis conductivity measurements show that as soon as the reaction occurs HCl is formed (Koster and Asmus, 1971). I see no other interpretation of these data than the dissociative electron transfer.

Symons: Well, I come back then to my first point if I may. This is a very long way round to get your trichloromethyl radical. You are now invoking hydrogen peroxide in the first case to get the hydroxyl radical, which is a tremendously reactive species - it's not going to wait around for carbon tetrachloride to come along and so on. You've got a lot of steps in the chain. Is there not a metal complex which can directly form $CCl_3^{\bullet}$?

Willson: Well, I think there must be but we've tried to look at the reaction of carbon tetrachloride, for instance, with a simple quinone electron donor of very low redox potential like anthrasemiquinone and we have not been able to observe it. This does not necessarily mean that it does not go: it just means that it is too slow for the pulse radiolysis technique. But the difficulty with these reactions is not knowing the polarity of the environment. In theory most of these reactions should occur because they are dissociative electron capture and therefore not equilibria. For instance, superoxide anion plus carbon tetrachloride should give O_2 plus the trichloromethyl radical plus chloride ion. This has not been observed in water as yet but it does occur in dimethyl sulphoxide. It depends very much on the polarity or the dielectric constant of the environment whether these reactions occur (Shenoy *et al.*, 1975).

Symons: In fact, if you're talking about a lipid medium, which I believe is the case for carbon tetrachloride, what your problem really is, is how to cope with the chloride ion because that's going to be very unhappy in the lipid medium: it wants an aqueous medium. I would suggest, if it does happen via a metal complex, that the chloride remains bound to the metal. In other words, that iron plus carbon tetrachloride goes to iron chloride plus trichloromethyl radical. That would overcome the solvation problem of the chloride ion and probably lower the redox potential.

Slater: Could I try to summarise what we feel about this. I think there is some good evidence now in the literature, that you can get a direct electron transfer between the P_{450}-iron and the carbon tetrachloride leading to the $CCl_3^{\cdot}$ and CCl_2 products. There is evidence that electron transfer can occur from the flavoprotein but not directly to carbon tetrachloride, as far as we are aware. For many years I've been postulating a diversion through a non-heme iron-sulphur complex. What we know from recent studies, and Dr Willson will summarise them, is that if we can produce radicals like superoxide or the hydroxyl radical, provided we have the right environment in terms of substances that can react with oxidising species like hydroxyl radical and become in the processes radicals that can react with carbon tetrachloride, then you have another route to trichloromethyl radical production. But your point about the iron complex is a very good one and I think my only conclusion at the moment is there seems to be a whole range of reactions that can actually generate trichloromethyl radical, either by dissociative electron capture, or by homolysis, or by reaction indirectly with secondary radicals. A study relevant to Professor Symon's question has been made by Hájak *et al.* (1980) who demonstrated a metal oxide induced redox chain addition of CCl_4 to a carbon-carbon double bond over the temperature range 76-200°C.

REFERENCES to Discussion

Akera, T. and Brody, T.M. (1968). *Molec. Pharmacol.* 4, 600-612.
Akera, T. and Brody, T.M. (1969). *Molec. Pharmacol.* 5, 605-614.
Akera, T. and Brody, T.M. (1970). *Molec. Pharmacol.* 6, 557-563.
Akera, T. and Brody, T.M. (1972). *Biochem. Pharmacol.* 21, 1403-1411.
Bahnemann, D. (1981). Ph.D. Thesis, Technical University of Berlin.
Hajek, M., Silhavy, P. and Malek, J. (1980). *Collection Czech. Chem. Commun.* 45, 3488-3501.
Koster, R. and Asmus, K.-D. (1971). *Z. Naturforsch.* 266, 1104-1108.
Levy, L. and Burbridge, T.N. (1967). *Biochem. Pharmacol.* 16, 1249-1260.
Shenoy, M.A., George, K.G., Singh, B.B. and Gopal-Ayengar, A.R. (1975). *Int. J. Radiat. Biol.* 28, 519-526.

Activation of Carbon Tetrachloride: Chemical Principles and Biological Significance

T.F. SLATER

INTRODUCTION

In this article I will concentrate upon work relating to the metabolic activation of carbon tetrachloride (CCl_4): this will allow me to discuss a number of concepts that are of general importance to biochemical pathology.

The administration of a single dose of CCl_4 to an adult rat (or to many other species of animal) produces a centrilobular necrosis and fatty degeneration of the liver (Cameron and Karunaratne, 1936). Since the early 1960s it has been realised that some so-called "protective agents" can have markedly beneficial effects on the extent of necrosis due to CCl_4-toxicity, whilst not affecting overmuch those cellular disturbances that lead to triglyceride accumulation (Rees and Spector, 1961; Rees and Shotlander, 1963). Moreover, it is well known that many agents can produce a fatty liver without associated liver necrosis (see Dianzani, 1978); fat accumulation in the liver is generally regarded as an essentially reversible phenomenon, whereas necrosis involves the irreversible death of a group of cells. These points are the main justification for considering that the pathways resulting in necrosis or fatty degeneration are distinguishable, at least to some extent, and may be experimentally investigated in separate ways. In this paper I will not consider those aspects related to the onset of fatty degeneration: a comprehensive and cogently argued review of that subject has been given by Dianzani (1978).

EARLY VIEWS ON THE BIOTRANSFORMATION OF $CHCl_3$ AND CCl_4

Most of the early studies in this area were directed towards an understanding of the necrogenic action of $CHCl_3$ on the liver. Detailed histopathological studies of this toxic action of $CHCl_3$ had been made by Wells (1908) and Whipple and Sperry (1909). In 1911 Muller made the interesting suggestion that $CHCl_3$ was toxic to the liver as a result of its conversion to phosgene:

$$2CHCl_3 + O_2 \longrightarrow 2COCl_2 + 2HCl$$

This reaction readily occurs, for example, in bright sunlight, and a small proportion of ethanol (0.5 - 1% v/v) is normally added to $CHCl_3$ to reduce the formation of $COCl_2$. The suggestion of Muller (1911) is of current interest in relation to recent demonstrations that both $CHCl_3$ and CCl_4 form small amounts of $COCl_2$ in liver microsomal suspensions (Mansuy *et al.*, 1977a; Pohl *et al.*, 1979; Shah *et al.*, 1979); the $COCl_2$ was identified by reacting it with an excess of cysteine to form a 2-oxo-thiazolidine-4-carboxylic acid:

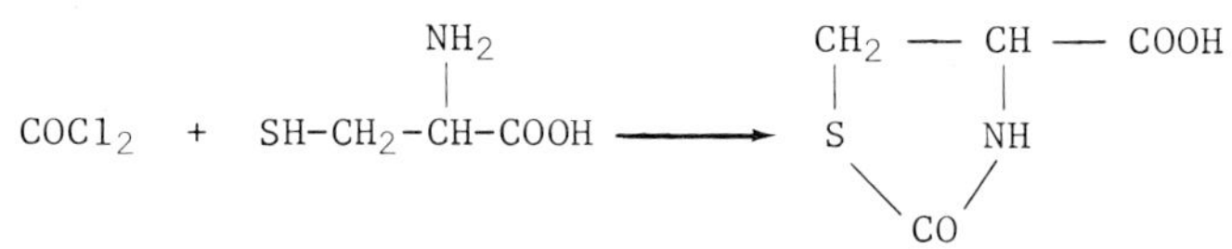

In addition, as will be discussed later in much more detail, the fast reaction technique of pulse radiolysis indicates that phosgene may arise from the following free radical reactions (Packer *et al.*, 1978):

$$CCl_3^{\bullet} + O_2 \longrightarrow CCl_3O_2^{\bullet} \ (+\ RH) \longrightarrow CCl_3O_2H + R^{\bullet}$$

$$CCl_3O_2H \longrightarrow COCl_2 + HOCl$$

Graham (1915) took the suggestion of Muller (1911) to a further stage by relating the toxicity of $CHCl_3$ to the production of hydrochloric acid, formed by rapid, spontaneous hydrolysis of phosgene:

$$CHCl_3 \longrightarrow COCl_2 \xrightarrow{H_2O} CO_2 + 2HCl$$

In this way $CHCl_3$ produces three molar proportions of HCl :

$$2CHCl_3 + O_2 \longrightarrow 2COCl_2 + 2HCl$$

$$2COCl_2 + 2H_2O \longrightarrow 2CO_2 + 4HCl$$

Graham (1915) concluded that the known order of liver toxicity demonstrated by CH_2Cl_2, $CHCl_3$ and CCl_4 was a result of the different molar proportions of HCl produced on hydrolysis. He reported that the intravenous injection of large amounts of alkaline solution could inhibit the development of necrosis caused by $CHCl_3$. The direct addition of even quite high concentrations of phosgene to microsomal suspensions, however, is not accompanied by disturbances characteristic of CCl_4-intoxication (e.g. depression of glucose-6-phosphatase activity; destruction of cytochrome P_{450}); it appears, in consequence, that phosgene *per se* is not a major contributor to such features of the overall injury (Waller and Recknagel, 1980).

The major advance in the understanding of the bioactivation of these compounds came through the work of Butler (1961) who suggested that CCl_4 toxicity was associated with the formation of the free radical trichloromethyl ($CCl_3^{\bullet}$). He was able to detect $CHCl_3$ in the expired air of dogs that had been dosed with CCl_4; the $CHCl_3$ presumably coming from a hydrogen-abstraction reaction:

$$CCl_3^{\bullet} + RH \longrightarrow CHCl_3 + R^{\bullet}$$

Moreover, Butler demonstrated that homogenates of mouse liver, heart, brain, lung, kidney and muscle could also produce $CHCl_3$ from CCl_4 during 24 h incubation at 37°C. Mouse liver homogenate that was pre-heated for 45 min at 100°C also formed some $CHCl_3$ from CCl_4, having approx. 30% the activity of fresh homogenate in this respect. Solutions of thiols (GSH, cysteine) and ascorbic acid were found to convert CCl_4 to $CHCl_3$ under the incubation conditions used. Butler's work pointed to a biotransformation of CCl_4 via a $CCl_3^{\bullet}$ free radical to a product $CHCl_3$; his results suggested that such a reaction pathway could occur in tissue homogenates by both enzymic and non-enzymic mechanisms.

Shortly after Butler's work, several other groups reported that CCl_4 and $CHCl_3$ are metabolised by liver samples *in vitro* and by rats *in vivo* with the production of CO_2 and, in the case of CCl_4, to $CHCl_3$; these studies are summarised by Recknagel (1967) and Slater (1972).

These metabolic studies were supplemented by experiments showing that $[^{14}C]CCl_4$ was covalently bound to liver cell fractions (e.g. phospholipids), and that at least some of the $[^{14}C,^{36}Cl]CCl_4$ bound in the proportions of $^{14}C/^{36}Cl$ of 1:3 (Reynolds, 1967 and Gordis, 1969; see Recknagel and Glende, 1973 for background references).

During the 1960s therefore, a considerable amount of evidence was collected to justify the view that CCl_4 (and $CHCl_3$) undergo metabolic biotransformation. The association between such a metabolism and the toxic properties of CCl_4 was clearly emphasised by Slater (1966a), Recknagel and Ghoshal (1966) and McLean and McLean (1966).

LIPID PEROXIDATION

Butler's suggestion that CCl_4 is metabolised in the liver to a free radical product ($CCl_3^{\bullet}$), which was responsible for a significant part of the subsequent damage, was seized upon quickly by several groups of investigators when it was found that CCl_4 stimulated lipid peroxidation, a free radical process, in liver samples. The first reports demonstrated this effect in liver homogenates (Comporti, 1964; Comporti *et al.*, 1965); the effect was confirmed in microsomes plus cell sap suspensions by Ghoshal and Recknagel (1965), and in washed microsomes provided with a source of NADPH (Slater, 1966b, 1967). A link between the liver toxicities of CCl_4 and of ethanol with lipid peroxidation had been suggested by Di Luzio and Costales (1965) on the basis of earlier work demonstrating protective action by various antioxidants (Hove, 1948, 1953; Gallagher, 1961; Di Luzio, 1963). In the context of the stimulation of lipid peroxidation by CCl_4 in liver cell fractions, it is germane to the story to mention the early work of Hove (1953), who showed that CCl_4 could exert a pro-oxidant effect on autoxidising lipid. The background to these developments is well summarised by Recknagel (1967).

The view that the stimulation of lipid peroxidation by CCl_4 resulted from a metabolic activation to $CCl_3^{\bullet}$, followed by initiation of the chain reaction by the action of $CCl_3^{\bullet}$ on polyunsaturated fatty acids

(PUFA), was strengthened (i) by the finding (Slater and Sawyer, 1970) that the stimulation was proportional to the square-root of the CCl_4 concentration, as expected for a free radical initiator; and (ii) that the stimulation found in a series of halogenomethanes was proportional to the bond dissociation energies required for free radical production (Slater and Sawyer, 1970). Activation of CCl_4 to $CCl_3^{\cdot}$ was suggested to involve the microsomal NADPH-cytochrome P_{450} electron transport chain (NADPH-P_{450} chain) because of (i) the increasing emphasis on the importance of this enzyme sequence in metabolising foreign substances (see Brodie *et al.*, 1958) at that time; (ii) the main localisation of the NADPH-P_{450} chain in liver tissue (for example, see a topical report by Knecht, 1966), the site of major damage caused by CCl_4; (iii) the known occurrence of free radical moieties in the endoplasmic reticulum, flavosemiquinones for example, that could act as sites for one-electron transfer (Slater, 1966a); and (iv) the increased toxicity of CCl_4 in rats that had been pre-treated with phenobarbital, a procedure known to induce cytochrome P_{450} (McLean and McLean, 1966).

Additional evidence in favour of a free radical process being important in the development of CCl_4-mediated liver injury came from studies with a number of agents that could protect against certain features of the injury. Many of these agents were well known antioxidants and/or free radical scavengers (see Recknagel, 1967; Slater, 1966a, 1978 for background references). It is now well recognised, however, that most if not all of such agents have more than one mode of action on complex biological systems *in vitro*, and especially on whole animals. To illustrate this latter point, the detailed analysis by Reddrop *et al.* (1981a,b) of the effects of promethazine on CCl_4-mediated liver injury *in vivo* can be cited. It is now clear that many factors such as decreased absorption of the toxic agent, changes in body temperature, interference with the lipid-protein membrane mosaic, oxidation of NADPH, etc., may play important roles in such protective effects, in addition to the underlying free radical scavenging action. A diagrammatic view of the variety of such mechanisms that can operate in protection is shown in Fig. 1.

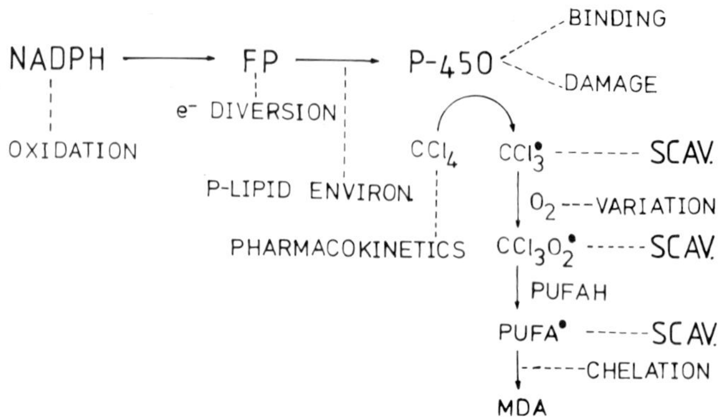

FIG. 1 This illustrates the variety of protective mechanisms that may operate in a situation where a toxic agent (e.g. CCl_4) is metabolically activated via cytochrome P_{450} to a free radical product that stimulates lipid peroxidation. Abbreviations: FP, flavoprotein; scav., free radical scavenger; PUFAH, polyunsaturated fatty acid; MDA, malonaldehyde. The protective mechanisms involve (i) oxidation of the reduced nucleotide (NADPH); (ii) diversion of electron flow from the flavoprotein into other pathways; (iii) changes in the phospholipid environment, including changes in fluidity, that affect the FP-P_{450} coupling; (iv) factors affecting the uptake, distribution and excretion of the toxic agent (called pharmacokinetic effects here); (v) competitive binding and/or destruction of P_{450}; (vi) scavenging of the activated free radical; (vii) variation in the O_2 tension that can affect the formation of more electrophilic species such as $CCl_3O_2^{\bullet}$; (viii) variation in the PUFA content; (ix) and effects on the peroxidative breakdown of the PUFA$^{\bullet}$ free radical to various products including MDA.

LOCUS OF ACTIVATION OF CCl_4

The ideas and developments discussed above led to the view in the late 1960s that CCl_4 was metabolised by the NADPH-P_{450} chain to a free radical product, the trichloromethyl radical; moreover, it was the general view that the locus of activation was cytochrome P_{450} itself. An interaction of CCl_4 with P_{450} to give a Type I difference spectrum had been demonstrated by McLean (1967), and a number of other studies were consistent with a P_{450}-locus (for example, see Glende, 1972; Suarez and Bhonsle, 1976; Villarruel *et al.*, 1977; Masuda and Murano, 1978). However, attempts to selectively block the P_{450}-site or the flavoprotein site with selective inhibitors (Slater and Sawyer, 1971) gave conflicting results that pointed to a locus of activation of CCl_4 (at least, an activation related to the stimulation of lipid

TABLE 1 Effects of free radical scavengers and other agents on various aspects of the interactions of CCl_4 with rat liver microsomes

Agent	Concn. (μM)	Lipid peroxidation (%)†	Aminopyrene demethylation (%)†	Covalent binding (%)†
Promethazine	10	15	90	85
Propyl gallate	10	15	133	88
Vitamin K_3	4	8	100	81
p-CMB	100	139	20	70
SKF.525A	200	74	40	148
Pyrazole	5×10^3	106	35	103
Dodecyl sulphate	10	143	76	69
DMSO	2.3×10^6	215	27*	112
Codeine	5×10^3	96	24	70
GSH	100	54	100	51
	500	37	-	13

*1.4 M. † Values are % of controls.

It can be seen that the agents illustrated have differing effects on (i) the CCl_4-stimulated lipid peroxidation; (ii) the demethylation of aminopyrene; and (iii) covalent binding of $^{14}C-CCl_4$ to microsomal protein. For experimental details see Slater (1972), Slater and Sawyer (1971) and Cheeseman (1982).

peroxidation) proximal to P_{450}. Many more inhibitors have been studied in this respect in the last few years and some of these data are given in Table 1. A comprehensive discussion concerning the locus of activation of CCl_4 on the NADPH-P_{450} chain has been given recently (Slater, 1981a). The conclusion reached (Slater, 1981a) was that (i) more than locus of activation may occur; one proximal to P_{450}, for instance, and one on P_{450} itself; (ii) different forms of P_{450} exist that are differentially susceptible to the inhibitors used and are differentially active in metabolising CCl_4 (see Head *et al.*, 1980; McCay *et al.*, 1980a) and/or (iii) the inhibitors used in the studies *in vitro* cause artificial routes of electron flow out from the NADPH-P_{450} chain. The overall situation becomes even more complex to analyse when the effects of the inhibitors on covalent binding from

$[^{14}C]CCl_4$ are considered (see Slater, 1981a); this aspect is referred to by Cheeseman (1982) in this symposium.

An early effect of CCl_4 *in vivo* in the rat was shown to be a destruction of NADPH (Slater *et al.*, 1964); this phenomenon appeared to be a genuine destruction rather than oxidation to $NADP^+$ since the total of NADPH + $NADP^+$ also decreased. A possible mechanism for this effect was suggested by the work of Slater and Jose (quoted in Slater, 1972) who produced $CCl_3^{\bullet}$ photochemically and found that this was associated with a rapid loss of NADPH. Since the decrease in NADPH *in vivo* is prevented by agents that attenuate necrosis (Slater *et al.*, 1966) it is possible that the decreased NADPH content is an important feature of the necrogenic series of reactions. Moreover, since the decrease in NADPH is about 30% of the total liver's content within 1-2 h of intoxication with CCl_4 (Slater *et al.*, 1964), and since only a similar proportion of liver cells become necrotic, then it may be that in the centrilobular regions of the liver lobules there is a virtual total destruction of NADPH, with all the serious consequences for cell metabolism that this would entail.

DEMONSTRATION OF THE FORMATION OF $CCl_3^{\bullet}$

It can be realised from the above discussion that, by the early 1970s, there were many references in the literature to the metabolic activation of CCl_4 to $CCl_3^{\bullet}$ by the NADPH-P_{450} chain. It was natural, therefore, to try to obtain substantial evidence for the formation of $CCl_3^{\bullet}$ by the liver NADPH-P_{450} chain both *in vitro* and *in vivo*. After all, the suggested occurrence of such a metabolic intermediate as proposed in many authoritative papers, and in numerous review lectures, is not a satisfactory substitute for fact.

Some reasonably convincing *indirect* evidence for the formation of $CCl_3^{\bullet}$ had been obtained: the formation of C_2Cl_6 as a by-product of the metabolism of CCl_4 (Fowler, 1969) is best seen as a free radical dimerisation process:

$$CCl_3^{\bullet} + CCl_3^{\bullet} \longrightarrow C_2Cl_6$$

Further, double-label radioisotope experiments with $[^{14}C,^{36}Cl]CCl_4$ gave results for covalent binding that were consistent with the fragment bound being $CCl_3^{\bullet}$ (Reynolds, 1967; Gordis, 1969).

Attempts to demonstrate the formation of $CCl_3^{\bullet}$ directly by electron spin resonance (ESR) spectroscopy were not successful, however. The reasons for this lack of success (for discussion and references see Ingall *et al.*, 1978) probably relate to the low steady-state concentration of $CCl_3^{\bullet}$ in biological systems due, in turn, to a low rate of production of the free radical, and a high chemical reactivity of $CCl_3^{\bullet}$ that leads to its rapid disappearance.

Thus, by the mid-1970s there was a compelling requirement to obtain hard evidence for the formation of $CCl_3^{\bullet}$ by the NADPH-P_{450} chain, and there was a similar requirement for quantitative kinetic data on the chemical reactivity of this presumed metabolic intermediate. To provide useful data on these aspects we turned to the technique of pulse radiolysis (see Willson and Slater, 1975; Willson, 1978).

PULSE RADIOLYSIS

Details of this technique and application to biologically important radical species can be found in Willson (1978) and will be elaborated in the following paper of this Symposium (Willson, 1982). Using pulse radiolysis it is possible to study the interactions of $CCl_3^{\bullet}$ with selected molecular species (e.g. amino acids, nucleotide bases, PUFA, scavengers, etc.), and to obtain quantitative rate data for such reactions. The $CCl_3^{\bullet}$ free radicals can be produced by the reactions shown in Fig. 2 involving (i) isopropanol-acetone-water mixtures; (ii) *t*-butanol and (iii) direct radiolysis (see Symons *et al.*, 1981) of pure CCl_4

When $CCl_3^{\bullet}$ was studied under *strictly anaerobic* conditions it was found (Packer *et al.*, 1978) that $CCl_3^{\bullet}$ is not chemically *very* reactive with most other molecular species tested, except dioxygen. A rapid reaction (approaching diffusion control) of $CCl_3^{\bullet}$ with dioxygen occurs, however, that yields a product substantially more reactive as an electrophile; the product has properties consistent with the $CCl_3O_2^{\bullet}$ peroxy-radical. Some values for the rate constants of $CCl_3O_2^{\bullet}$ with various substances are shown in Table 2. It can be seen that

(a)

$$H_2O \rightsquigarrow e^-_{aq},\ OH^\bullet,\ H^\bullet \qquad \text{(i)}$$

$$CCl_4 + e^-_{aq} \longrightarrow CCl_3^\bullet + Cl^- \qquad \text{(ii)}$$

$$OH^\bullet + (CH_3)_3COH \longrightarrow (CH_3)_2\text{-}C(^\bullet CH_2)\text{-}OH + H_2O \qquad \text{(iii)}$$

(b)

$$H_2O \rightsquigarrow e^-_{aq},\ OH^\bullet,\ H^\bullet \qquad \text{(iv)}$$

$$H^\bullet \text{ or } OH^\bullet + CH_3CHOH\,CH_3 \longrightarrow (CH_3)_2\,\overset{\bullet}{C}(OH) + H_2 \text{ (or } H_2O) \qquad \text{(v)}$$

$$e^-_{aq} + CH_3CO\,CH_3 \longrightarrow CH_3\overset{\bullet}{\overline{CO}}\,CH_3 \qquad \text{(vi)}$$

$$CH_3\overset{\bullet}{\overline{CO}}\,CH_3 + H_2O \longrightarrow (CH_3)_3\,\overset{\bullet}{C}\,(OH) + OH^- \qquad \text{(vii)}$$

$$(CH_3)_2\,\overset{\bullet}{C}\,(OH) + CCl_4 \longrightarrow (CH_3)_2\,CO + CCl_3^\bullet + Cl^- + H^+ \qquad \text{(viii)}$$

FIG. 2 Pulse radiolysis of CCl_4 in (a) aqueous *t*-butanol and (b) aqueous acetone and isopropanol. Reactions (i) and (iv) show the production of free radicals and the hydrated electron by high energy irradiation of water. In (iii) the $OH^\cdot$ are removed by reaction with *t*-butanol; the yield of $H^\cdot$ from (i) is small under these conditions. In (v) the product is the isopropanol radical that interacts with CCl_4 as shown in (viii).

decreasing the number of chlorine atoms in $(CH_3)_{3-n}Hal_nO_2^\cdot$ decreases reactivity (Packer *et al.*, 1980). It is also important to note the very rapid reaction of $CCl_3O_2^\cdot$ with some amino acids, and with so-called selective singlet oxygen quenchers such as β-carotene and diphenylfuran (Packer *et al.*, 1981).

The work with pulse radiolysis has led to the view (see Slater, 1981b) that the local concentration of dioxygen in the region of CCl_4 activation may be of critical importance in deciding whether the activated product $CCl_3^\cdot$ goes via covalent binding or, after reaction with O_2, initiates lipid peroxidation (Fig. 3). Clearly, the formation of *two* relatively reactive species ($CCl_3^\cdot$ and $CCl_3O_2^\cdot$) may help substantially in understanding the different effects of metabolic

TABLE 2 Rate constants for some reactions of $CCl_3O_2^{\bullet}$ and related free radicals with various biologically interesting compounds.

	pH	Rate of reaction M^{-1} s^{-1}			
		$CCl_3O_2^{\bullet}$	$CCl_2HO_2^{\bullet}$	$CClH_2O_2^{\bullet}$	$CH_3O_2^{\bullet}$
Promethazine	7	5×10^8	6.7×10^6	3.6×10^7	no reaction detected
Ascorbic acid	7	2×10^8	2.6×10^8	9×10^7	2.2×10^6
Cysteine	12	5×10^7			
Tyrosine	12	1.6×10^8			
Tryptophan	7	10^8			
Arachidonic acid	7	6×10^6			
β-carotene	7	1.5×10^9			
Diphenylfuran	7	6×10^7			

The data are from Packer *et al.* (1978, 1980, 1981) and Slater (1981a).

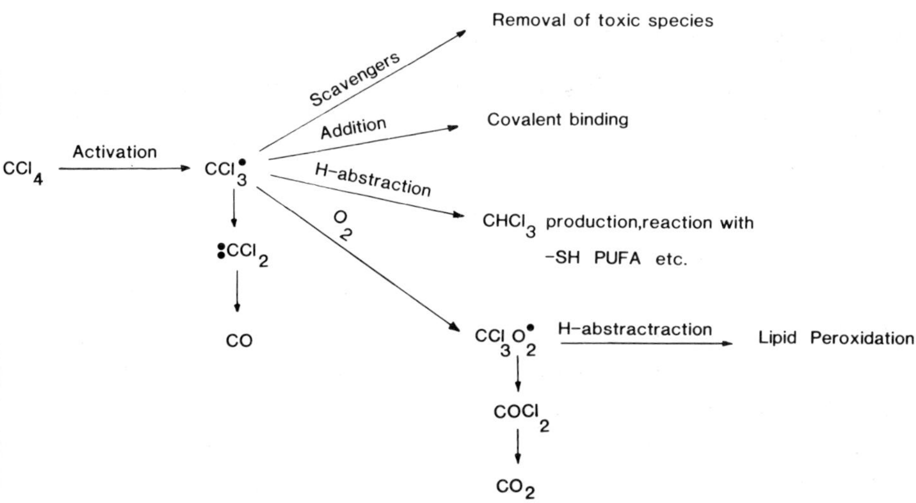

FIG. 3 The activation of CCl_4 to the trichloromethyl free radical ($CCl_3^{\bullet}$) is shown followed by a variety of reactions including (a) the addition of oxygen to yield the trichloromethyl peroxy radical; (b) dechlorination via the carbene to carbon monoxide; and (c) covalent binding. Since the reactions with O_2 is very rapid, then the relative proportions of the different pathways shown will have a strong dependence on the local O_2 concentration.

inhibitors on covalent binding and on the stimulation of lipid peroxidation (see Cheeseman, 1982).

SPIN TRAPPING OF $CCl_3^{\cdot}$

Although direct ESR spectroscopy of liver samples was not successful in demonstrating the occurrence of $CCl_3^{\cdot}$ as a metabolic intermediate (see above), the development of spin trapping techniques afforded new hope (for review of this technique see Jantzen, 1980). Our first efforts with this technique commenced in 1976 in collaborative work with Professor Anton Stier. In those early studies we used methylnitroso-propane (MNP) as the trap, and we found a strong triplet ESR signal shortly after adding CCl_4 to a microsome suspension containing NADPH (Fig. 4); no significant signal occurred without CCl_4, or in the absence of NADPH, and a much smaller response was obtained with $CHCl_3$. However, the triplet signal was not affected by using $[^{13}C]CCl_4$ in place of $^{12}CCl_4$ and this led us to the conclusion that we had not trapped $CCl_3^{\cdot}$ itself but a secondary lipid radical or even $CCl_3O_2^{\cdot}$ (Ingall *et al.*, 1978). Attempts conclusively to trap $CCl_3^{\cdot}$ after generating it anaerobically by high energy radiation gave a product that showed ^{13}C-splitting (Ingall *et al.*, 1978) and a narrow nitrogen hyperfine structure. It is realised now, however, that the product was an acyl adduct derived from $CCl_3^{\cdot}$ and MNP by degradative reactions (see Janzen, 1980; Symons *et al.*, 1981).

The early work with MNP was interesting, however, in showing that some features of the CCl_4-microsomal interaction could be studied by spin trap techniques. The triplet formed by CCl_4-microsomal mixtures is probably due to a lipid-MNP adduct as a closely similar spectrum is obtained on incubating lipoxygenase with arachidonic acid and MNP (Fig. 4).

McCay's group introduced the use of the spin trap phenyl-butylnitrone (PBN) for studying CCl_4-mediated reactions (for review see McCay *et al.*, 1980b) and we have now used this spin trap extensively. Our evidence is consistent with that of Poyer *et al.* (1980) in showing that a PBN-CCl_3 adduct can be trapped in liver microsomes plus NADPH plus CCl_4; the product shows satisfactory splitting with ^{13}C-substitution (Poyer *et al.*, 1980; Tomasi *et al.*, 1980). Confirmatory

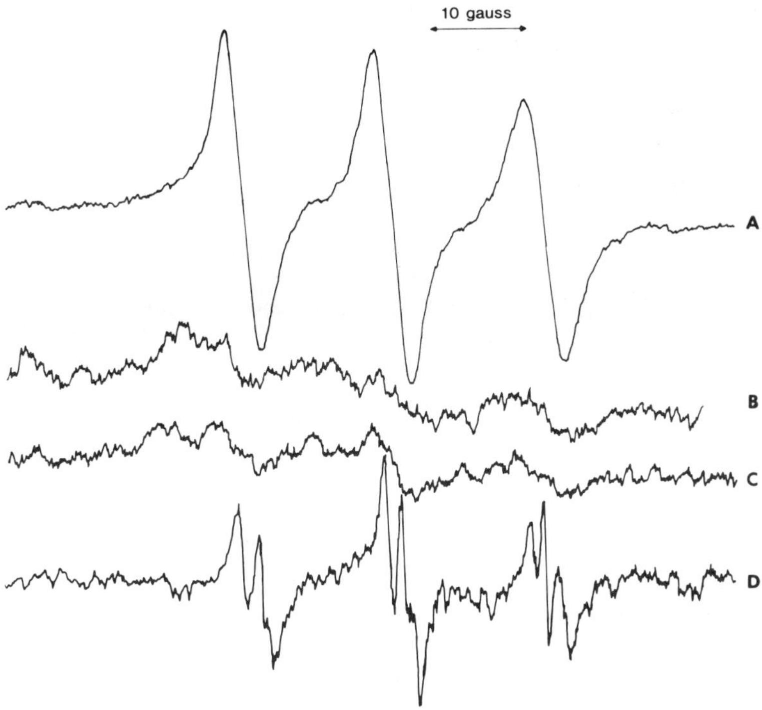

FIG. 4 Spin trapping experiments with 2-methyl-2-nitrosopropane (MNP). In (A), liver microsomes were incubated with MNP and CCl_4 for 5 min at 37°C in the presence of an NADPH-generating stock (see Ingall *et al.*, 1978). In (B), the CCl_4 was omitted, and in (C) $CHCl_3$ was used in place of CCl_4. The MNP was freshly prepared as a solution (8.5 mg/ml) in acetone; the CCl_4 (5 μl) was added to 0.4 ml of NADPH-stock, 0.4 ml of microsomes (equivalent to 3.8 g liver from a male rat induced for 7 d with phenobarbital) and 0.05 ml MNP. After 5 min at 37°C, the suspension was extracted with 2 volumes of Methanol:Chloroform (1:2) and the chloroform layer used for ESR analysis. The ESR conditions (Varian E-9) were: power, 200 mW; modulation, 0.6 Gauss; range, 100 Gauss; receiver gain in (a) 10^4, (b) 2.5×10^4 and (c) 2.5×10^4. Experiment (D) shows results for an experiment in which MNP was incubated with linoleic acid and soya bean lipoxygenase for 2 min at room temperature. The ESR conditions were: power, 25 mW; modulation, 2 Gauss; receiver gain, 10^6. Spectrum (A) shows a very broad triplet without significant hydrogen-hyperfine components; it can be considered as an envelope of a number of contributory signals. The lipoxygenase-linoleic acid spectrum (D) shows a similar nitrogen-hyperfine splitting to (B) but there are easily recognisable hydrogen-hyperfine components, and an additional signal that is not readily identifiable. Spectrum (B) shows that with short incubation times there is no significant signal from the trap alone; Spectrum (C) shows that $CHCl_3$ does not react in the same way as CCl_4. Spectra (A-C) are unpublished experiments with Professor A. Stier and Dr. S. Finch performed in 1976; Spectrum (D) is unpublished data from work with Dr A. Tomasi.

evidence has been obtained from experiments on the radiolysis of CCl_4 (Symons *et al.*, 1981).

In addition, our combination of spin trapping with $CCl_3^{\cdot}$ generation by high energy radiation shows quite unequivocally that the $CCl_3^{\cdot}$-PBN adduct is the major form trapped in aerobic microsomes in isolated hepatocytes and *in vivo*. Although CCl_3O_2-PBN can be trapped in artificial model systems (Tomasi *et al.*, 1980) it seems that the reactivity of $CCl_3O_2^{\cdot}$ with neighbouring biomolecules, the impracticability of obtaining high local concentrations of PBN in biological systems compatible with normal metabolism, and the relative rate constants for the $CCl_3O_2^{\cdot}$-biomolecule and $CCl_3O_2^{\cdot}$-PBN interactions (see Packer *et al.*, 1978, 1980; Tomasi *et al.*, 1980) all make the trapping of $CCl_3O_2^{\cdot}$ unfavourable in biomembrane systems. More detailed data on the spin trapping of $CCl_3^{\cdot}$ and $CCl_3O_2^{\cdot}$ can be found in the recent papers by Symons *et al.* (1981) and Albano *et al.* (1982).

REACTIVITY OF $CCl_3^{\cdot}$ AND $CCl_3O_2^{\cdot}$

The spin trap studies outlined above have demonstrated that $CCl_3^{\cdot}$ is formed in liver microsomes and in liver *in vivo*; the pulse radiolysis data emphasise the rapid interaction of $CCl_3^{\cdot}$ with dioxygen to yield the substantially more electrophilic free radical $CCl_3O_2^{\cdot}$. These two free radical products of the activation of CCl_4 can exert damaging effects on neighbouring enzymes and cell components in a variety of ways:

Covalent Binding. Both $CCl_3^{\cdot}$ and $CCl_3O_2^{\cdot}$ can be expected to covalently bind to neighbouring molecules (e.g. across double bonds, or to S- and N-atoms). The covalent binding of $CCl_3O_2^{\cdot}$ would result in a product (CCl_3-O-O-X) that probably would not survive normal work up procedures giving, in practical terms, major covalent binding from $CCl_3^{\cdot}$. A *possibility*, however, is that two $CCl_3O_2^{\cdot}$ species can interact to go via an intermediate tetroxide, yielding the breakdown product $CCl_3O^{\cdot}$ that could potentially give a stable covalently bound product:

$$2CCl_3O_2^{\cdot} \longrightarrow CCl_3O_2\text{-}O_2\text{-}CCl_3 \longrightarrow 2\ CCl_3O^{\cdot} + O_2$$

and an excited oxygen species. For discussion of such tetroxide reactions see Bartlett and Guaraldi (1967) and Ingold (1973). Covalent binding may occur, therefore, through a variety of mechanisms, and could be a significant contribution to overall cell injury (for background references see Reynolds and Yee, 1967; de Toranzo *et al.*, 1977; Gillette, 1980).

Lipid Peroxidation. The pulse radiolysis data show clearly that $CCl_3O_2^{\cdot}$ is much more effective than $CCl_3^{\cdot}$ in abstracting an $H^{\cdot}$-atom from PUFA to initiate peroxidation. This is not to say that $CCl_3^{\cdot}$ itself cannot initiate peroxidation but only that it is much less reactive and, in consequence, can diffuse further allowing wider scope for covalent binding reactions. A most important feature of lipid peroxidation is the production of secondary and tertiary breakdown products (e.g. reactive aldehydes and peroxides) that can diffuse and extend an essentially local injury to distant sites; this aspect is considered in more detail later.

Nucleotide Destruction. As discussed previously, one of the earliest disturbances observed in liver *in vivo* during CCl_4 intoxication is a destruction of NADPH (Slater *et al.*, 1964). The loss of NADPH could arise by free radical attack, including covalent binding, or by oxidative damage due to lipid peroxides (Lotscher *et al.*, 1979).

Thiol-oxidation. Electrophilic species like $CCl_3O_2^{\cdot}$ can interact with thiols (especially thiol anions) to yield thiyl radicals that can dimerise to give the disulphide:

$$RS\bar{:} + CCl_3O_2^{\cdot} \longrightarrow RS^{\cdot} + CCl_3O_2\bar{:}$$

$$2RS^{\cdot} \longrightarrow RSSR$$

Secondary effects on thiols can arise from interactions with aldehydic products of peroxidation (see Schauenstein *et al.*, 1977).

Membrane Fluidity. Lipid peroxidation can result in changes in membrane fluidity as a result of the changing proportions of $C_{20:4}$ to other fatty acids that occur during peroxidation, and because bifunctional products of peroxidation (e.g. malonaldehyde) can cross-link membrane proteins. Some effects of peroxidation on microsomal membrane fluidity as measured by an ESR spin label technique have been reported (Dobretsov *et al.*, 1977; Slater, 1979).

Damage to Cytochrome P_{450}. The metabolism of CCl_4 by the NADPH-P_{450} chain is associated with a destruction of P_{450} (Glende, 1972; Ugazio *et al.*, 1973). A number of other toxic agents that are activated by P_{450} also produce a destruction of the hemoprotein (for review see De Matteis, 1978). Interesting model experiments on iron porphyrin-halogenomethane interactions have been described by Mansuy *et al.* (1977b) and by Brault *et al.* (1980); these experiments are relevant to the proposal that an important intermediate of the metabolism of CCl_4 by P_{450} is the carbene CCl_2 (Ahr *et al.*, 1980). The substantial decrease in the NADPH-cytochrome P_{450} system produced by CCl_4 could have a number of interesting and important consequences. Firstly, it can render the animal much less susceptible to a further dose of CCl_4 (or any toxic agent requiring activation by the P_{450}-route), as shown clearly by Glende (1972) and Ugazio *et al.* (1973). Secondly, it can result in larger exposure times to agents, both endogenous and exogenous, that are normally metabolised and detoxified by the liver. Thirdly, and especially in situations where CCl_4 is given repeatedly, there may be severe disturbance in the conversion of cholesterol to bile acids that could contribute to the cirrhogenic effects of chronic dosing with CCl_4.

CARBENE INTERMEDIATES

To the damaging intermediates of CCl_4 metabolism already discussed ($CCl_3^{\bullet}$, $CCl_3O_2^{\bullet}$ and possibly $CCl_3O^{\bullet}$) can now be added the carbene derivative CCl_2. In one proposed scheme (Ahr *et al.*, 1980) the carbene is shown as being formed from a $CCl_3^{\bullet}$ species in close juxtaposition to the Fe-prophyrin ring of P_{450}.

$$(Fe^{3+}\text{-porph}) \text{ --- } CCl_3 \longrightarrow (Fe^{2+}\text{-porph}) \text{ --- } CCl_2$$

Liberation of CCl_2 would be followed by rapid hydrolysis to give carbon monoxide. For other data on the formation of carbon monoxide during lipid peroxidation in liver microsomes, probably involving haem breakdown, see De Matteis *et al.* (1977) and Guzelian and Swisher (1979). Since carbon monoxide is not a significant product of CCl_4 metabolism under aerobic conditions, it would seem as if carbene release is not of *major* importance in CCl_4 activation. However, the formation of a P_{450}-carbene complex may be relevant to the destruction of P_{450} that occurs during CCl_4 metabolism (see Poli *et al.*, 1981).

TISSUE DISTRIBUTION OF INJURY DUE TO CCl_4

In the adult rat the necrosis produced by a sub-lethal dose of CCl_4 is mainly restricted to the centrilobular zone of the liver lobules. This tissue and cellular distribution of injury due to CCl_4 mirrors the distribution of cytochrome P_{450}, which is mainly found in the liver (see Benedetto *et al.*, 1981) and which is concentrated in the centrilobular cells of the liver (Gooding *et al.*, 1978). This relationship between the site of injury and a relative abundance of P_{450} may reflect (i) a major role for P_{450} in the activation of CCl_4 as already discussed, and (ii) a role for P_{450} in propagating lipid peroxidation through a peroxidatic-type activity (Svingen *et al.*, 1979). An activation of CCl_4 proximal to P_{450} may function in stimulating lipid peroxidation through such a peroxidatic-linked propagation (Fig. 5).

CCl_4 also causes tissue disturbances outside the liver but these extrahepatic injuries are small in comparison to the *extent* of the centrilobular necrosis in the liver.

The extent of the injury produced by CCl_4 in various tissues of the rat probably depends on a considerable number of cellular factors including: (a) the concentration of P_{450} in the endoplasmic reticulum, (b) the activity of the NADPH-flavoprotein (FP) which may initiate peroxidation by one-electron donation, and which acts as the reducing source for P_{450}, (c) the co-operativity between the flavoprotein and P_{450}, which reflects membrane fluidity and protein conformational effects, (d) the local concentration of $C_{20:4}$ fatty acid and other susceptible PUFA around the site of initiation, (e) the local concentration of dioxygen that can function as a substrate for competing P_{450}-mixed function oxidase activity, and to convert $CCl_3^{\bullet}$ to the more electrophilic $CCl_3O_2^{\bullet}$, (f) the local supply of NADPH, necessary for reduction of the flavoprotein, (g) the local concentration of

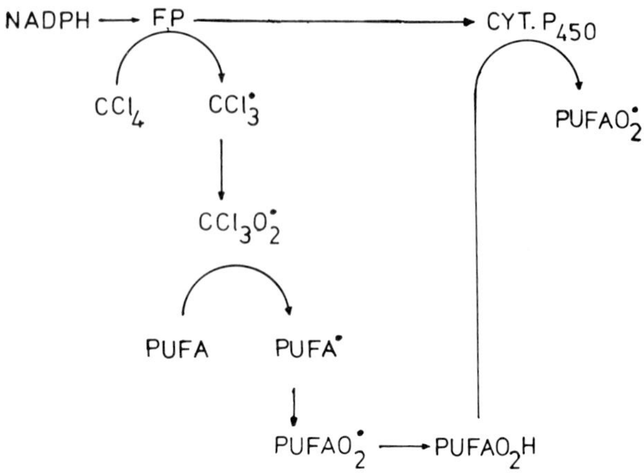

FIG. 5 Activation of CCl_4 by interaction with the NADPH-P_{450} electron transport chain. Initiation is shown in this figure at the flavoprotein (FP) site but this is not intended to indicate a unique interaction of flavoprotein with CCl_4, only that a reaction near to the FP site may occur (i.e. proximal to P_{450}). The initiation stage results in the formation of $CCl_3^{\bullet}$ radicals followed by interaction with O_2 to give the more electrophilic species $CCl_3O_2^{\bullet}$. This then interacts with polyunsaturated fatty acid (PUFA) and propagation of lipid peroxidation is shown involving P_{450}. The scheme is intended to indicate how different components of the NADPH-P_{450} chain can participate in an overall peroxidative sequence. It is also quite possible to consider initiation and propagation occurring at P_{450}, and similarly for the FP-site.

endogenous (or in experimental conditions, exogenous) antioxidant that can attenuate the peroxidative reactions, (h) the availability of reactions that compete with PUFA for the $CCl_3O_2^{\bullet}$ reactive species, and thereby diminish the rate and possibly the extent of initiation.

Normal adult rat liver possesses relatively high contents of NADPH, PUFA in the endoplasmic reticulum, NADPH-flavoprotein (FP) and cytochrome P_{450}; it also receives a rich supply of oxygenated blood. Moreover, there is normally a good co-operativity between the flavoprotein and P_{450} in the adult rat as evidenced by the wide range and relatively high activities of drug metabolism. If we represent the stimulation of lipid peroxidation as a function f of the variables just outlined, then a functional relationship can be written as below:

$$\text{stimulation of peroxidation} = f\left[\frac{\text{FP} \times \text{P}_{450} \times \text{PUFA} \times \text{NADPH} \times \text{Co-operativity}}{\text{body temperature} \times \text{antioxidant} \times \text{competing reactions}}\right]$$

I must strees, however, in case it is not immediately obvious, that the exact mathematical relationships amongst the components of this function are not defined at the present time; the function f, can be used, therefore, only in a qualitative sense.

By inspection of the above function it can be considered that the addition of CCl_4 to adult rat *liver* microsomes results in an increase of peroxidation because many factors are in favour of appreciable metabolic activation, initiation and propagation of peroxidation such that the natural defence mechanisms (i.e. antioxidant) are comparatively easily overwhelmed. With other tissues, however, such as brain or testis or lung, one or more of the "advantageous factors" may be severely restrictive so that a significant CCl_4-stimulation of peroxidation does not occur. Examples of such limiting features may be the low P_{450} activity (see Brown *et al.*, 1969; Strobel *et al.*, 1978; Sultatos and Vesell, 1980) and increased antioxidant levels (see Ahmed and Slater, 1981) reported in hepatic tumours, the low $C_{20:4}$ fatty acid content of some microsomal membranes (see Gurr and James, 1975; Ahmed and Slater, 1981) and the low NADPH content of many extra-hepatic tissues (see Long, 1961).

Some data on the tissue variability in some of the components discussed above are given in Table 3.

An important factor to consider in extra-hepatic tissues like lung, testis, etc. is that components such as P_{450} may be localised to only one cell type, which can be a minor proportion of the total cellular architecture. In such cases, the "advantageous factors" for a CCl_4-stimulation of lipid peroxidation will probably only operate in such specialised cell types, such as the Clara cell in the lung (Longo *et al.*, 1978; Serabjit-Singh *et al.*, 1980; Boyd *et al.*, 1980).

What is not known is whether the local concentration of antioxidant in extra-hepatic tissues, tumours and experimentally modified cells is normally near to a critical level such that relatively small changes in antioxidant concentration could result in corresponding

TABLE 3 Relative distributions (liver 100%) of various microsomal components in different rat tissues.

Tissue	P_{450}	NADPH cyt.c reductase	NADPH ADP/Fe^{2+}-lipid peroxidation	Covalent binding [^{14}C]CCl_4	$C_{20:4}$	Spin trap adduct formation
Liver	100	100	100	100	100	100
Kidney	15	36	13	6	106	2
Lung	8	45	8	2	43	1
Testis	9	17	13	0.5	42	5
Brain	6	21	21	3	34	3

Covalent binding is of [^{14}C]CCl_4 to microsomal protein; $C_{20:4}$ represents the distribution of arachidonic acid; spin trap adduct formation refers to the production of a CCl_3-phenyl butylnitrone adduct on incubating microsomes in the presence of NADPH, CCl_4 and spin trap. For experimental details see Benedetto *et al.* (1981).

changes in lipid peroxidation. The data of Burlakova (1975) suggest that appreciable fluctuations of antioxidant content occur with modifications of the cell cycle and this, in turn, indicates that, in some cell types at least, lipid peroxidation may primarily reflect the local status of the antioxidant content. Artificial modification of other factors in the peroxidation function f (such as increasing O_2, PUFA or initiator radical concentration) would then be expected to overwhelm a delicately balanced system.

Glutathione is a major contributor to the control of lipid peroxidation in intact hepatocytes (see Hogberg and Kristoferson, 1977), presumably through roles in GSH-peroxidases and transferases, and by direct reaction with aldehydes (see Schauenstein *et al.*, 1977). In addition, liver cell supernatant contains an inhibitor of the CCl_4-stimulated lipid peroxidation (Kamataki *et al.*, 1977) that is distinct from GSH peroxidase.

It should, of course, be borne in mind in such discussion that whilst an antioxidant may considerably retard peroxidation for a variable period of time (depending on its local concentration, its effectiveness as a scavenger, and the relative rate of production of the damaging species) it will eventually be consumed unless naturally produced in biosynthetic reactions, or regenerated by "repair processes" involving reaction with other pools of antioxidant. In the latter context, the "repair" of vitamin E radical by reaction with vitamin C is noteworthy (Packer *et al.*, 1979).

SPREADING CONSEQUENCES OF THE LESION

The primary effects of $CCl_3^{\bullet}$ and $CCl_3O_2^{\bullet}$ will be determined by their radii of diffusion, which will be small, from the loci of formation of these free radical species (Slater, 1976). In addition, the immediate effects will be a function of the local dioxygen concentration that governs the electrophilicity of the parent radical. Thus the immediate impact of CCl_4 activation is restricted to a lobular site, due to the centrilobular distribution of P_{450}, and the related intralobular heterogenous distributions of GSH (Smith *et al.*, 1979) and O_2; to a cellular site since P_{450} and the NADPH-flavoprotein are essentially restricted to endoplasmic reticulum; and to a very localised sphere of diffusion in those membranes by the high chemical reactivity of the free radical products. Because $CCl_3O_2^{\bullet}$ is very reactive then one cannot expect it to leave the endoplasmic reticulum membrane and, in consequence, a direct interaction with DNA in mammalian cell nuclei is unlikely. In fact, the testing of CCl_4 for mutagenicity by the Ames test has been generally unsuccessful (see McCann *et al.*, 1975; Fishbein, 1976; Uehleke *et al.*, 1977). Secondarily-derived radicals, of lower reactivity than $CCl_3O_2^{\bullet}$ may be able to diffuse to DNA, and to react with it but the overall rate of reaction from such minor pathways of CCl_4-activation is likely to be very low.

Initiation of peroxidation by $CCl_3O_2^{\bullet}$ in the endoplasmic reticulum is accompanied by the production of a wide variety of aldehydes as reported here at this meeting by Esterbauer (1982). These aldehydes have long enough biological life-times to diffuse away from the site of formation and to cause pathological disturbances at a considerable distance. An indication of the complexity of aldehydic products formed during CCl_4-stimulated lipid peroxidation is given in Fig. 6. A detailed description of the patterns of aldehyde production in lipid peroxidation is given by Esterbauer in this symposium (see also Esterbauer *et al.*, 1982).

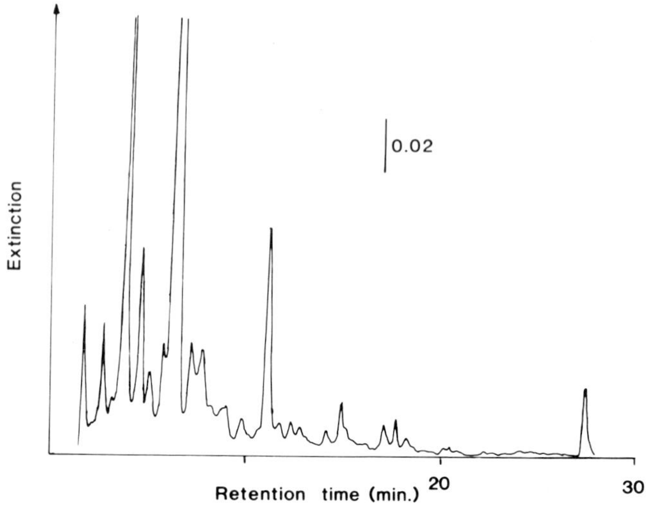

FIG. 6 Separation of the dinitrophenyldydrazine derivatives of non-polar carbonyls by high pressure liquid chromatography (detector wavelength 378 nm). The carbonyls were produced by incubation of rat liver microsomes with an NADPH-generating stock solution and ADP/Fe^{2+} (for details see Esterbauer *et al.*, 1982); incubation time, 5 min at 37°C. The figure shows a complex variety of non-polar products, and similar complexity was observed in the polar carbonyl group. Many different carbonyl products can also be obtained on incubating microsomes with CCl_4, or with ascorbate/Fe^{2+}. The spectrum shown here is an unpublished study by Professor H. Esterbauer, Dr. K. Cheeseman and the author. Full details and background references to this type of carbonyl separation can be found in articles by Esterbauer (1982) and Esterbauer *et al.* (1982). I am indebted to Professor Hermann Esterbauer for invaluable advice and practical expertise in this area of study.

A major finding (Benedetti *et al.*, 1980) was the isolation of 4-hydroxynonenal as a biologically active product of microsomal lipid peroxidation. This aldehyde has been shown by Dianzani and colleagues (personal communication) to inhibit adenyl cyclase at μM concentration, and thus can affect a wide range of associated reactions. An important task for future studies will be to obtain reliable quantitative information on the tissue contents of such aldehydes during the early stages of CCl_4-intoxication. Such studies will be complicated, however, by any metabolism of the aldehydic products that occurs, and by the interaction of the aldehydes with cellular components (e.g. with amino and thiol groups). In consequence a value obtained for "free aldehydes" in the cellular cytosol can be expected to reflect only a minimum value for the actual production of such compounds.

Other products of lipid peroxidation include lipid peroxides of varying molecular weight; at low concentration these can influence the prostaglandin cascade (Hemler *et al.*, 1979).

More recent work has also implicated disturbances of the microsomal calcium pump during CCl_4-intoxication (Lowrey *et al.*, 1981) but whether this is a primary lesion (due to CCl_4-activation products) or is secondary to damage to adenyl cyclase and ionic transport by products of lipid peroxidation is not yet clear. It can be seen clearly, therefore, how such diffusible products of a spatially restricted primary lesion can cause widespread cellular malfunction through such interactions with the cellular secondary messenger systems.

SUMMARY

Covalent binding and a stimulation of lipid peroxidation in liver microsomes can be detected within minutes of an oral dosing with CCl_4 (see Recknagel and Glende, 1973). A significant decrease in total liver NADPH has occurred by 1 h post-dosing (Slater *et al.*, 1964), whilst the rate of protein synthesis is also decreased early in the injury (Smuckler *et al.*, 1962).

Significant arguments have been made in favour of covalent binding, lipid peroxidation or protein synthesis, each being of major importance in the ensuing development of liver necrosis. However, in each case, telling points against such unicausal views of liver injury have also been made. In the case of protein synthesis it is known that some substances (for example, ethionine) can cause profound falls in the rate of protein synthesis but this does not result in necrosis (see Villa-Trevino *et al.*, 1963; Ugazio and Lombardi, 1965; Dianzani, 1978). With lipid peroxidation, de Toranzo *et al.* (1978) have reported that, in certain strains of mice, CCl_4 produces liver necrosis but no detectable lipid peroxidation. On the other hand, Recknagel and Glende (1973) have summarised evidence that favours lipid peroxidation as a major event rather than covalent binding; Mitchell *et al.* (1979) have argued that lipid peroxidation often occurs as a result, rather than the cause, of liver necrosis. Perhaps an explanation of these seeming conflicts is that the *relative* extents of the various processes vary somewhat according to the precise reaction conditions, and the type of tissue sample used. And that it is a *combination* of damaging events, which may have variable extents from one to another, that overwhelms the organised behaviour of the cell and its protective mechanisms. In this sense, covalent binding will be responsible for one set of damaging reactions; lipid peroxidation, depression of protein synthesis, decrease of NADPH, etc. for others. This concept may be likened to a polycausal view of cell injury by an agent such as CCl_4 that quite evidently disturbs the cell in many ways.

An important point to consider is that the effect of CCl_4 on cells in a liver lobule will not be an "all-or-none" case of either cell death (necrosis) or undamaged cells. Rather, there can be expected to be a range of injurious phenomena covering cell death in centrilobular regions especially, to relatively minor perturbations in the periportal zone, with differing degrees of injury in between. If this concept is valid then it means that some cells not lethally damaged by CCl_4 will be severely depressed in their rates of protein synthesis, and will have some modification in cell membrane behaviour due to failures in protein replacement and to some products of lipid peroxidation. If the depression of protein synthesis is commensurate with the turnover times of such membrane proteins as calmodulin, clathrin, receptor glycoproteins, adenyl cyclase, hormone receptors, etc. then the response of the cell to its surroundings will be profoundly modified. Moreover, if such disturbances are long lasting, due to chronic exposure to the toxic agent, then one can expect significant changes in DNA expression as a result of membrane-hormone (or second messenger) interactions. Such changes in DNA expression may contribute to the increased cell proliferation and fibrosis, observed after repeated exposure to agents like CCl_4.

ACKNOWLEDGEMENTS

I am grateful to the Cancer Research Campaign, the Medical Research Council, the Science Research Council, the National Foundation for Cancer Research, Ciba-Geigy Ltd. and The Wellcome Foundation for financial help in the studies reported here, which have taken place over a considerable period of time. I am also indebted to Professor M.A. Dianzani, Professor H. Esterbauer, Professor A. Stier, Dr. G. Poli and Dr. K. Cheeseman for much helpful advice.

REFERENCES

Ahmed, S.M. and Slater, T.F. (1981). "Recent Advances in Lipid Peroxidation and Tissue Injury". (Eds. T.F. Slater and A. Garner), Brunel University, Biochemistry Department, London.

Ahr, H.J., King, L.J., Naistainczyk, W. and Ullrich, V. (1980). *Biochem. Pharmacol.* 29, 2855-2861.

Albano, E., Slater, T.F., Symons, M. and Tomasi, A. (1982). *Biochem. J.* (Submitted).

Bartlett, P.D. and Guaraldi, G. (1967). *J. Am. Chem. Soc.* 89, 4799-4801.

Benedetti, A., Comporti, M. and Esterbauer, H. (1980). *Biochim. Biophys. Acta* 620, 281-296.

Benedetto, C., Dianzani, M.U., Ahmed, M., Cheeseman, K., Connelly, C. and Slater, T.F. (1981). *Biochim. Biophys. Acta* (In press).

Boyd, M.R., Statham, C.N. and Longo, N.S. (1980). *J. Pharmacol. Exp. Ther.* 212, 109-114.

Brault, D., Bizet, C., Morliers, P., Rougee, M., Land, E.J., Santus, L. and Swallow, A.J. (1980). *J. Am. Chem. Soc.* 102, 1015-1020.

Brodie, B.B., Gillette, J.R. and La Du, B.N. (1958). *In* "Annual Review of Biochemistry" (Eds. J.M. Luck, F.W. Allen and G. Mackinnly) Vol. 27, pp.427-454, Annual Reviews Inc., Palo Alto, California.

Brown, H.D., Morris, H.P., Chattopadhyay, S.K., Patel, A.B. and Pennington, S.N. (1969). *Experientia* 25, 358-359.

Burlakova, E.B. (1975). *Russ. Chem. Rev.* 44, 871-880.

Butler, T.C. (1961). *J. Pharmacol. Exp. Ther.* 134, 311-319.

Cameron, G.R. and Karunaratne, W.A.E. (1936). *J. Pathol. Bacteriol.* 42, 1-21.

Cheeseman, K. (1982). *In* "Free Radicals, Lipid Peroxidation and Cancer" (Eds. D.C.H. McBrien and T.F. Slater) pp.197-214 , Academic Press, London.

Comporti, M. (1964). *Boll. Soc. Ital. Biol. Sper.* 41, 222-225.

Comporti, M., Saccocci, C. and Dianzani, M.U. (1965). *Enzymologia* 29, 185-205.

De Matteis, F. (1978). *In* "Haem and Haemoproteins" (Eds. F. de Matteis and N. Aldridge) pp.95-127, Springer, FRG.

De Matteis, F., Gibbs, A.H. and Unseld, A. (1977). *Biochem. J.* 168, 417-422.

De Toranzo, E.G.D., Diaz Gomez, M.I. and Castro, J.A. (1978). *Res. Commun. Chem. Pathol. Pharmacol.* 19, 347-352.

Dianzani, M.U. (1978). *In* "Biochemical Mechanisms of Liver Injury" (Ed. T.F. Slater), pp.45-95. Academic Press, London.

Di Luzio, N.R. (1963). *Physiologist* 6, 169.

Di Luzio, N.R. and Costales, F. (1965). *Exp. Mol. Pathol.* 4, 141-154.

Dobretsov, G.E., Borschevskaya, T.A., Petrov, V.A. and Vladimirov, Y.A. (1977). *FEBS Lett.* 84, 125-128.

Esterbauer, H. (1982). *In* "Free Radicals, Lipid Peroxidation and Cancer" (Eds. D.C.H. McBrien and T.F. Slater), pp.101-128. Academic Press, London.

Esterbauer, H., Cheeseman, K., Dianzani, M.U., Poli, G. and Slater, T.F. (1982). *Chem. Biol. Interact.* (Submitted).

Fishbein, L. (1976). *Mutat. Res.* 32, 267-308.
Fowler, J.S.L. (1969). *Br. J. Pharmacol.* 37, 733-737.
Gallagher, J.S.L. (1961). *Nature (London)* 192, 881-882.
Ghoshal, A.K. and Recknagel, R.O. (1965). *Life Sci.* 4, 1521-1530.
Gillette, J.R. (1980). *In* "Microsomes, Drug Oxidations, and Chemical Carcinogenesis" (Eds. M.J. Coon, A.H. Conney, R.W. Estabrook, H.V. Gelboin, J.R. Gillette and P.J. O'Brien), Vol. II, pp.777-788. Academic Press, New York.
Glende, E.A. (1972). *Biochem. Pharmacol.* 21, 1697-1702.
Gooding, P.E., Chayen, J., Sawyer, B. and Slater, T.F. (1978). *Chem. Biol. Interact.* 20, 299-310.
Gordis, E. (1969). *J. Clin. Invest.* 48, 203-209.
Graham, E.A. (1915). *J. Exp. Med.* 22, 48-75.
Gurr, M.I. and James, A.T. (1975). "Lipid Biochemistry", 2nd Ed. Chapman and Hall, London.
Guzelian, P.S. and Swisher, R.W. (1979). *Biochem. J.* 184, 481-489.
Head, B., Moody, D.E., Woo, C.H. and Smuckler, E.A. (1980). *Fed. Proc.* 39, 1015.
Hemler, M.E., Cook, H.W. and Lands, W.E.M. (1979). *Arch. Biochem. Biophys.* 193, 340-345.
Hogberg, J. and Kristoferson, A. (1977). *Eur. J. Biochem.* 74, 77-82.
Hove, E.L. (1948). *Arch. Biochem. Biophys.* 17, 467-473.
Hove, E.L. (1953). *J. Nutr.* 51, 609-622.
Ingall, A., Lott, K.A.K., Slater, T.F., Finch, S. and Stier, A. (1978). *Biochem. Soc. Trans.* 6, 962-964.
Ingold, K.U. (1973). *In* "Free Radicals" (Ed. J.K. Kochi) Vol. 1, pp.37-112. Wiley-Interscience, New York.
Janzen, E.G. (1980). *In* "Free Radicals in Biology" (Ed. W.A. Pryor) Vol. 4, pp.116-154. Academic Press, New York.
Kamataki, T., Sugita, O., Kitada, M., Naminohara, S. and Kitagawa, H. (1977). *Res. Commun. Chem. Pathol. Pharmacol.* 17, 265-273.
Knecht, M. (1966). *Z. Naturforsch.* Teil. B:21, 799-801.
Long, C. (Ed.) (1961). *In* "Biochemists' Handbook", E. and F. Spon, London.
Longo, N., Statham, C., Sasame, H. and Boyd, M. (1978). *Fed. Proc.* 37, 505.
Lotscher, H.R., Winterhalter, K.H., Carafoli, E. and Richter, C. (1979). *Proc. Natl. Acad. Sci. USA* 76, 4340-4344.
Lowrey, K., Glende, E.A. and Recknagel, R.O. (1981). *Biochem. Pharmacol.* 30, 135-140.
Mansuy, D., Beaune, P., Cresteil, T., Lange, M. and Leroux, J.-P. (1977a). *Biochem. Biophys. Res. Commun.* 79, 513-517.
Mansuy, D., Lange, M., Chottara, J.C., Guerin, P., Morliere, P., Brault, D. and Rougee, M. (1977b). *J. Chem. Soc. Commun.* 648-649.
Masuda, Y. and Murano, T. (1978). *Biochem. Pharmacol.* 27, 1983-1985.
McCann, J., Choi, E., Yamasaki, E. and Ames, B.N. (1975). *Proc. Natl. Acad. Sci. USA* 72, 5135-5139.
McCay, P.B., Noguchi, R., Lai, E.K. and Fong, K.-L. (1980a). *Fed. Proc.* 39, 612.
McCay, P.B., Noguchi, T., Fong, K.-L., Lai, E.K. and Poyer, J.L. (1980b). *In* "Free Radicals in Biology" (Ed. W.A. Pryor), Vol. IV, pp.155-186, Academic Press, New York.
McLean, A.E.M. (1967). *Biochem. Pharmacol.* 16, 2030-2033.

McLean, A.E.M. and McLean, E.K. (1966). *Biochem. J.* 100, 564-571.
Mitchell, J.R., Smith, C.V., Lauterburg, B.H. and Horning, E.C. (1979). *Gastroenterology* 77, A.28.
Muller, R. (1911). *Z. Exp. Pathol. Ther.* 9, 103-125.
Packer, J.E., Slater, T.F. and Willson, R.L. (1978). *Life Sci.* 23, 2617-2620.
Packer, J.E., Slater, T.F. and Willson, R.L. (1979). *Nature (London)* 278, 737-738.
Packer, J.E., Willson, R.L., Bahnemann, D. and Asmus, K.-D. (1980). *J. Chem. Soc., Perkin Trans.* 2, 296-299.
Packer, J.E., Mahood, J.S., Mora-Arellano, V.O., Slater, T.F., Willson, R.L. and Wolfenden, B.S. (1981). *Biochem. Biophys. Res. Commun.* 98, 901-906.
Pohl, L.R., George, J.W., Martin, J.L. and Krishna, G. (1979). *Toxicol. Appl. Pharmacol.* 48, Abstracts of the 18th Annual Meeting of the Society of Toxicology, A219.
Poli, G., Cheeseman, K., Slater, T.F. and Dianzani, M.U. (1981). *Chem. Biol. Interact.*
Poyer, J.L., McCay, P.B., Lai, E.K., Janzen, E.G. and Davis, E.R. (1980). *Biochem. Biophys. Res. Commun.* 94, 1154-1160.
Recknagel, R.O. (1967). *Pharmacol. Rev.* 19, 145-208.
Recknagel, R.O. and Ghoshal, A.K. (1966). *Lab. Invest.* 15, 132-146.
Recknagel, R.O. and Glende, E.A. (1973). *Crit. Rev. Toxicol.* 2, 263-297.
Reddrop, C.J., Riess, W. and Slater, T.F. (1981a). *Biochem. Pharmacol.* 30, 1443-1447.
Reddrop, C., Riess, W. and Slater, T.F. (1981b). *Biochem. Pharmacol.* 30, 1449-1455.
Rees, K.R. and Spector, W.G. (1961). *Nature (London)* 190, 821-822.
Rees, K.R. and Shotlander, V.L. (1963). *Proc. Roy. Soc. (London) Ser. B.* 157, 517-535.
Reynolds, E.S. (1967). *J. Pharmacol. Exp. Ther.* 155, 117-126.
Reynolds, E.S. and Yee, A.G. (1967). *Lab. Invest.* 16, 591-603.
Schauenstein, E., Esterbauer, H. and Zollner, H. (1977). *In* "Aldehydes in Biological Systems", Pion Ltd., London.
Serabjit-Singh, C.J., Wolf, C.R., Philpot, R.M. and Plopper, C.G. (1980). *Science* 207, 1496-1470.
Shah, H., Hartman, S.P. and Weinhouser, S. (1979). *Cancer Res.* 39, 3942-3947.
Slater, T.F. (1966a). *Nature (London)* 209, 36-40.
Slater, T.F. (1966b). *Biochem. J.* 101, 16-17p.
Slater, T.F. (1967). Proc. 4th FEBS Meeting, Oslo, Abstract 216.
Slater, T.F. (1972). "Free Radical Mechanisms in Tissue Injury", Pion Ltd., London.
Slater, T.F. (1976). *In* "Recent Advances in Biochemical Pathology: Toxic Liver Injury" (Eds. M.U. Dianzani, G. Ugazio and L.M. Sena), pp.381-390. Minerva Medica, Torino.
Slater, T.F. (Ed.) (1978). "Biochemical Mechanisms of Liver Injury", Academic Press, London.
Slater, T.F. (1979). *In* "Submolecular Biology and Cancer" (Eds. G.E.W. Wolstenholme, D.W. Fitzsimons and J. Whelan), pp.301-321, Excerpta Medica, Amsterdam.
Slater, T.F. (1981a). "Recent Advances in Lipid Peroxidation and Tissue Injury" (Eds. T.F. Slater and A. Garner), Brunel University Biochemistry Department, London.

Slater, T.F. (1981b). *In* "Biological Reactive Intermediates" (Eds. R. Snyder, D.V. Parke, J. Kocsis, D.J. Jollow and G.G. Gibson), (in press). Plenum Publishing Co., New York.
Slater, T.F. and Sawyer, B.C. (1970). *FEBS Lett.* 11, 132-136.
Slater, T.F. and Sawyer, B.C. (1971). *Biochem. J.* 123, 815-821.
Slater, T.F., Strauli, U.D. and Sawyer, B.C. (1964). *Biochem. J.* 93, 260-266.
Slater, T.F., Sawyer, B.C. and Strauli, U.D. (1966). *Biochem. Pharmacol.* 15, 1273-1278.
Smith, M.T., Loveridge, N., Wills, E.D. and Chayen, J. (1979). *Biochem. J.* 182, 103-108.
Smuckler, E.A., Iseri, O.A. and Benditt, E.P. (1962). *J. Exp. Med.* 116, 55-72.
Strobel, H.W., Dignam, J.D., Saine, S.E., Fang, W.-F. and Fennell, P.M. (1978). *Mol. Cell. Biochem.* 22, 70-91.
Suarez, K.A. and Bhonsle, P. (1976). *Toxicol. Appl. Pharmacol.* 37, 23-27.
Sultatos, L.G. and Vesell, E.S. (1980). *Proc. Natl. Acad. Sci. USA* 77, 600-603.
Svingen, B.A., Buege, J.A., O'Neal, F.O. and Aust, S.D. (1979). *J. Biol. Chem.* 254, 5892-5899.
Symons, M.C.R., Albano, E., Slater, T.F. and Tomasi, A. (1981). *Radiat. Phys. Chem.*
Tomasi, A., Albano, E., Lott, K.A.K. and Slater, T.F. (1980). *FEBS Lett.* 122, 303-306.
Uehleke, H., Werner, T., Greim, H. and Kramer, M. (1977). *Xenobiotica* 7, 393-400.
Ugazio, G. and Lombardi, B. (1965). *Lab. Invest.* 14, 711-719.
Ugazio, G., Koch, R.R. and Recknagel, R.O. (1973). *Exp. Mol. Pathol.* 18, 281-289.
Villarruel, M. del C., de Toranzo, E.G.D. and Castro, J.A. (1977). *Toxicol. Appl. Pharmacol.* 41, 337-344.
Villa-Trevino, S., Shull, K.H. and Farber, E. (1963). *J. Biol. Chem.* 238, 1757-1763.
Waller, R.L. and Recknagel, R.O. (1980). *Fed. Proc.* 39, 612.
Wells, H.G. (1908). *Arch. Intern. Med.* 1, 589-601.
Whipple, G.H. and Sperry, J.A. (1909). *In* "Liver Necrosis and Repair". Bulletin of the Johns Hopkins Hospital No.222, pp.278-289.
Willson, R.L. (1978). *In* "Biochemical Mechanisms of Liver Injury" (Ed. T.F. Slater), pp.123-224. Academic Press, London.
Willson, R.L. (1982). *In* "Free Radicals, Lipid Peroxidation and Cancer" (Eds. D.C.H. McBrien and T.F. Slater), pp.275-303. Academic Press, London.
Willson, R.L. and Slater, T.F. (1975). *In* "Fast Processes in Radiation Chemistry and Biology" (Eds. G.E. Adams, E.M. Fielden and B.D. Michael), pp.147-161. John Wiley, New York.

DISCUSSION

Adams: I think you established the case for the multiple causality very well indeed but is there any evidence for the role of the OH radical or is this purely speculative? It is very difficult to imagine how that could be produced by carbon tetrachloride.

Slater: The evidence is very indirect. It is based on the following sequence: carbon tetrachloride produces a rapid destruction of P_{450}, resulting in electrons tending to leave the chain more easily from the flavoprotein locus, then, in the presence of oxygen, superoxide can be produced. At the same time the membrane is highly disorganised and all sorts of new interactions become available, especially in terms of metal contamination in isolated microsomes. So I think the superoxide that's produced can, in the presence of metals, be taken to produce at least some hydroxyl radicals. That is the argument, I have no evidence for it, but such suggestions are in the literature.

Adams: That argument is used sometimes in other contexts.

Mason: I was curious about this mechanism because we have evidence against the involvement of cytochrome P_{450} in CCl_4-induced lipid peroxidation, because CO does not diminish carbon tetrachloride induced lipid peroxidation which you would expect to happen if cytochrome P_{450} destruction was indirectly causing lipid peroxidation (Wolf *et al.*, 1980).

Slater: I would not say that P_{450} destruction was causing lipid peroxidation, that would be one contribution. What I imagine myself, and this a purely personal view, is that carbon tetrachloride can interact with various components of the microsomal electron-transport chain, and depending on your own experimental conditions, on contamination with iron, on oxygen levels, on the pre-treatment giving induction and so on, you favour one particular pathway over the others. It does not mean to say that you close them all down, relative to one, but you change the proportions and what I suspect happens at least in systems where P_{450} is rapidly depleted, like *in vivo*, is that you do change electron pathways significantly. But I would not say that P_{450} destruction is the cause of the lipid peroxidation, far from it.

Mason: Well, if it were the cause then I would expect lipid peroxidation induced by carbon tetrachloride to be CO inhibitable, which it is not, as you yourself have shown.

Slater: Yes indeed.

Esterbauer: Are there any quantitative or semi-quantitative data for carbon tetrachloride. For instance, how much is bound as CCl_3, how much is converted to CO_2 and chloroform and what is the loss of polyunsaturated fatty acids (arachidonic acid and linoleic acid) in absolute amounts?

Slater: Yes, there is a huge amount of data on these points. Several groups measured the changes in polyunsaturated fatty acids, McCay's group in Oklahoma for instance, Professor Dianzani's group in Turin, and Comporti's group in Siena, who demonstrated a preferential effect on the phosphatidyl ethanolamine class, for example. Then in relation to the overall production of CO_2 and chloroform or covalent binding of ^{14}C-CCl_3 there are considerable data going back quite a long time. Reynold's work on covalent binding is very good in this respect. What we have done recently with Colin Reddrop (Reddrop *et al.*, 1980a,b, 1981a,b) is to develop very sensitive and extremely accurate methods for following chloroform expiration and chloroform levels in blood, of animals exposed to very low concentrations of carbon tetrachloride. So we have data on that. The overall conclusion is that when you give carbon tetrachloride to an uninduced adult male intact rat the expiry of chloroform and carbon dioxide is really quite a low proportion of the dose of CCl_4. If you induce the rat you can get a much bigger expiry of chloroform. So the overall conversion rate is quite low in the intact animal, but it does depend very much on the species, the sex, on the age, on the dietary treatment, the level of anti-oxidant and on the dose that is given (because chloroform production from the intact rat is very easily saturated by carbon tetrachloride dosing, so it plateaus out at a very low carbon tetrachloride administered dose). All of these data are available in the literature. It is very hard to give you an answer in a few words other than to say the conversion of CCl_4 to $CHCl_3$ and CO_2 is quite small.

Asmus: I would like to add some data just from the purely chemical point of view since it also was asked how much CO_2 was produced (Monig, 1980; Monig, J. and Asmus, K.-D,, to be published). If we take carbon tetrachloride, reduce it, let the $CCl_3^{\bullet}$ radical react with oxygen, and the only other solute present in solution is something which can provide a hydrogen atom, say an alcohol, then the $CCl_3O_2^{\cdot}$ radical breaks down completely to carbon dioxide and chloride. This means you get a Cl^-/CO_2 ratio of 4:1 with respect to the carbon tetrachloride or 3:1 with respect to the $CCl_3O_2^{\cdot}$. Now we don't know really what the mechanism is but you mentioned that the $CCl_3O_2^{\cdot}$ abstracts a hydrogen atom. But this seems to be a rather slow reaction. So in some systems you may have a chance of a radical radical reaction, and if two of these peroxy radicals meet they can eliminate oxygen and produce an alkoxy radical which will be even more reactive. The alkoxy radical once it abstracts a hydrogen atom forms CCl_3OH, which will immediately break down to HCl and phosgene and the latter could then hydrolyse to CO_2.

Slater: Well, I am very interested in that, because the reason I simply put up the $CCl_3O_2^{\cdot}$ was on the assumption that it abstracts an electron and then protonates very fast to give CCl_3O_2H. But the possibility that peroxy radicals (such as $CCl_3O_2^{\cdot}$) forming a tetroxide ($CCl_3O_2O_2CCl_3$) and then breaking down to the alkoxy radical ($CCl_3O^{\cdot}$) is something that has interested us, because it has really quite profound implications for studies on covalent binding, in the sense that I feel that the covalent binding from the peroxy radical would not survive the work up procedures that we normally use. But covalent binding from an alkoxy radical may well survive, and nobody as far as I am aware, has ever looked to see if in the covalent binding of carbon tetrachloride there is any oxygen inserted at the same time. We are looking very hard at that because we could also expect to see activated oxygen from the tetroxide breakdown.

Asmus: In this respect it might even be interesting to compare these results with the results from chloroform (Monig, 1980). If you reduce chloroform, eliminate one chloride and produce the $CCl_2HO_2^{\cdot}$ radical, this could undergo the same sequence, i.e. radical-radical reaction, elimination of oxygen and production of an alkoxy radical. But if that abstracts an hydrogen atom and breaks down you would not get phosgene. You were talking about the reduced effect you see in the case of chloroform. I wonder whether this is relevant?

Slater: Only for lipid peroxidation.

Asmus: But this reaction sequence would leave out the phosgene.

Slater: Phosgene has been detected after chloroform and CCl_4 dosing but I think the production rate of phosgene is really quite low and not sufficient to account for the main features of the liver injury. I think it is an interesting pathway, but not of major significance overall in terms of the biological effects of CCl_4.

Asmus: These are just possible pathways which I would like to suggest from the pulse radiolysis and gamma-radiolysis work. But it would certainly go along with a number of your observations.

Slater: Well, what we suspect is that chloroform is metabolised essentially in a different way from carbon tetrachloride, and I think this relates also to Professor Stier's work with halothane. I feel that you should consider my remarks today to be basically directed towards carbon tetrachloride because I think the problems of chloroform metabolism and toxicity are a different story.

REFERENCES to Discussion

Monig, J. (1980). Diploma Thesis, Technical University of Berlin.

Reddrop, C.J., Reiss, W. and Slater, T.F. (1980a). *J. Chromatog.* 192, 375-386.

Reddrop, C.J., Reiss, W. and Slater, T.F. (1980b). *J. Chromatog.* 193, 71-82.

Reddrop, C.J., Reiss, W. and Slater, T.F. (1981a). *Biochem. Pharmacol.* 30, 1443-1447.

Reddrop, C.J., Reiss, W. and Slater, T.F. (1981b). *Biochem. Pharmacol.* 30, 1449-1455.

Wolf, C.R., Harrelson, W.G., Jr., Nastainczyk, W.M., Philpot, R.M., Kalyanaraman, B. and Mason, R.P. (1980). *Mol. Pharmacol.* 18, 553-558.

Iron and Hydroxyl Free Radicals in Enzyme Inactivation and Cancer

R.L. WILLSON

INTRODUCTION: FREE RADICALS, RADIATION AND CANCER

Since 1973 a large number of cancer patients have been treated with the drugs metronidazole (Flagyl) or misonidazole (Ro 07-0582) in combination with radiation therapy (Foster and Willson, 1973; Urtasun *et al.*, 1976; Adams *et al.*, 1976). Clinical trials, taking place in several centres, particularly in the United States and the United Kingdom have attracted international interest and the possible wider use of these drugs in combination with established cytotoxic agents such as adriamycin and melphelan is being actively considered (Sutherland, 1974; Foster and Willson, 1976; Foster *et al.*, 1976; Rose *et al.*, 1980).

As often seems the case in cancer research, serendipity has undoubtedly played a part in these developments. In the context of the present meeting however, it is particularly encouraging that the clinical use of these drugs (originally synthesised for other purposes) has stemmed directly from fundamental free radical studies *in vitro*. In this contribution I will first outline these studies briefly and then describe some of the "mechanistic spin offs" which are currently being applied to our investigation into the possible role of free radicals in carcinogenesis.

It is now generally appreciated that:

(a) radiation exposure can cause cancer,

(b) radiation exposure produces free radicals,

(c) free radicals can be formed in biological systems by processes other than radiation exposure.

Clearly these facts do not imply that free radicals are responsible for radiation-induced cancers let alone cancers generally. Unfortunately the very manner in which cancers develop over a protracted time-scale has meant that the identification of any role for free radicals in carcinogenesis (an event which may take place in less than a millisecond) is extremely difficult. As in the case of viruses, the presence of free radicals in tumour tissue neither implies their involvement in neoplastic growth nor, more importantly, in carcinogenesis. However, a strong case has been established for a role for free radicals in other forms of radiation injury more accessible to study, for example cellular toxicity and damage to DNA and enzymes. It is not unreasonable to assume therefore that they are also involved in radiation-induced carcinogenesis. Several questions immediately arise.

Are free radicals in any way responsible for cancers induced by agents other than radiation?

If so, which free radicals are involved and how are they formed?

What factors affect their numbers and what are their actions?

Can their actions be modified: if so, how?

Are additional factors also necessary for carcinogenesis?

It is in an attempt to answer these questions that current pulse radiolysis and associated stationary state biochemical studies are being undertaken at Brunel.

As a working hypothesis cancer is considered as but one form of free radical induced tissue injury: in this instance oxidative subcellular injury which usually leads to cell death is limited but not sufficiently so as to prevent one or more cells and their progeny being permanently affected (Willson, 1977a,b, 1979a,b) (Fig. 1).

RADIOSENSITISER DEVELOPMENT: A STIMULATOR OF FREE RADICAL RESEARCH

The rationale for initially using metronidazole and misonidazole as adjunctive agents in cancer therapy was based on the long established fact that if cells are deprived of oxygen they are generally much more resistant to radiation killing. This is true of both normal and malignant cells. The cells of normal tissue, however, are usually

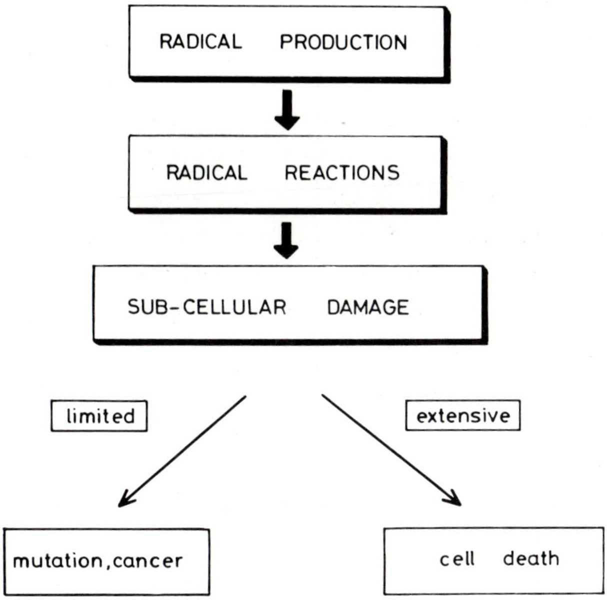

FIG. 1 Cancer as a result of limited sub-cellular damage.

well supplied with oxygen, whereas in poorly vascularised tumour tissue hypoxic cells may be present. Some of these hypoxic cells will remain viable after treatment with the radiation doses that the normal tissue surrounding the tumour can tolerate. By the mid 1950s several trials were being undertaken in which patients were subjected to three atmospheres of oxygen at the time of radiation treatment. It was hoped to increase the oxygen concentration in the blood and thereby decrease the fraction of hypoxic tumour cells that might be present. Results were equivocal, however, and the possibility of finding drugs which could be administered to patients more conveniently and which only sensitised hypoxic cells began to be seriously considered. A chemical was needed which on the one hand sensitised like oxygen but on the other hand was metabolised more slowly, enabling it to diffuse into those regions of the tumour that oxygen might not reach.

Fortunately, a considerable literature had accumulated concerning substances which would sensitise cellular systems to the lethal effects of radiation or protect them from it. A number of mechanistic models for the sensitising action had and have since been proposed. Two in particular have provided a considerable stimulus in the search for clinically useful compounds.

(a) The "radical fixation versus repair" model in which a radical formed on a vital molecule by oxidative attack can be repaired by hydrogen or electron donation from a reducing substance or alternatively be further oxidised by a sensitising agent so "fixing" the damage (Alexander and Charlesby, 1955; Alper, 1956; Howard-Flanders, 1958; Willson and Emmerson, 1970; Asquith *et al.*, 1954), e.g.

$$OH^{\bullet} + TH \longrightarrow T^{\bullet} + H_2O$$

$$T^{\bullet} + RSH \longrightarrow TH + RS^{\bullet} \quad \text{(repair)}$$

$$T^{\bullet} + O_2 \longrightarrow TO_2^{\bullet} \text{ or } T^{\bullet +} + O_2^{\bullet -} \quad \text{(fixation)}$$

(b) The "charge recombination" model in which a radical-cation formed on a vital molecule may interact to some extent with an electron adduct so regenerating the original molecule: alternatively, the electron adduct may react with a sensitiser of high electron affinity to form an adduct less likely to donate its electron to the critical radical-cation, e.g.

$$TH + X \xrightarrow{\text{radiation}} TH^{\bullet +} + X^{\bullet -}$$

then $$TH^{\bullet +} + X^{\bullet -} \longrightarrow TH + X$$

$$X^{\bullet -} + O_2 \rightleftharpoons X + O_2^{\bullet -}$$

or less likely $$TH^{\bullet +} + O_2^{\bullet -} \longrightarrow TH + O_2$$

The probability of repair will depnd on the relative one electron oxidation couple $E_7^{\frac{1}{2}}$ $(O_2/O_2^{\bullet -})$ - $E_7^{\frac{1}{2}}$ $(X/X^{\bullet -})$ (Adams, 1968; Willson *et al.*, 1974).

Clearly both models have much in common: in both instances the sensitiser is credited with oxidising properties. A knowledge of fundamental data concerning free radical reactions involving biological molecules and likely sensitising agents is thus a necessary pre-requisite for any systematic study.

It was fortunate that this resurgence of interest in radiosensitising drugs coincided with the development of the pulse radiolysis technique. Whereas much of the earlier information concerning free radical reactions had been derived by interpolation of product analysis data, it now became possible to observe the radical reactions directly, at least in solution. A catalogue of valuable data concerning a wide variety of potential radiosensitisers quickly accumulated. Many compounds, including nitric oxide, several stable nitroxide free radicals, quinones and conjugated carbonyls, chosen on the basis of their ability to enter into free radical reactions, were subsequently shown to selectively sensitize hypoxic bacteria to radiation killing. In 1970 sensitisation of mammalian cells by *p*-nitroacetophenone (PNAP) was reported (Asquith *et al.*, 1970). Pulse radiolysis studies had shown that tetranitromethane and nitrobenzene reacted readily with several organic radicals (Asmus *et al.*, 1964, 1966). Experiments with PNAP (chosen initially not because it was a nitro compound but because of an interest in acetophenones containing electron attracting groups) showed that it too could readily accept an electron from a variety of electron adducts ($X^{\cdot -}$) as well as oxidise other organic radicals. Studies with other nitro compounds quickly followed and led to the suggestion of the possible clinical usefulness of metronidazole (Foster and Willson, 1973). At the same time a pulse radiolysis method for measuring the relative one-electron oxidation potential of chemicals able to oxidise organic free radicals was reported (Patel and Willson, 1973). Although metronidazole was shown to be less electron affinic than *p*-nitroacetophenone it was argued that its favourable pharmacology and toxicology would outweigh this possible disadvantage (Willson *et al.*, 1974).

Animal studies were soon undertaken and preliminary trials with patients with brain tumours began in Canada later that year. Studies with other nitroimidazoles quickly followed. One such compound, Ro 07-0582 (which like metronidazole had been synthesised initially as a possible antitrichomonal drug and was later given the name misonidazole), was shown to be particularly active in the sense that a drug concentration lower than that for metronidazole was required for a similar degree of reactivity *in vitro*. Animal studies showed that the drug was also active *in vivo* and although its toxicology was less favourable than metronidazole clinical trials were begun at several centres and continue today (Asquith *et al.*, 1974; Adams *et al.*, 1980).

A large number of related nitro compounds have since been screened *in vitro* and their activities have been found to correlate well with their one electron oxidation potential as measured by pulse radiolysis (Adams *et al.*, 1979). Clearly such a correlation does not necessarily prove that the models on which the nitro compounds were originally chosen are correct; indeed, results on the chemotherapeutic action of the drugs suggest that the formation of toxic products on reduction may also be important. They do, however, provide encouragement for a fundamental approach at the molecular level to cancer associated problems and illustrate the potential value of the pulse radiolysis technique in the study of free radical mediated damage (Willson, 1977a,b, 1979a.b; Wardman, 1977; Adams and Wardman, 1977). In the long term, perhaps more significantly, they have also provided impetus for a reassessment of the role of iron and other metals in carcinogenesis (Willson, 1976a,b,c, 1977a,b, 1979a,b).

During a study of the metabolism of metronidazole by anaerobic bacteria of the rat caecum it was observed that oxygen and several compounds which reacted with sulphydryl compounds or complexed iron inhibited the reduction of the drug. Although the observation could be adequately explained by the involvement of iron and SH-containing enzymes, a direct interaction of sulphydryl and nitro compounds in the presence of iron could not be ruled out (Willson and Searle, 1975; Searle and Willson, 1976). The possibility that some sensitising agents acted by reducing the concentration of endogenous SH compounds and thus the probability of radical repair had often been considered but had been thought unlikely in the case of nitro compounds: no reaction had been observed between PNAP and cysteamine or metronidazole and dithiothreitol for example. When metronidazole was incubated with cysteine, under nitrogen, little if any reduction was apparent. However, in the presence of ferrous ions the drug was reduced exponentially and a strong colour formed immediately the component solutions were mixed. Kinetic studies indicated this to be due to a drug-iron-cysteine complex which was slowly reduced to a weakly coloured ferrous-sulphydryl complex with the formation of free radicals (Willson, 1977a,b,c; Bahnemann *et al.*, 1978) as shown in the following scheme:

$$Fe^{2+}(RS^-)_2 + RNO_2 \rightleftharpoons [Fe^{3+}(RS^-)_2 \text{ ---- } RNO_2^{\cdot -}]$$

$$[Fe^{3+}(RS^-)_2 \text{ ---- } RNO_2^{\cdot -}] + RS^- \longrightarrow Fe^{2+}(RS^-)_2 + RNO_2^{\cdot -} + RS^{\cdot}$$

Control experiments showed, surprisingly, that a similar intense colour also formed in the absence of the drug if traces of oxygen were present. Stopped-flow experiments confirmed that the rate of appearance of the colour was exceptionally rapid (for 125 μM oxygen, a half life of approx 20 ms was measured). A search of the literature revealed that a similar colour had been observed nearly a century earlier (Baumann, 1884; Mathews and Walker, 1909). However, although the iron-catalysed oxidation of sulphydryl compounds was well known the formation of this coloured complex seemed to have received little attention. The very speed of the reaction and the fact that by analogy with metronidazole, superoxide ($O_2^{\cdot -}$) might be formed and thence by way of hydrogen peroxide, hydroxyl radicals, was particularly stimulating.

Hydroxyl radicals formed by iron-catalysed reactions would have the same damaging properties as hydroxyl radicals produced by radiation exposure, that is provided they are generated in the vicinity of vital molecules.

$$Fe^{2+}(RS^-)_2 + O_2 \rightleftharpoons [Fe^{3+}(RS^-)_2 \text{ --- } O_2^{\cdot -}]$$

$$[Fe^{3+}(RS^-)_2 \text{ --- } O_2^{\cdot -}] + RS^- \longrightarrow Fe^{2+}(RS^-)_2 + O_2^{\cdot -} + RS^{\cdot}$$

$$Fe^{2+}(RS^-)_2 + O_2^{\cdot -} + 2H^+ \longrightarrow Fe^{3+}(RS^-)_2 + H_2O_2$$

$$Fe^{2+}(RS^-)_2 + H_2O_2 \longrightarrow Fe^{3+}(RS^-)_2 + OH^{\cdot} + OH^-$$

$$OH^{\cdot} + \text{target} \longrightarrow \text{damage}$$

PULSE RADIOLYSIS STUDIES OF FREE RADICAL REACTIONS

Several accounts of pulse radiolysis equipment are now available (see Willson, 1979a). Briefly, the technique can be considered as the high energy analogue of flash photolysis where the flash lamp is replaced by a pulsed radiation source, such as a linear accelerator. Since many radicals are highly coloured and absorb at wavelengths different from those of the molecule from which they are derived, kinetic absorption spectroscopy is the most commonly used analytical technique. An outline plan of the Brunel Equipment is shown (Fig. 2).

The basis of the specificity of the technique relies on the fact that ionising radiation is often absorbed throughout the irradiated system, the extent of absorption in particular components depending

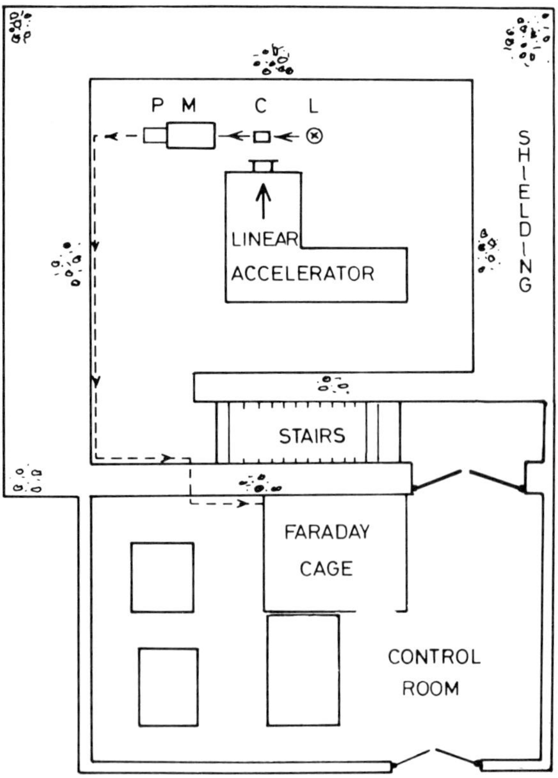

FIG. 2 The Brunel University pulse radiolysis facility with Lower Irradiation Laboratory housing the linear accelerator, analysing light (L), sample cell (C), monochromator (M) and photomultiplier (P). The Faraday cage in the Upper Control Room contains equipment for data collection, storage and processing.

only on their weight fraction. (This is unlike the case with visible or ultraviolet light when the energy is absorbed in discrete chromophoric groups.) Thus in many biological systems most of the radiation is absorbed by water and as a result some molecules are ionised. Thus following a 200 ns radiation pulse the majority of free radicals present in solution (typically, 1-10 μM concentration) are solvated electrons (e^-aq) and hydroxyl radicals ($OH^\bullet$) formed according to:

$$H_2O \xrightarrow[\text{ionisation}]{\text{radiation}} H_2O^{\bullet +} + e^- \xrightarrow{H_2O} H^+ + OH^\bullet + e^-aq$$

The hydroxyl radical is an extremely strong oxidant and the hydrated electron an extremely strong reducing agent. These species will react with other solutes present in the system, the extent depending on the rate of reaction of the species with a particular solute and its concentration.

Fortunately, several solutes are specific in their reactions with radicals, reacting rapidly with $OH^\bullet$ and slowly with e^-aq or *vice versa*. Thus by irradiating compounds of interest in the presence of suitably high concentrations of selective free radical scavengers of this type the reactions of the radicals can be effectively controlled. The absorption spectra of a wide variety of free radicals and their rates of reaction with other radicals and solutes can be readily measured. In the context of tissue injury it is in the study of electron transfer reactions that the technique has perhaps made its greatest contribution. Data concerning the rates at which free radicals donate or accept an electron from other solutes has been valuable in interpreting the manner in which substances such as paraquat, carbon tetrachloride, phenthiazines and quinone and nitro-compounds may interact with cellular systems, the proviso being that information concerning reactions occurring in an *aqueous* medium *in vitro* may not be relevant always to the *in vivo* situation.

NUCLEOPHILIC RADICALS: ONE-ELECTRON OXIDATION POTENTIALS AND ELECTRON CASCADES

The ease with which consecutive electron transfer reactions can take place in neutral aqueous solution can be readily demonstrated by pulse radiolysis (Adams *et al.*, 1968; Adams and Willson, 1973; Willson,

1970, 1977b; Packer *et al.*, 1979). The hydrated electron reacts rapidly with a variety of molecules. In a system containing different solutes A, B, C and D, each of which reacts at a near diffusion-controlled rate with the reducing species and which are present in concentrations such that A >> B >> C >> D the electron adduct $A^{\bullet -}$ will be formed initially. However, subsequent electron transfer reactions may occur with $A^{\bullet -}$ reacting with B to form $B^{\bullet -}$ and so until eventually $D^{\bullet -}$ is formed (Fig. 3).

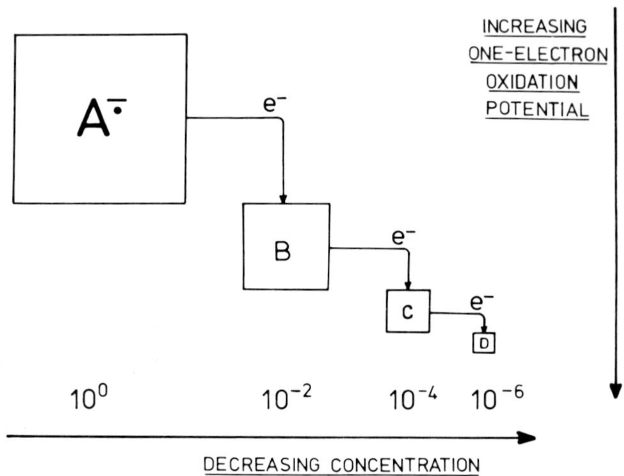

FIG. 3 Sequential electron transfer from solute in highest concentration but of lowest one-electron oxidation potential.

Whether or not such a sequence of reactions or "electron cascade" occurs depends on the concentrations of the solutes present and the rate constants of the forward and reverse reactions of the individual electron transfer processes. These are themselves dependent on the one-electron oxidation potentials (E^1_7) of the couples involved. The pulse radiolysis technique has proved to be particularly useful for the measurement of these potentials. During radiosensitisation studies in the early 1970s a rapid reaction of the semiquinone of anthraquinone2,6,disulphonate with oxygen was observed due to the following reaction.

$$AQ^{\bullet -} + O_2 \longrightarrow AQ + O_2^{\bullet -}$$

With benzoquinone, however, the reverse reaction was apparent:

$$BQ^{\cdot -} + O_2 \longrightarrow BQ + O_2^{\cdot -}$$

Further studies with other quinones established that such reactions were indeed equilibrium processes, e.g.

$$DQ^{\cdot -} + O_2 \rightleftharpoons DQ + O_2^{\cdot -}$$

In the case of duroquinone measurement of the height of the absorptions at different quinone and oxygen concentrations (Fig. 4) enabled the equilibrium constant and hence the relative one-electron oxidation potential

$$\Delta E_7^1 = E_7^1\ (DQ/DQ^{\cdot -}) - E_7^1\ (O_2/O_2^{\cdot -}) = -0.095\ V.$$

to be calculated (Willson, 1970; Patel and Willson, 1973).

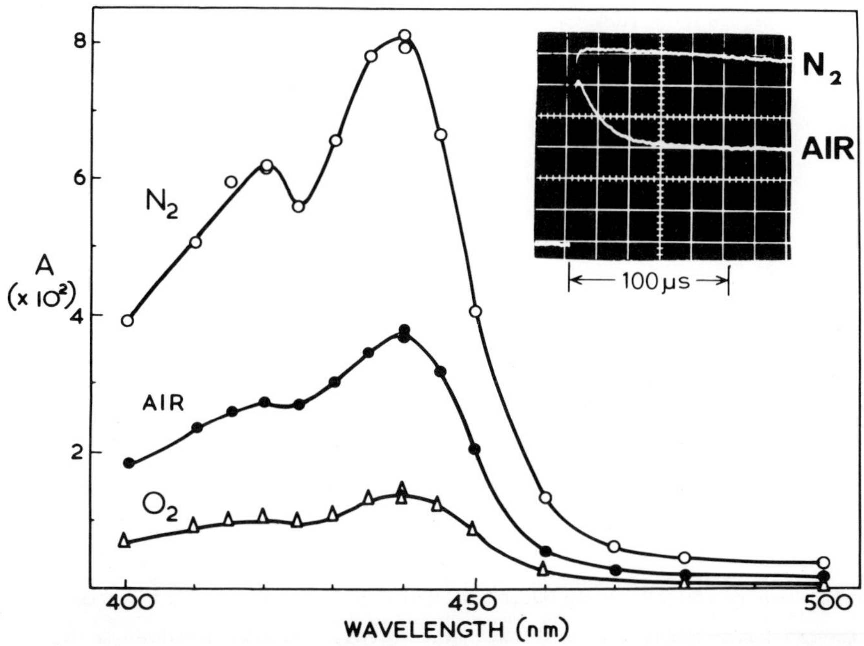

FIG. 4 Transient absorption spectra 100 μs after pulse radiolysis of a neutral aqueous-isopropanol-acetone solution of duroquinone, saturated with nitrogen (O), air (●) and oxygen (Δ).

It was later pointed out that a value of E_7^1 ($DQ/DQ^{\cdot -}$) = 0.25 V could be derived from published spectroscopic data and using the above relative value an absolute value for E_7^1 ($O_2/O_2^{\cdot -}$) = 0.16 V could be calculated (Wood, 1974).

TABLE 1 One-electron oxidation potentials determined by pulse radiolysis

Compound	E_7^1
cyt. c	0.26 V.*
benzoquinone	0.1
2,methyl benzoquinone	0.02
2,3,dimethyl benzoquinone	- 0.07
oxygen (1M)	- 0.16
2,3,5,trimethyl benzoquinone	- 0.17
4,nitropyridine	- 0.19
duroquinone	- 0.24*
FAD	- 0.24
adriamycin	- 0.29
riboflavin	- 0.29
benzyl viologen	- 0.35*
p. nitroacetophenone (PNAP)	- 0.36
misonidazole	- 0.38
anthraquinone 2 sulphonate	- 0.38
methyl viologen (paraquat)	- 0.45*
nitrobenzene	- 0.49
metronidazole	- 0.49
NAD^+	- 0.93

*crossed checked by other methods.

Many other one-electron oxidation potentials (see Table 1) have since been measured using this pulse radiolysis equilibrium method (Ilan *et al.*, 1974, 1976; Meisel and Neta, 1975a,b; Wardman and Clarke, 1976; Anderson, 1976; Wardman, 1977; Farrington *et al.*, 1980; Anderson, 1980; Svingen and Powis, 1981).

Using such values equilibrium constants, K_c, for a particular redox couple can be calculated using the formulae:

$$E_7^1 .F = \Delta G = -RT\ln K_c$$

where F and R are the Faraday and Gas constants respectively.

Several studies have indicated that the larger the difference in the oxidation potentials of a reacting solute and those of a series of electron acceptors or donors of a related structure, the greater the rate constant for the transfer reaction (Rao and Hayon, 1973; Wardman and Clarke, 1976). For example, the rate constant for the reaction of the electron adduct of metronidazole with oxygen is greater than that for misonidazole is greater than that for PNAP.

HYDROXYL AND RELATED ELECTROPHILIC RADICALS: ABTS A NEW REFERENCE COMPOUND

The possible role of electrophilic species as ultimate carcinogens has been the subject of much discussion. Many free radicals are electrophilic. Although in the last decade considerable interest has surrounded the reaction of the superoxide radical, $O_2^{\bullet -}$ there is now a growing acceptance that the highly electrophilic hydroxyl radical, $OH^{\bullet}$, or peroxyl radicals, $RO_2^{\bullet}$, are the more likely damaging species in many biological systems. These radicals generally absorb in the ultraviolet where their direct observation is usually difficult. Nevertheless, their reactions can be conveniently studied by pulse radiolysis, either directly by following the formation of an absorbing product as in the case of phenylalanine, or indirectly by using a reference compound as a competing solute. Several substances have been used as references in this way including phenylalanine itself, and ferrocyanide and thiocyanate ions (Willson *et al.*, 1971). Recently, prompted by a report of its use as a reference chromophore in peroxidase studies, we have found that the dye ABTS (2,2' azino-di-[3-ethylbenzthiazoline-6-sulphonate]) is well suited for pulse competition studies (Childs and Bardsley, 1975). It reacts rapidly with several electrophilic free radicals. Although in the case of $OH^{\bullet}$ some radical addition is indicated, simple electron transfer with the formation of a long-lived radical-cation with a high extinction coefficient predominates in many instances (Fig. 5) (B. Wolfenden and R.L. Willson, unpublished).

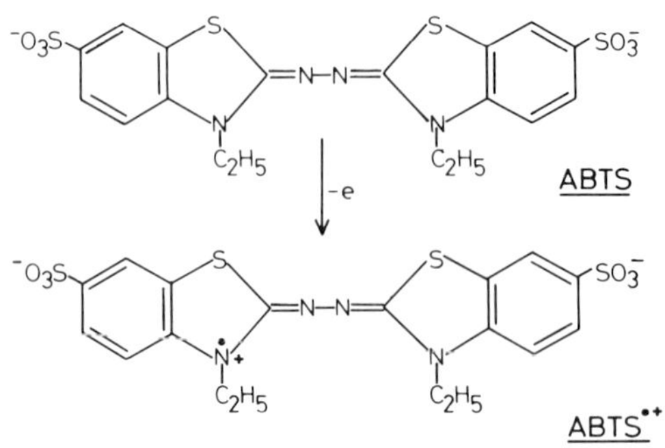

FIG. 5 Structure of the new reference compound ABTS (see text).

From measurements of the rate of formation of the cation on pulse radiolysis of solutions of the dye at different concentrations and saturated with nitrous oxide the absolute rate constant $k = 1.2 \times 10^{10}\ M^{-1}s.^{-1}$ of the following reaction has been measured (Fig. 6).

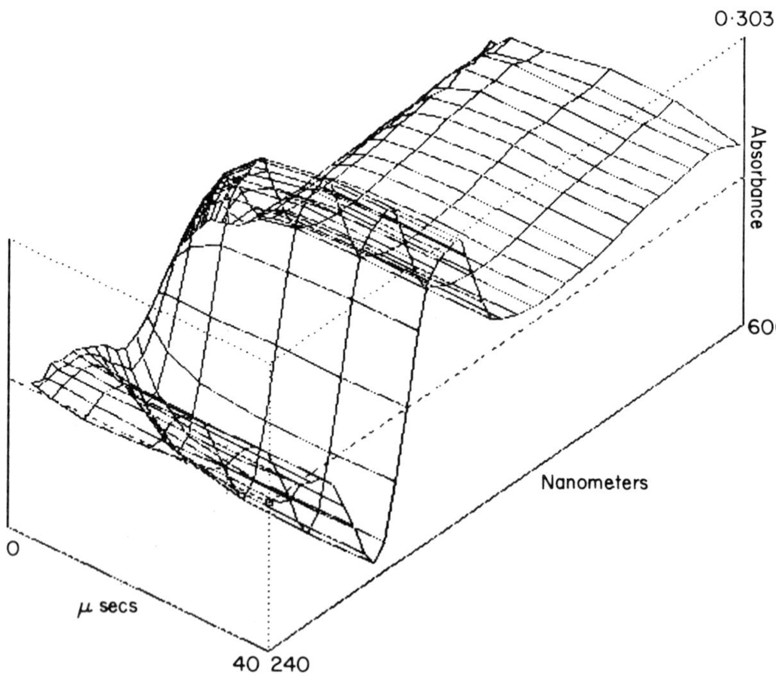

FIG. 6 Three dimensional absorption spectrum (time, absorption, wavelength) of the product of the reaction of $OH^{\cdot}$ with ABTS attributed principally to the radical-cation $ABTS^{\cdot+}$.

$$OH^{\bullet} + ABTS \longrightarrow OH^{-} + ABTS^{\bullet +} \quad (\lambda\ max = 415\ nm)$$

In the presence of other solutes which react with $OH^{\bullet}$ according to

$$OH^{\bullet} + S \longrightarrow \text{products with no absorption at 415 nm}$$

simple competition can be observed. A typical kinetic plot is shown (Fig. 7).

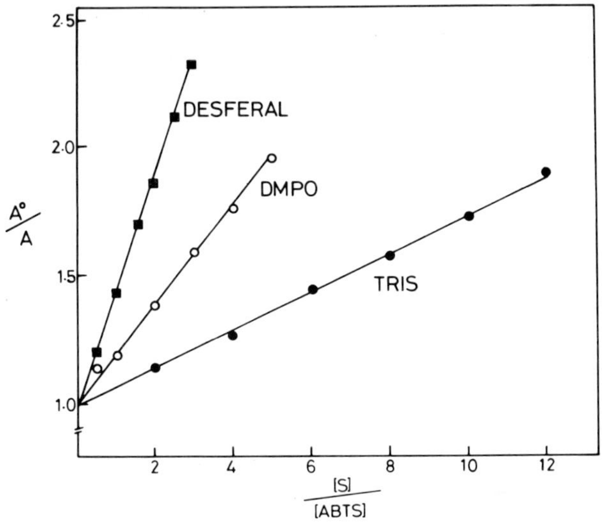

FIG. 7 Typical competition plots for the reaction of $OH^{\bullet}$ with ABTS and other solutes.

Some rate constants for the reaction of $OH^{\bullet}$ determined using this method along with values determined by other methods in parenthesis are given in Table 2. Rate constants for the reaction of the peroxy radicals derived from carbon tetrachloride and from halothane ($CCl_3O_2^{\bullet}$ and $CF_3CHClO_2^{\bullet}$ respectively) have been determined similarly. In the case of halothane ($CF_3CHClBr$) and ABTS the rate of formation of the radical-cation on pulse radiolysis of air-saturated solutions containing excess *t*-butanol was first order for dye concentration over the range 100–300 μM in agreement with the following scheme.

$$e^{-}_{aq} + CF_3CHClBr \longrightarrow CF_3CHCl^{\bullet}$$

$$CF_3CHCl^{\bullet} + O_2 \longrightarrow CF_3CHClO_2^{\bullet}$$

$$CF_3CHClO_2^{\bullet} + ABTS \longrightarrow CF_3CHClO_2^{-} + ABTS^{\bullet +} \quad (k = 3.9 \times 10^8 M^{-1} s^{-1}).$$

TABLE 2 Rate constants for the reaction with $OH^{\bullet}$

	K	($10^9\ M^{-1}s^{-1}$)
Methanol	1.0	(0.9)
Ethanol	1.9	(1.85)
Isopropanol	1.9	(2.1)
t-butanol	0.6	(0.52)
Acetone	0.13	(0.10)
Formate	3.5	(3.5)
Thymine	5.5	(5.4)
Phenyl alanine	6.4	(6.4)
Desferal	5.3	(-)

At higher ABTS concentrations (3 and 4 mM) however, the rate of formation remained almost constant in agreement with the reaction of the halogen radical with oxygen becoming the rate determining step and $k = 1.5 \times 10^9\ M^{-1}s^{-1}$ (J.Monig and R.L. Willson, unpublished). A similar phenomenon has been observed in studies of the reaction of the $CCl_3O_2^{\bullet}$ with the phenothiazine metiazinic acid where $k = 3.3 \times 10^9\ M^{-1}s^{-1}$ was determined for the analogous reaction of $CCl_3^{\bullet}$ and oxygen (Bahnemann, 1981).

PROTECTION BY REDUCING SUBSTANCES AND MULTIPLE ELECTRON TRANSFER COCKTAILS

If electrophilic radicals are responsible for some forms of tissue injury it is not surprising that nucleophilic compounds may not only provide a target for damage but may also serve as protective agents. This will only be so if the damage is unimportant because the compounds are present to excess. Compounds such as cysteine, cysteamine, ascorbate, phenothiazines and various phenols clearly fall into this category. The amino acids tryptophan and methionine may also have a role in this respect since they both react rapidly with $OH^{\bullet}$ and recently have also been found to react rapidly with $CCl_3O_2^{\bullet}$ to form absorbing products (J. Monig and R.L. Willson, unpublished).

Studies have also shown that, as in the case of nucleophilic radicals, electrophilic radicals can also enter into sequential electron transfer reactions but in this instance the radical is the electron acceptor. For example, the individual reactions of the following sequence have been characterised (Asmus *et al.*, 1979; Packer *et al.*, 1979; Mahood *et al.*, 1980).

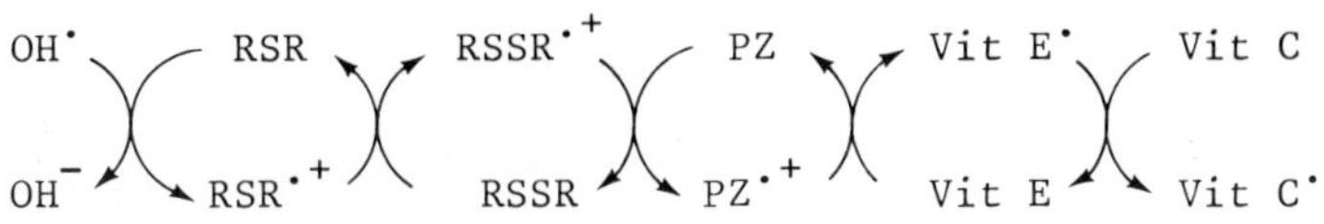

The net reaction is thus:

$$OH^{\bullet} + \text{Vit C} \longrightarrow \text{Vit C}^{\bullet} + OH^{-}$$

Such processes clearly suggest a basis for the design of protective cocktails. Provided ascorbic acid for instance is present in high concentration other compounds such as vitamin E or phenothiazines may need only be present in low concentration to contribute to a protective effect. Such processes may help to overcome a steric or solubility barrier and may explain why only frank vitamin C and not E deficiency has been observed in man.

LOWER ELECTROPHILICITY AND GREATER SPECIFICITY BUT POSSIBLY GREATER DAMAGE

It is sometimes assumed that the greater the electrophilicity of a radical the greater its damaging potential. It can easily be demonstrated that in a multicomponent system this is not necessarily the case (Fig. 8).

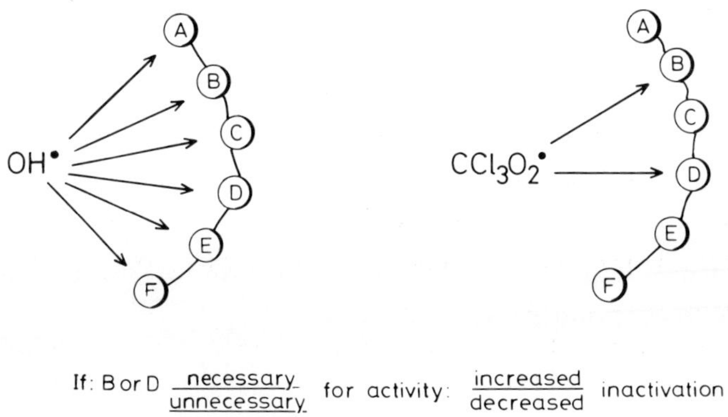

FIG. 8 Enzyme inactivation by free radicals. Specificity of $CCl_3O_2^{\bullet}$ compared to $OH^{\bullet}$

If one compares for example reactions of $OH^{\bullet}$ and the much less reactive $CCl_3O_2^{\bullet}$ with an enzyme, $OH^{\bullet}$ will react readily with many residues whereas the peroxy radical is likely to react only with cysteine, tryptophan and methionine moieties (Packer *et al.*, 1980). Thus, if none of these moieties is essential for activity a decreased extent of damage will result. If, on the other hand, one or more is essential then increased inactivation may occur. For example, in the case of lysozyme, on irradiation in nitrous oxide saturated solutions considerable inactivation occurs (Fig. 9). This is attributed to the reactions:

$$e^-_{aq} + N_2O \longrightarrow OH^{\bullet} + OH^- + N_2$$

$$OH^{\bullet} + \text{lysozyme} \longrightarrow \text{inactivation}$$

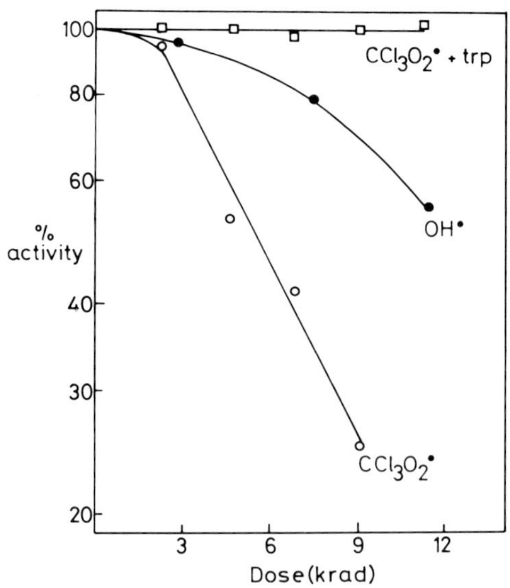

FIG. 9 Inactivation of lysozyme by $OH^{\bullet}$ and $CCl_3O_2^{\bullet}$, and protection by isopropanol and acetone and by tryptophan (see text).

With air saturated solutions in the presence of isopropanol and acetone the superoxide radical is formed and little inactivation occurs:

$$e^-_{aq} + CH_3COCH_3 + H_2O \longrightarrow CH_3COHCH_3^{\bullet} + OH^-$$

$$OH^{\bullet} + CH_3CHOHCH_3 \longrightarrow CH_3COHCH_3^{\bullet} + H_2O$$

$$CH_3COHCH_3^{\bullet} + O_2 + OH^- \longrightarrow CH_3COCH_3 + O_2^{\bullet -} + H_2O$$

$$O_2^{\bullet -} + \text{lysozyme} \longrightarrow \text{slow (no inactivation)}$$

When 10^{-2} M CCl_4 is also present, however, the extent of damage is even greater than for $OH^{\bullet}$ due to the formation of $CCl_3O_2^{\bullet}$. Furthermore, if the common amino acids are added separately to this irradiated system tryptophan, methionine and cysteine (1 mM) protect completely and histidine to a less extent (Fig. 9) (J. Taylor, G. Thomson and R.L. Willson, unpublished).

$$CH_3COHCH_3^{\bullet} + CCl_4 \longrightarrow CH_3COCH_3 + H^+ + Cl^- + CCl_3^{\bullet}$$

$$CCl_3^{\bullet} + O_2 \longrightarrow CCl_3O_2^{\bullet}$$

$$CCl_3O_2^{\bullet} + \text{lysozyme} \longrightarrow \text{inactivation}$$

$$CCl_3O_2^{\bullet} + \text{tryptophan} \longrightarrow \text{protection}$$

PROTECTION BY OXIDISING SUBSTANCES: ELECTRON TRANSFER SHUNTS INVOLVING NAD^+ AND THE CRUCIAL ROLE OF OXYGEN

In the studies with lysozyme described above increased inactivation of the enzyme does not occur if only low concentrations of CCl_4 are present. On the other hand, at high CCl_4 to O_2 ratios the reaction with CCl_4 predominates and damaging $CCl_3O_2^{\bullet}$ rather than $O_2^{\bullet -}$ is formed. In the presence of NAD^+ (10^{-2} M), however, the coenzyme can compete effectively for the isopropanol radical giving rise to $NAD^{\bullet}$. This $NAD^{\bullet}$ reacts rapidly with oxygen forming $O_2^{\bullet -}$ but only slowly if at all with CCl_4 and protection is again observed (Fig. 10).

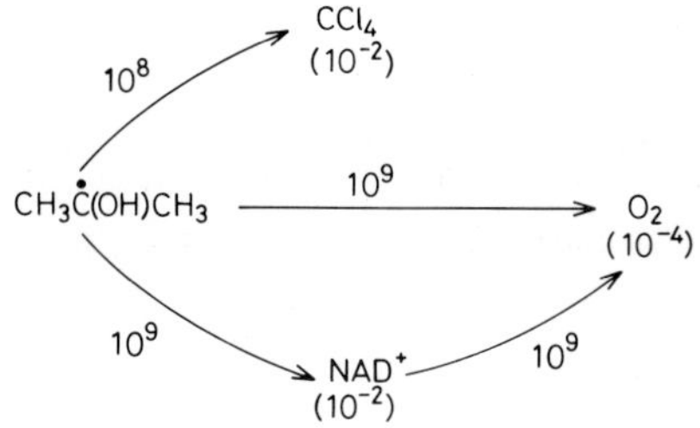

FIG. 10 Scheme for the protective action of NAD^+ (see text).

A similar effect has been observed when metronidazole rather than NAD^+ is added to the system, and also when cytochrome C reduction rather than lysozyme inactivation is used as the end point (J. Monig and R.L. Willson, unpublished).

IRON AND HYDROXYL RADICAL PRODUCTION: DIFFICULTIES OF IDENTIFICATION USING SPIN TRAPS

The role of "decompartmentalised" i.e. "ill-placed" or "misplaced" iron in some forms of tissue injury was discussed at length at the CIBA Symposium on Iron Metabolism in 1976. A considerable amount of further evidence has since emerged supporting the formation of $OH^\bullet$ in the iron-catalysed oxidation of cysteine by a mechanism similar to that already described (Searle and Willson, 1975; Willson, 1977a,b, 1979a,b; Bahnemann *et al.*, 1978). The formation of $OH^\bullet$ and $O_2^{\bullet -}$ in the iron-catalysed oxidation of thioglycollate had in fact been postulated some twenty years earlier and more recently evidence had been published indicating their formation in the autoxidation of other sulphydryl compounds (Lanfrom and Nielson, 1957; Misra, 1974). With dithiothreitol, for example, $OH^\bullet$ scavengers inhibited the autoxidation but not the coupled reduction of the dye nitroblue tertrazolium (NBT). Superoxide dismutase on the other hand did inhibit dye reduction and a similar inhibition has since been observed with the iron-cysteine system (K.A. Cheeseman, personal communication). The oxidation of NADPH on incubation with dithiothreitol and ferrous iron has also been reported and again the production of $OH^\bullet$ has been implicated (Baccanari, 1978).

Recently, A.J.F. Searle and A. Tomasi at Brunel (personal communication) have confirmed unequivocally that $OH^\bullet$ can be produced in the iron-cysteine-oxygen system. When a solution containing cysteine (125 mM) ferrous sulphate (12.5 μM) and the spin trap 5,5 dimethyl-1-pyrroline-1-oxide (DMPO) (200 mM), in the presence of HCl/Tris buffer (25 mM, pH 7.4) was examined by electron spin resonance spectroscopy, a spectrum previously assigned to the DMPO-OH adduct was observed (Fig. 11). No signal was observed when oxygen was absent or excess zinc was present. The fact that the radical was due directly to the production of $OH^\bullet$ and not to the reactions:

$$Fe^{3+}\text{ complex} + DMPO \longrightarrow Fe^{2+}\text{ complex} + DMPO^{\cdot +}$$

$$DMPO^{\cdot +} + H_2O \longrightarrow DMPO\text{-}OH^{\cdot} + H^{+}$$

was confirmed with the finding that in the presence of excess isopropanol (2 M) the DMPO-OH$^{\cdot}$ signal was replaced by a signal with a large contribution attributable principally to the DMPO-isopropanol radical adduct.

In view of the large number of reactions that might occur in these systems the fact that the ESR signals could be detected only after a careful choice of solute concentrations is not surprising. The spin trap must be in sufficiently high concentration to compete effectively with cysteine and the Tris buffer for OH$^{\cdot}$ and, when isopropanol is present, with oxygen for the isopropanol radical. Furthermore, the nitroxide free radical adduct must itself react sufficiently slowly with the iron-cysteine complex or with the isopropanol radical to allow it to be formed in a detectable steady state concentration.

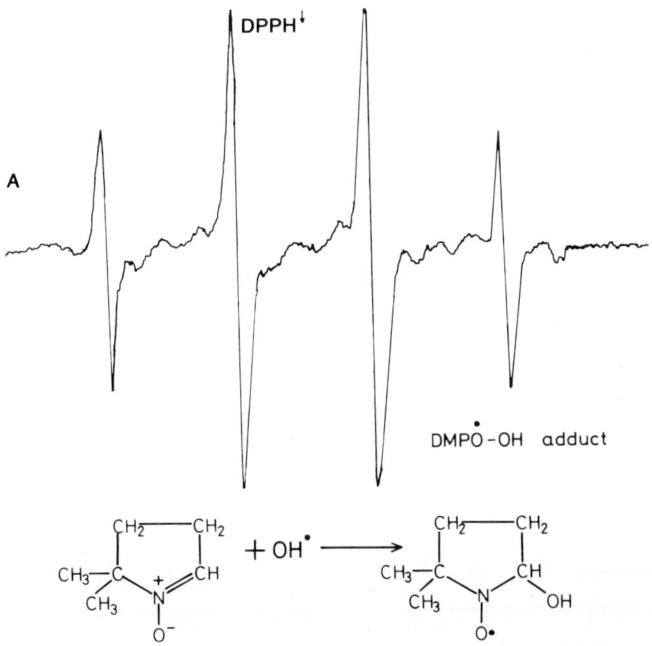

FIG. 11 Structure of the spin trap DMPO, the nitroxide radical formed by OH$^{\cdot}$ addition and the ESR spectrum observed with a DMPO solution containing iron and cysteine, attributed to the nitroxide.

The rates of reaction of several nitroxide radicals with organic radicals have already been determined by pulse radiolysis and further work is currently in progress to obtain data relevant to spin trapping studies. The rates of reaction of DMPO with $OH^•$ and the isopropanol radical have been determined by competition with ABTS and *p*-nitroacetophenone respectively (V. Mora, B. Wolfenden and R.L. Willson, unpublished results).

$$OH^• + RS^- \longrightarrow OH^- + RS^• \quad (k = 4\times10^{10}\ M^{-1}s^{-1})$$

$$OH^• + TRIS \longrightarrow \text{products} \quad (k = 3.3\times10^{8}\ M^{-1}s^{-1})$$

$$OH^• + DMPO \longrightarrow DMPO-OH^• \quad (k = 2.3\times10^{9}\ M^{-1}s^{-1})$$

$$OH^• + CH_3CHOH\ CH_3 \longrightarrow CH_3C(OH)CH_3^• + H_2O \quad (k = 2.1\times10^{9}\ M^{-1}s^{-1})$$

$$CH_3C(OH)\ CH_3^• + O_2 \longrightarrow CH_3C(OH)CH_3(O_2^•) \quad (k = 4\times10^{9}\ M^{-1}s^{-1})$$

$$CH_3C(OH)CH_3^• + DMPO \longrightarrow CH_3C(OH)CH_3 - DMPO^• \quad (k = 5.4\times10^{7}\ M^{-1}s^{-1})$$

$$CH_3C(OH)CH_3\text{-}DMPO^• + RS^- \longrightarrow \text{products}$$

$$CH_3C(OH)CH_3\text{-}DMPO^• + CH_3C(OH)CH_3^• \longrightarrow \text{products}$$

A value of $k_{OH+DMPO} = 2.7 \times 10^9\ M^{-1}s^{-1}$ has also been determined by ESR competition studies (Marriott *et al.*, 1980).

ILL-PLACED IRON AS A CO-CARCINOGEN

In the healthy cell the potent catalytic activity of iron is well controlled. The metal is compartmentalised by incorporation into macromolecular structures such as haemoglobin, the cytochromes or ferritin or bound to proteins such as transferrin. However, in disease, as a result of structural disorder or through the action of a chemical or virus, iron may reach sites to which it does not normally have access. Abnormal damaging oxidation reactions with free radical formation may result. If such reactions take place near critical molecules, for example DNA, the effects could be similar to those produced by exposure to ionising radiation and cancer or other tissue disorders could result (Willson, 1977a,b).

The present interest at Brunel in the role of iron in carcinogenesis has been stimulated considerably by the writings of Adrian

Albert. In his book "Selective Toxicity" (Albert, 1973), he describes how, in his studies with hydroxyquinoine (oxine), he found the chemical to be non-toxic to *Staphylococcus aureus* suspended in distilled water. If, however, cells were suspended in meat broth medium, or in water containing ferrous sulphate, considerable toxicity was evident after only three minutes. Furthermore, if zinc was added in large excess compared to iron, it had a protective effect. Albert proposed that oxine acted as a cooperative chelating agent, the 1:1 and 1:2 iron complex catalysing the oxidation of essential SH groups, and the 1:3 complex facilitating transport across the cell membrane. If other "inert" metals such as zinc were present in large excess compared to iron then, provided the stability constant of the "inert" complex was greater or approximately equal to that of iron, the "inert" metal would have a protective action.

A large number of other examples illustrating the importance of metal chelation were also given. Compounds such as EDTA had long been used in horticulture to assist the growth of fruit trees and iron-fastidious plants, such as rhododendrons, on alkaline soil. As long ago as 1947 the toxic action of the encephalomyelitis virus had been ascribed to it having the ability to transport iron across the blood-brain barrier which is normally impervious to the metal (Racker and Krimsky, 1947).

Thus the presence of foreign substances in tissue could have a marked effect on metal distribution: ill placement of iron could well occur (Fig. 12). If the resultant damage is extensive the cells may die. If, however, such damage is limited a cell may survive but not without some heritable change taking place. A foreign molecule C, for example, may be covalently grafted onto a sensitive target such as DNA by a free radical mechanism

$$\text{DNA} \xrightarrow{\text{free radicals}} \text{DNA}^{\bullet}$$

$$\text{C} \xrightarrow{\text{free radicals}} \text{C}^{\bullet}$$

$$\text{DNA}^{\bullet} + \text{C}^{\bullet} \longrightarrow \text{DNA-C}$$

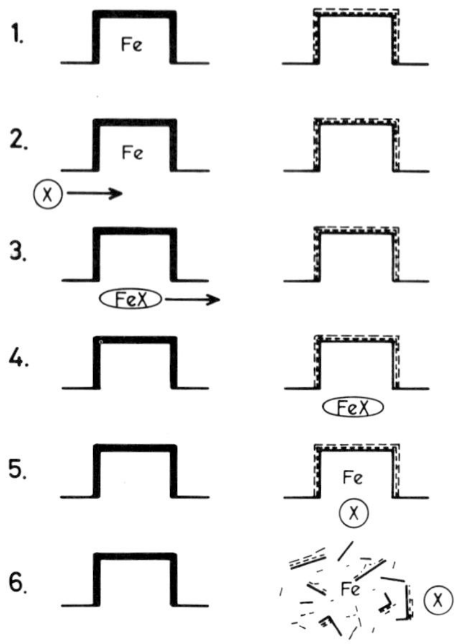

FIG. 12 Iron decompartmentalisation and ill-placement leading to free radical damage. An agent X transports iron from a "safe site" to a "sensitive site" which is subsequently destroyed.

We have seen how the spin trap DMPO can react readily with organic free radicals to form relatively stable nitroxide free radicals. Reaction of a DNA radical with the stable nitroxide free radical triacetonamine-N-oxyl has been observed directly by pulse radiolysis. Stationary studies using radioactive material have indicated that DNA-nitroxide adducts are formed (Willson and Emmerson, 1970).

Space does not permit the development of these arguments more fully. Other evidence on the role of decompartmentalised iron in carcinogenesis and in the action of some chemotherapeutic drugs such as metronidazole and bleomycin and the possible protective role of zinc has been published (Willson, 1976a,b, 1977a,b). Considerable encouragement has recently been provided by the *in vitro* studies with DNA and bleomycin which have shown that the drug's action involves an iron drug complex and the formation of free radicals. The zinc complex was inactive (Lown and Sim, 1977, and this Symposium).

$$BLM + Fe^{2+} \longrightarrow (BLM)Fe^{2+}$$

$$(BLM)Fe^{2+} + O_2 \longrightarrow (BLM)Fe^{3+} + O_2{}^{\bullet -}$$

$$(BLM)Fe^{2+} + H^+ + O_2{}^{\bullet -} \longrightarrow (BLM)Fe^{3+} + H_2O_2$$

$$(BLM)Fe^{2+} + H_2O_2 \longrightarrow (BLM)Fe^{3+} \quad OH^{\bullet} + OH^-$$

$$OH^{\bullet} + DNA \longrightarrow \text{damage}$$

Several cancers have long been associated with previous infection, and the fact that bleomycin is produced by cultures of *Streptomyces verticillus* may have wide implications. The possible role of malarial infection and the Epstein-Barr virus in the aetiology of Burkitt's lymphoma, for example, has attracted considerable interest, but unequical evidence for a causal relationship along classical molecular biological lines has not been forthcoming (Burkitt, 1962; Dalldorf *et al.*, 1964; de The *et al.*, 1978).

A free radical mediated process of carcinogenesis seems well worthy of consideration. Infection by the malarial parasite leads to disturbance in iron metabolism and hydrogen peroxide production has also been observed (Etkin and Eaton, 1975; Eckman and Eaton, 1979; Friedman 1979). In health, biochemistry undoubtedly rules; structure and order prevail. In disease, molecular anarchy can occur; countless simple reactions can take place governed only by the rules of basic chemistry.

ACKNOWLEDGEMENTS

The Brunel Free Radical Research Group is indebted to the Cancer Research Campaign, the International Atomic Energy Agency, the Medical Research Council, the National Foundation for Cancer Research and the Wellcome Foundation for financial support. I am indebted to my colleagues Dieter Asmus, Detlef Bahnemann, Jeff Mahood, Jorg Monig, Victor Mora, John Packer, Andy Searle, Michel Schaefer, Trevor Slater, Aldo Tomasi, John Taylor, Gavin Thomson and Brian Wolfenden for permission to refer to unpublished results.

REFERENCES

Adams, G.E. (1968). *In* "Radiation Chemistry of Aqueous Solutions" (Ed. G. Stein) pp.241-258, Interscience, London.

Adams, G.E. and Wardman, P. (1977). *In* "Free Radicals in Biology" (Ed. W.A. Pryor) Vol.3, pp.53-95, Academic Press, New York.

Adams, G.E. and Willson, R.L. (1973). *In* "Advances in Radiation Research. Biology and Medicine" (Ed. J.F. Duplon and A. Chapiro), pp.199-215, Gordon and Breach, New York.

Adams, G.E., Michael, B.D. and Willson, R.L. (1968). *Adv. Chem. Ser.* 71, 289-308.

Adams, G.E., Dische, S., Fowler, J.F. and Thomlinson, R.H. (1976). *Lancet* (i) 186-188.

Adams, G.E., Clarke, E.D., Flockhart, I.R., Jacob, R.S., Shemi, D.S., Stratford, I.J., Wardman, P., Watts, M.E., Parrick, J., Wallace, R.G. and Smithen, C.E. (1979). *Int. J. Radiat. Biol.* 35, 133-150, 151-160.

Adams, G.E., Ahmed, I., Fielden, E.M., O'Neill, P. and Stratford, I.J. (1980). *Cancer Clin. Trials* 3, 37-42.

Albert, A. (1973). "Selective Toxicity" 5th Ed. Chapman and Hall, London.

Alexander, P. and Charlesby, A. (1955). *In* "Radiobiology Symposium, Liege" (Eds. Z.M. Bacq and P. Alexander), pp.49-60. Butterworths Scientific Publications, London.

Alper, T. (1956). *Radiat. Res.* 5, 573-586.

Anderson, R.F. (1976). *Ber. Bunsenges. Phys. Chem.* 969-972.

Anderson, R.F. (1980). *Biochem. Biophys. Acta* 590, 277-281.

Asmus, K.D., Henglein, A., Ebert, M. and Keene, J.P. (1964). *Ber. Bunsenges. Phys. Chem.* 68, 657-663.

Asmus, K.D., Wigger, A. and Henglein, A. (1966). *Ber. Bunsenges. Phys. Chem.* 68, 862-868.

Asmus, K.D., Bahnemann, D., Monig, J., Searle, A. and Willson, R.L. (1979). *In* "Studies in Physical and Theoretical Chemistry" Vol.6, (Eds. H.E. Edwards, S. Navaratnam, B.J. Parsons and G.O. Phillips), pp.39-47. Elsevier, Amsterdam.

Asquith, J.C., Foster, J.L., Willson, R.L., Ings, R. and McFadzean, J.A. (1974). *Br. J. Radiol.* 47, 474-481.

Asquith, J.C., Watts, M.E., Patel, K., Smithen, C.E. and Adams, G.E. (1974). *Radiat. Res.* 60, 108-118.

Asquith, J.C., Willson, R.L. and Adams, G.E. (1970). *Abst. IV. Int. Congr. Radiat. Res., Evian, France.* p.11.

Baccanari, D.P. (1978). *Arch. Biochem. Biophys.* 191, 351-357.

Bahnemann, D. (1981). Ph.D. Thesis. Technical University, West Berlin.

Bahnemann, D., Basaga, H., Dunlop, J.R., Searle, A.J.F. and Willson, R.L. (1978). *Br. J. Cancer Supp.* III, 16-19.

Baumann, E. (1884). *Z. Physiol. Chem.* 8, 299-305.

Burkitt, D.P. (1969). *J. Natl. Cancer Inst.* 42, 19-28.

Childs, R.E. and Bardsley, W.G. (1975). *Biochem. J.* 145, 93-103.

Dalldorf, G., Linsell, C.A., Barhart, F.E. and Martyn, R. (1964). *Perspect. Biol. Med.* 7, 435-449.

de The, G., Geser, A., Day, N.E., Tukei, P.M., Williams, E.H., Beri, D.P., Smith, P.G., Dean, A.G., Bornkamm, G.W., Feorino, P. and Henle, W. (1978). *Nature (London)* 274, 756-761.

Eckman, J.R. and Eaton, J.W. (1979). *Nature (London)* 278, 754-756.

Etkin, N.L. and Eaton, J.W. (1975). *In* "Erythrocyte structure and Function" (Ed. G.J. Brewer), pp.219-232. Liss, New York.

Farrington, J.A., Land, E.J. and Swallow, A.J. (1980). *Biochim. Biophys. Acta* 590, 273-276.

Foster, J.L., Conroy, P.J., Searle, A.J. and Willson, R.L. (1976). *Br. J. Cancer* 33, 485-490.
Foster, J.L. and Willson, R.L. (1973). *Br. J. Radiol.* 46, 234-235.
Foster, J.L. and Willson, R.L. (1976). *In* "Chemotherapy" Vol.7 (Eds. K. Hellmann and T.A. Connors), pp.215-222. Plenum, New York.
Friedman, M.J. (1979). *Nature (London)* 280, 245-247.
Howard-Flanders, P. (1958). *Adv. Biol. Med. Phys.* 6, 553-603.
Ilan, Y.A., Meisel, D. and Czapski, G. (1974). *Isr. J. Chem.* 12, 891-895.
Ilan, Y.A., Czapski, G. and Meisel, D. (1976). *Biochim. Biophys. Acta* 430, 209-224.
Lanfrom, H. and Nielson, S.O. (1957). *J. Am. Chem. Soc.* 79, 1966-1970.
Lown, J.W. and Sim, S. (1977). *Biochem. Biophys. Res. Commun.* 77, 1150-1157.
Mahood, J.S., Packer, J.E., Searle, A.J.F., Willson, R.L. and Wolfenden, B.S. (1980). *In* "Phenothiazines and Structurally Related Drugs" (Eds. E. Usdin, H. Eckert and I.S. Forrest), pp.103-106. Elsevier, Amsterdam.
Marriott, P.R., Perkins, M.J. and Griller, D. (1980). *Can. J. Chem.* 58, 803-807.
Mathews, A.P. and Walker, S. (1909). *J. Biol. Chem.* 6, 299-312.
Meisel, D. and Neta, P. (1975a). *J. Am. Chem. Soc.* 97, 5198-1203.
Meisel, D. and Neta, P. (1975b). *J. Phys. Chem.* 79, 2459-2461.
Misra, H.P. (1974). *J. Biol. Chem.* 249, 2151-2155.
Packer, J.E., Slater, T.F. and Willson, R.L. (1978). *Life Sci.* 23, 2617-2620.
Packer, J.E., Slater, T.F. and Willson, R.L. (1979). *Nature (London)* 278, 737-738.
Packer, J.E., Mahood, J.S., Willson, R.L. and Wolfenden, B.S. (1980). *Int. J. Radiat. Biol.* 39, 135-141.
Patel, K.B. and Willson, R.L. (1973). *J. Chem. Soc. Faraday Trans. 1* 69, 814-825.
Rao, P.S. and Hayon, E. (1973). *Nature (London)* 243, 344-346.
Racker, E. and Krimsky, I. (1947). *J. Exp. Med.* 85, 715-727.
Rose, C.M., Millar, J.L., Peacock, J.H., Phelps, T.A. and Stephens, T.C. (1980). *In* "Radiation Sensitisers: Their Use in the Clinical Management of Cancer" (Ed. L. Brady), pp.250-257. Mason, New York.
Searle, A.J.F. and Willson, R.L. (1975). *Nature (London)* 255, 498-500.
Searle, A.J.F. and Willson, R.L. (1976). *Xenobiotica* 6, 457-464.
Sutherland, R.M. (1974). *Cancer Res.* 34, 3501-3503.
Svingen, B.A. and Powis, G. (1981). *Arch. Biochem. Biophys.* 209, 119-126.
Untasun, R., Band, P., Chapman, J.D., Feldstein, M.L., Meike, B. and Fryer, C. (1976). *New Engl. J. Med.* 294, 1399-1400.
Wardman, P. (1977). *Curr. Top. Radiat. Res. Q.* 11, 347-398.
Wardman, P. and Clarke, E.D. (1976a). *J. Chem. Soc. Faraday Trans. 1* 72, 1377-1390.
Wardman, P. and Clarke, E.D. (1976b). *Biochem. Biophys. Res. Commun.* 69, 942-949.
Willson, R.L. (1970). *Chem. Commun.* 1005.
Willson, R.L. (1976a). *Panminerva Med.* 18, 391-402.
Willson, R.L. (1976b). *Lancet* (i), 1407.
Willson, R.L. (1976c). *Lancet* (i), 304-305.

Willson, R.L. (1977a). *In* "Iron Metabolism" Ciba Foundation Symposium 51, pp.331-354. Excerpta Medica, Amsterdam.
Willson, R.L. (1977b). *Chem. Ind.* 183-193.
Willson, R.L. (1977c). *In* "Metronidazole" (Ed. S.M. Finegold), pp.147-175. Excerpta Medica, Amsterdam.
Willson, R.L. (1979a). *In* Biochemical Mechanisms of Liver Injury" (Ed. T.F. Slater), pp.123-224. Academic Press, New York.
Willson, R.L. (1979b). *In* "Oxygen Free Radicals and Tissue Damage", Ciba Foundation Symposium 65, pp.19-42. Excerpta Medica, Amsterdam.
Willson, R.L., Cramp, W.A. and Ing, R.M.J. (1974). *Int. J. Radiat. Biol.* 26, 557-569.
Willson, R.L. and Emmerson, P.T. (1970). *In* "Radiation Protection and Sensitisation" (Eds. M. Quintiliani and H. Moroson), pp.73-79. Taylor and Francis, London.
Willson, R.L., Greenstock, C.L., Adams, G.E., Wageman, R. and Dorfman, L.M. (1971). *Int. J. Radiat. Phys. Chem.* 3, 211-220.
Willson, R.L. and Searle, A.J.F. (1975). *Nature (London)* 255, 498-500.
Wood, P.M. (1974). *FEBS Lett.* 44, 22-24.

DISCUSSION

Lohmann: You emphasise the importance of iron. Have you ever tried copper too, and why do you think the zinc is not effective at all?

Willson: We have tried other metals as catalysts for the reduction of metronidazole and other nitro-compounds. Indeed, copper does catalyse this reaction, but it is much, much slower. The reason zinc is ineffective is because it cannot readily undergo one electron redox changes. Zinc (1) and zinc (111) do not normally exist, and from a redox point of view, zinc is relatively inert.

Lohmann: On one of your slides you showed the vitamin c radical. Have you ever observed it?

Willson: Yes, we have looked at the reaction of ascorbic acid with a number of different radicals. Ascorbic acid will repair a simple organic radical, for example, an alcohol radical. It will also interact with radical cations from dGMP, from phenothiazines and probably from thio ethers.

Lohmann: In the absorption spectrum of duroquinone there was a shoulder, what is it due to? The main peak should be π-π* transition, normally one expects a shoulder due to an n-α* transition to appear at a longer wave length.

Willson: I cannot explain it I'm afraid, but it is certainly there with all the quinones we have studied. In a paper I published in 1973 I distinctly drew a reference line on all of the spectra to show

how the main peak and the shoulder shifted depending on the substituent groups.

Asmus: I would like to ask a question concerning the formation of the radical cation of ABTS. You mentioned that it has a very high rate constant of about 10^{10} $M^{-1}s^{-1}$ and then you showed that the centre of oxidation was the nitrogen. How sure are you that you are really producing the nitrogen centred radical cation? You have several other centres there. The sulphur could be a centre, and there are even more sites of attack for the $OH^{\bullet}$ radical. As we know, the $OH^{\bullet}$ radical likes to go for any centre of relatively high electron density.

Willson: This was the species suggested to be formed by the action of peroxidase and the diagram was cribbed directly from this paper. I agree with you that it would be better to draw a dot in a circle covering much of the molecule.

Asmus: Have you any evidence for $OH^{\bullet}$ attack on the aromatic part of the molecule?

Willson: Yes. The yields of $ABTS^{\bullet +}$ from $OH^{\bullet}$ were slightly lower than from Br_2^-, or other electrophilic radicals suggesting another site of attack.

Reactive Oxygen Species Leading to Lipid Peroxidation and DNA Lesions Implicated in the Cytotoxic Action of Certain Antitumour Antibiotics

J.W. LOWN, A.V. JOSHUA and H.-H. CHEN

INTRODUCTION

One of the hazards of life in an oxygen-rich environment is the toxicity of molecular oxygen and its derivatives, superoxide anion $O_2^{\cdot -}$, singlet oxygen, hydrogen peroxide and especially the hydroxyl radical (Calvin, 1969; Fridovich, 1974, 1977). Cellular defence mechanisms have evolved consisting of metalloenzymes; superoxide dismutases (which remove $O_2^{\cdot -}$) which function in tandem with catalases and peroxidases (to remove H_2O_2) and thereby prevent the generation of the more damaging $OH^{\cdot}$ (Fig. 1) (Fridovich, 1972, 1977). It is becoming

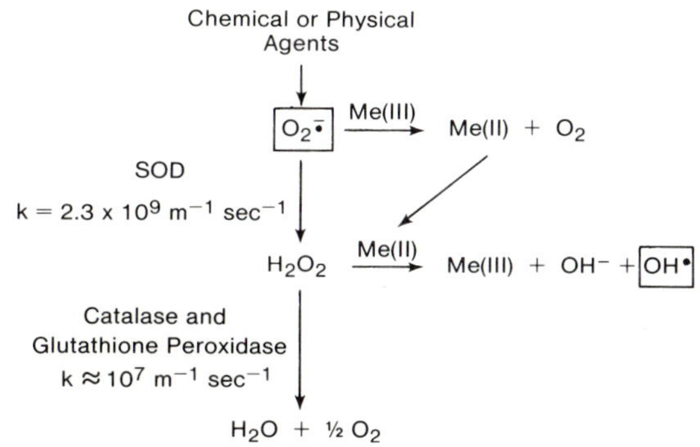

Uncatalyzed Reactions of Superoxide

$HO_2^{\cdot} + HO_2^{\cdot} \longrightarrow H_2O_2 + O_2 \quad k = 7.6 \times 10^5\ m^{-1}\ sec^{-1}$

$HO_2^{\cdot} + O_2^{\cdot -} + H^+ \longrightarrow H_2O_2 + O_2 \quad k = 8.5 \times 10^7\ m^{-1}\ sec^{-1}$

$O_2^{\cdot -} + O_2^{\cdot -} + 2H^+ \longrightarrow H_2O_2 + O_2 \quad k = 0.4\ m^{-1}\ sec^{-1}$

FIG. 1 Defence mechanisms against cellular oxygen toxicity.

recognised that certain disease states including cancer are associated with the breakdown of these defence mechanisms (McCord, 1974; Overley and Buettner, 1979; Peters and Seymour, 1978). Moreover, some of these reactive oxygen species are implicated in the molecular mechanisms of action of certain clinically effective antineoplastic agents (Cone *et al.*, 1976; Tomasz, 1976; Lown *et al.*, 1976, 1977, 1979; White and White, 1968).

This paper discusses the evidence in two such cases. The first of these cases involves the glycopeptide antibiotics bleomycin (BLM) and tallysomycin (TLM) (Fig. 2) where $O_2^{\cdot -}$, H_2O_2, and $OH^{\cdot}$ are implicated in the primary cytotoxic action (Sausville *et al.*, 1976; Lown and Sim, 1977). The second case involves anthracyclines, where reactive oxygen species are implicated in a critical secondary cardiotoxicity (Goodman and Hochstein, 1977; Lown *et al.*, 1977; Bachur *et al.*, 1979).

MATERIALS AND METHODS

BLM-A_2, BLM-B_2 and TLM-A were obtained from Bristol Laboratories, Syracuse, N.Y. TLM E_{1a} (Cu-complex) and TLM E_{1b} (Cu-complex) were kindly supplied by Dr. H. Kawaguchi, Bristol-Banyu Research Institute, Tokyo. Daunorubicin was from CalBiochem, La Jolla, CA. Adriamycin was obtained from the National Cancer Institute, NIH. The additional modified anthracyclines were prepared at SRI International, Menlo Park, CA. Superoxide dismutase (EC.1.15.1.1) was from Sigma Chemical Co., St. Louis, MO, and catalase (beef liver) was from Aldrich Chemical Co., Milwaukee, Wl. PM2-CCC-DNA was prepared as described previously (Morgan and Pulleyblank, 1974). Phenyl N-*tert*-butyl nitrone was from Aldrich and ethidium bromide, NADPH and disodium EDTA from Sigma.

Ethidium Fluorescence Determination of Superoxide Anion Generation by Nicking of PM2-CCC-DNA by Reductively Activated Antibiotics

The fluorometric methods of measuring strand breaking of PM2-CCC-DNA and its inhibition by selected enzymes and free radical scavengers have been described (Cone *et al.*, 1976; Morgan and Pulleyblank, 1974). The conversion of PM2-CCC-DNA to PM2-OC-DNA results in a 30% increase in fluorescence in an assay solution containing 20 mM potassium phosphate (pH 11.8) 0.2 mM EDTA and 0.5 μg/ml ethidium bromide and 100%

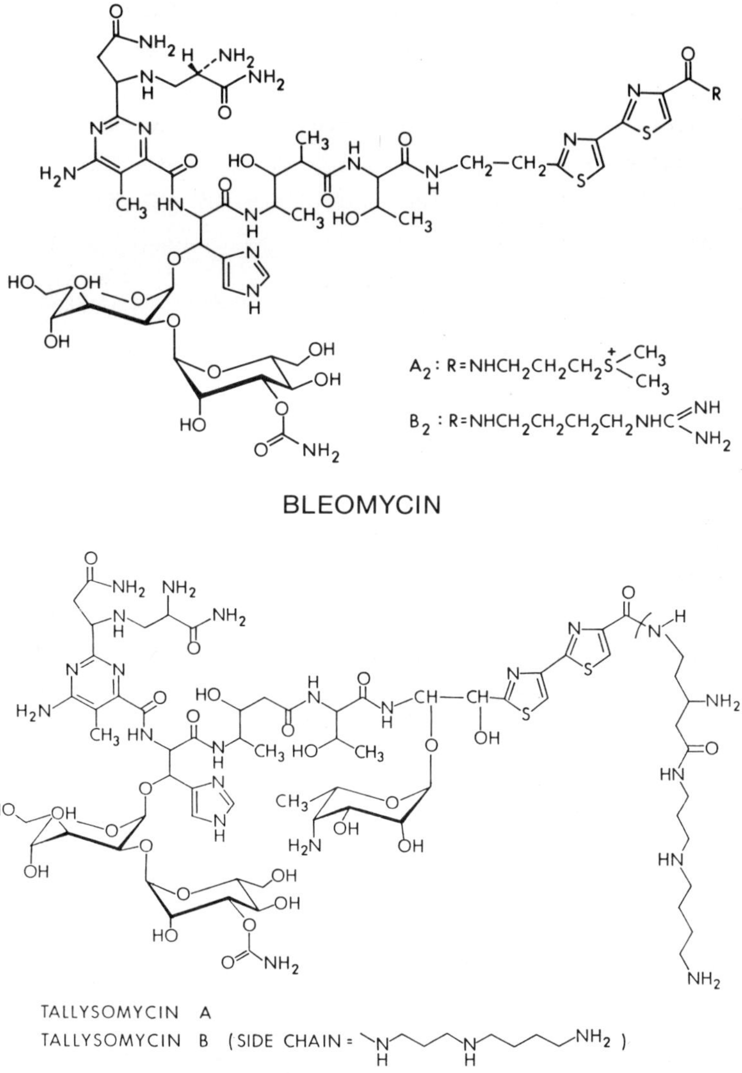

FIG. 2 The structures of bleomycin and tallysomycin

loss of fluorescence after a heating and cooling cycle (96°C for 4 min, then 23°C for 5 min) since the strands are now separate. The reactions were performed at 37°C in a volume of 200 µl containing potassium phosphate (pH 7.0), 1.02 A_{260} units of PM2-CCC-DNA (88% CCC) and other components as indicated in the legends to Figs 3 and 4.

Electrochemistry

Both DC and differential pulse polarographic studies were performed using Princeton Applied Research Equipment as described previously (Lown *et al.*, 1979; Rao *et al.*, 1977, 1978). The temperature was 37.5°C and all potentials were measured with respect to aqueous standard calomel electrode (S.C.E.). Solutions of the antibiotics were 1.0×10^{-4} M in aqueous solution with 10^{-2} M KCl and 10^{-2} M phosphate buffer (pH 7.2).

EPR Detection and Spin Trapping of Radical Species Generated from Antibiotics under Atmospheric Oxidation

EPR spectra were obtained using a Bruker ER-400 EPR spectrometer with a Varian V-3601 12 inch magnet and VFR Hall effect controller. Hyperfine couplings were obtained by comparison with peroxylamine disulfonate (spacing 13.0 G). Solutions contained 1.53×10^{-4} M antibiotic, 80 mM potassium phosphate buffer (pH 8.0), 80 mM phenyl-N-*tert*-butyl nitrone (PBN) and 5.37×10^{-4} M of appropriate reducing agent (Lown *et al.*, 1978).

RESULTS

Glycopeptide Antibiotics Bleomycin and Tallysomycin

A freshly prepared 2×10^{-6} M $FeSO_4$ solution nicks 30-50% PM2-CCC-DNA in 30 min at 37°C. Addition of 5×10^{-6} M BLM or TLM enhances the rate of DNA scission to 80-90% within 20 min (Fig. 3). Freshly prepared 5×10^{-5} M solutions of either BLM or TLM are capable of nicking up to 70% CCC-DNA in 20 min at pH 9.0, but are relatively slow at pH 7 and both antibiotics lose their nicking properties on prolonged exposure to air. The nicking ability can be restored to BLM and TLM by the addition and sequestration of 2×10^{-6} M $FeSO_4$. Alternatively continuous re-reduction of the trace of iron present in BLM or TLM by addition of 2×10^{-4} NADPH restores the original DNA nicking capacity. Careful exclusion of O_2 from the system severely retards DNA scission (Lown and Sim, 1977).

The cleavage of DNA by the glycopeptide antibiotic sequestered iron is inhibited by (i) superoxide dismutase, (ii) catalase, more efficiently by the two enzymes together, and (iii) free radical scavengers such as isopropyl alcohol, mannitol or sodium benzoate (Fig. 4).

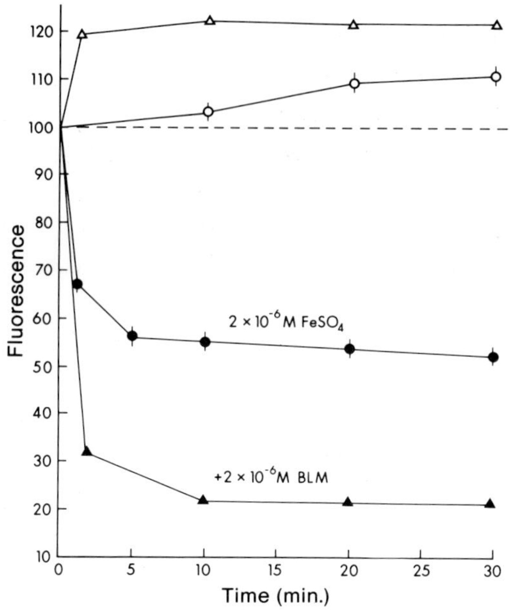

FIG. 3 Single strand scission of PM2-CCC-DNA by BLM in the presence of Fe(II) ion and its selective inhibition. Reactions were performed as described in methods with the following additional components: (ϕ) 2 x 10^{-6} M $FeSO_4$, (Δ) 2 x 10^{-6} M BLM.

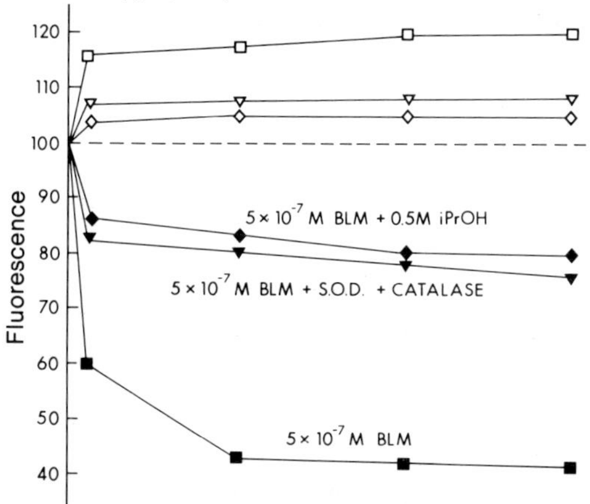

FIG. 4 Single strand scission of PM2-CCC-DNA by BLM in the presence of Fe(II) and its selective inhibition. Reactions were performed as described in methods with the following additional components: (□) 5 x 10^{-7} M BLM, (▽) 5 x 10^{-7} M BLM + 0.4 mg/ml superoxide dismutase and 0.08 mg/ml catalase, (◊) 5 x 10^{-7} M BLM and 0.5 M isopropyl alcohol.

For BLM the efficiency of DNA nicking increases from pH 4.7 (no nicking) with three pH optima at 9.3, 10.6 and 11.2. In the case of TLM only two pH optima are distinguished, 9.6 and 11.2. TLM binds sufficiently strongly to DNA to suppress the ethidium fluorescence and the binding increases from pH 7.0 to pH 4.7. Incubation of topo-isomerase relaxed PM2-CCC-DNA with BLM and TLM (6.66×10^{-5} M and 4.8×10^{-5} M respectively) for 3 h at 37°C (pH 7.0) and subsequent treatment with endonuclease VI neither caused an increase in fluorescence (assayed at pH 8.0) nor any appreciable cleavage (assayed at pH 11.8) (Lown and Joshua, 1980).

The copper-free TLM-E_{1a} in which the spermidine portion of the side chain of TLM-A has been degraded by spermidine oxidase to a 1,3-diaminopropane grouping (Konishi *et al.*, 1977) shows less binding to DNA compared with both TLM-A and TLM-A-Cu^{2+} as evidenced by suppression of the ethidium fluorescence. TLM-A and TLM-E_{1a} at a concentration of 4.8×10^{-5} M suppressed the fluorescence of PM2-CCC-DNA by 19% and 5.5% respectively (Fig. 5). Under similar conditions TLM-A-Cu^{2+} and TLM-E_{1a}-Cu^{2+} suppressed the fluorescence by 18% and 5% respectively. TLM-E_{1a} (1.9×10^{-5} M) in the presence of 4×10^{-6} M $FeSO_4$ nicks 86% PM2-CCC-DNA at 37°C (pH 7.0) in 30 min. The nicking was suppressed by the same selective enzyme and chemical inhibitors as for the parent antibiotic.

Incubation of the spin-trap PBN with BLM, TLM or TLM-E_{1a} in the presence of NADPH for 16 h produced the spin adduct PBN-OH, identified by its characteristic epr spectrum consisting of a triplet of doublets $a^N = 16.0$ G, $a^H_\beta = 3.4$ G, and $g = 2.0061$ (Fig. 6). Inclusion of catalase and superoxide dismutase in the reaction mixture almost completely suppressed the formation of the $OH^\bullet$ spin adduct (Lown and Joshua, 1980).

The electrochemical data on 1:1 BLM complexes of selected metal ions of biological interest are summarised in Table 1.

Anthracycline Antibiotics Adriamycin, Daunorubicin and Derivatives

The structures of anthracycline antibiotics are shown in Fig. 7. Daunorubicin (No.3 in Fig. 7) at a concentration of 4.5×10^{-5} M at pH 7.2, 37°C causes 90% single strand scission of PM2-CCC-DNA in

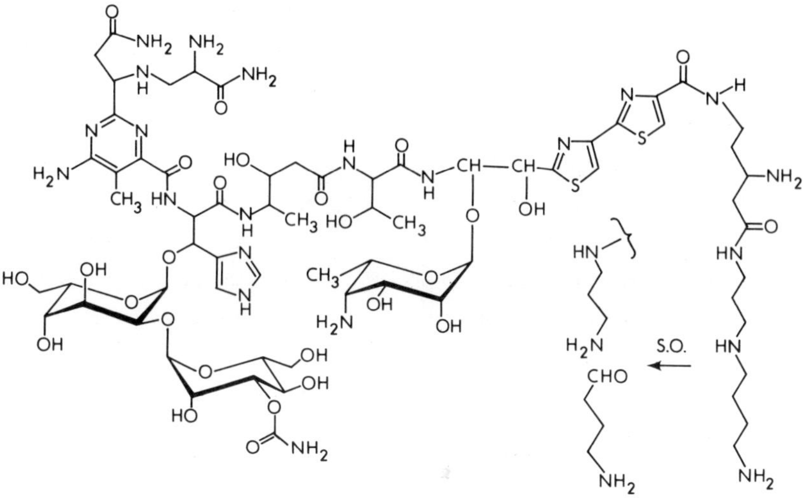

TALLYSOMYCIN A
TALLYSOMYCIN E_{1a} (Side chain truncated by Spermidine Oxidase [S.O.] from Serratia Marcescens).

	DNA BINDING[1]	DNA SCISSION[2]
TLM-A	19%	83%
TLM-Ela	5.5%	86%

1. Estimated by suppression of ethidium fluorescence for 4.8×10^{-5} M antibiotic
2. Determined for 1.92×10^{-5} M antibiotic, 37°, pH7 in 30 min.

FIG. 5 Enzyme modification of tallysomycin and its effects on DNA interaction.

TABLE 1 Characteristics of bleomycin-metal complexes

Complex	E^{1}_{o} (pH 7) volts*	Binding constant** (K_b)
BLM Fe(111)	+0.27	$10^{14.9}$
BLM Cu(11)	+0.196	$10^{13.8}$
BLM Cd(11)	-0.035	$10^{2.67}$
BLM Zn(11)	-0.501	10^{4}
BLM Ga(111)	-0.64	$10^{4.7}$

*NADPH/NADP couple at -0.30 volts is capable of reducing Fe, Cu and Cd complexes. **Computed from electrochemical data. Sequence indicates Fe may replace other metals from BLM complexes.

$$BLM.Fe^{2+} + O_2 \longrightarrow BLM.Fe^{3+} + O_2^{\bullet-}$$
$$BLM.Fe^{2+} + O_2^{\bullet-} \xrightarrow{2H^+} BLM.Fe^{3+} + H_2O_2$$
$$BLM.Fe^{2+} + H_2O_2 \longrightarrow BLM.Fe^{3+} + \dot{O}H + \bar{O}H$$

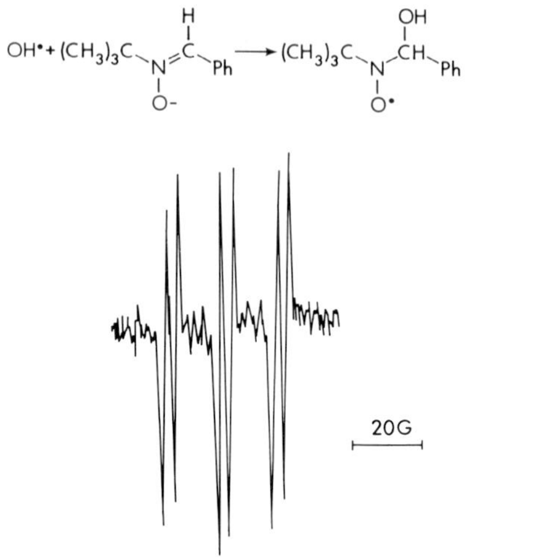

FIG. 6 Spin trapping of hydroxyl radical from oxidation of bleomycin. PBN incubated with BLM for 16 h (for conditions see text) produces the spin adduct PBN-OH. Its characteristic epr spectrum is shown.

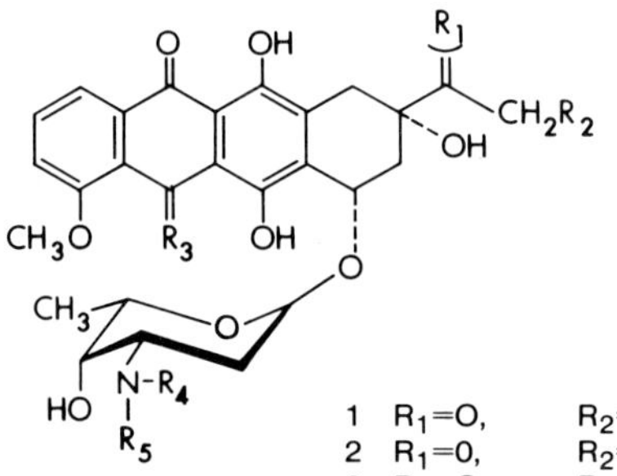

1	R_1=O,	R_2=H,	R_3=O,	$R_4=CH_3$,	$R_5=CH_3$
2	R_1=0,	R_2=OH,	R_3=O,	R_4=H,	R_5=H
3	R_1=O,	R_2=H,	R_3=O,	R_4=H,	R_5=H
4	R_1=O,	R_2=OH,	R_3=O,	$R_4=CH_3$,	$R_5=CH_3$
5	R_1=O,	R_2=H,	R_3=O,	R_4,	$R_5 = -[CH_2]_5$
6	R_1=O,	R_2=H,	R_3=O,	$R_4=CH_2Ph$,	R_5=H
7	R_1=O,	R_2=H,	R_3=O,	R_4,	$R_5 = -[CH_2]_2 O[CH_2]_2-$
8	R_1=H, OH,	R_2=H,	R_3=NH,	R_4=H,	R_5=H
9	R_1=O,	R_2=H,	R_3=NH,	R_4=H,	R_5=H
10	R_1=O,	R_2=H,	R_3=O,	$R_4=CH_2Ph$,	$R_5=CH_2Ph$
11	R_1=O,	R_2=H,	R_3=NH,	$R_4=CH_2Ph$,	$R_5=CH_2Ph$

FIG. 7 Structures of anthracycline antibiotics

75 min. 5-Imino-daunorubicin (No.9 in Fig. 7) under comparable conditions causes only 50% scission (Lown *et al.*, 1979a) while 13-dihydro-5-iminodaunorubicin (No.8 in Fig. 7), N,N-dibenzyl-5-imino-daunorubicin (No.11 in Fig. 7) gave 43, 10, and 0% DNA scission under comparable conditions. N,N-Dimethyl-daunorubicin (No.1 in Fig. 7) was highly effective giving 90% DNA scission in 75 min. The results of the other anthracyclines leading to intermediate extents of generation of reactive oxygen species are given in Table 2.

All anthracyclines show an initial reduction around -0.65 V (quinone or modified quinone). A process near -1.15 V appears to be associated with the side chain. Compounds with substituents on the sugar moiety have essentially the same reduction potential as daunorubicin, while those with 5-imino substituted chromophores are more difficult to reduce than daunorubicin.

Results on the extents of interaction of the anthracyclines with DNA, the inhibition of macromolecular synthesis (DNA and RNA) in leukaemia L1210 cells, cardiotoxicity data in rats, relative extents of oxygen consumption by rat liver microsomal activation, the aglycone group redox potentials and the relative extents of generation of reactive oxygen species as measured by the degree of DNA scission under standard conditions are given in Table 2 (Lown *et al.*, 1981).

DISCUSSION

Glycopeptides Bleomycin and Tallysomycin are Antitumour Antibiotics in which Oxygen Species are Involved in their Antineoplastic Action

BLM isolated from *streptomyces* (Umezawa *et al.*, 1975, 1976) and TLM isolated from *actinomycetes* (Kawaguchi *et al.*, 1977) are glycopeptides containing a number of heterocyclic centres. In the form of "blenoxane" a mixture of BLM-A_2 and BLM-B_2 the former is widely used clinically in the treatment of squamous cell carcinoma, Hodgkin's disease, malignant lymphoma and testicular carcinoma (Umezawa *et al.*, 1975, 1976). The principal side-effect of BLM is pulmonary toxicity and TLM is of interest because it shows a lower level of pulmonary toxicity. Considerable evidence has accumulated that DNA is the principal target of BLM in its antineoplastic action (Umezawa 1975, 1976). The evidence from this paper and the results of other workers (Sauseville *et al.*, 1976) suggest BLM functions by migrating to the

TABLE 2 Comparison of biological test data for anthracyclines with generation of reactive oxygen species

Anthra-cycline (numbered as in Fig. 7)	ΔTm ^{o}C	Inhib.of synth. in L1210 cells[a]		Activity against P388 leukaemia, mice q 4d, 5, 9, 13 % T/C (mg/kg)[b]	Cardiotoxicity Zbinden MCCD in rats min.cum. cardiotoxic dose mg/kg[c]	O_2 consumption rat liver microsomes as % activity of adriamycin[d]	$E_{\frac{1}{2}}$,V DC polarogram 50% CH_3CN	Reoxidation of reduced species CV,500 mV/s	Relative generation of reactive oxygen species 75 min 45 μm drug
		DNA ED_{50}μm	RNA ED_{50}μm						
1	17.5	0.62	0.12	186(2.4)	6	145	-0.65	>95	90
2	13.4	1.5	0.58	159(8)	11	100	-0.64	63	88
3	11.2	0.66	0.33	132(8)	14	109	-0.64	67	90
4	15.3	0.67	0.064	167(10)	11-16	108	-0.64	>95	90
5	16.4	0.62	0.03	191(6.2)	-	88	-0.655	e	87
6	10.2	1.6	0.17	184(18.8)	-	87	-0.65	e	73
7	23.3	0.35	0.0103	187(0.2)	-	25	-0.654	75	55
8	3.3	4.0	5.6	-	-	11	-0.72	10	43
9	6.25	1.6	1.3	130(3)	64	8.2	-0.70	13	55
10	1.4	>100	10	208(38)	125	0.5	-0.65	e	10
11	-0.8	>1000	160	101(5-150)	-	-	-0.745	e	0

[a] ΔTM and ED_{50} values from Tong *et al.* (1979a,b) were determined by the method of G. Tong *et al.* (1976). [b] Assays arranged through the Drug Research and Development Program, Division of Cancer Treatment, National Cancer Institute - BDF and CDF mice were injected i.p. on days 1-9 or days 5, 9, 10 with the specified drug dose. See Geran *et al.* (1972). T/C is the ratio of average survival times of treated mice to untreated controls in percent (Tong *et al.*, 1979a,b). [c] Cardiotoxicity in rats assay described in Zbinden *et al.* (1978). [d] Reference: Gordon *et al.* (1980). [e] Compound insoluble in water.

cell nucleus where Fe III is sequestered in a hexacoordinate structure at one end of the molecule. The binding constants given in Table 1 indicate iron would be capable of displacing other metals. The selective quenching of the fluorescence characteristic of the bithiazole moiety upon adding DNA (Povirk *et al.*, 1979, 1981) gives evidence for binding of the antibiotic to its cell target by intercalation of the latter group in a sequence selective fashion (Takeshita *et al.*, 1979). The fact that the spermidine oxidase degraded TLM-A still binds to DNA supports this view but the fact that the binding is thereby decreased shows that the β-lysine-spermidine group provides additional binding. Since TLM-E_{1a} is still capable of nicking DNA this experiment confirms that the iron is not chelated in this portion of the molecule. Once bound the sequestered Fe(III) undergoes a cycle of redox steps (Fig. 8). The electrochemical data of Table 1 demonstrate Fe(III) reduction is compatible with biological reductants such as NADH (see also Dabrowiak and Santillo, 1979). Interaction of BLM Fe(II) or TLM Fe(II) with O_2 generates reactive oxygen species which are identified by the selective enzymatic inhibition as $O_2^{\cdot -}$, and H_2O_2 and by the spin-trapping experiments as $HO^{\cdot}$

The latter extremely reactive species when generated in close proximity to DNA is known to lead to strand scission (Dizdaroglu *et*

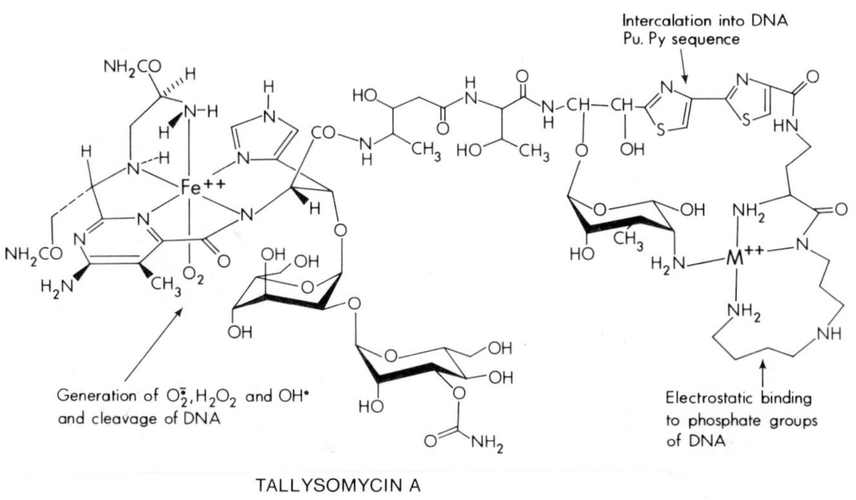

FIG. 8 The mechanism of tallysomycin action.

al., 1975). The above data permit us to propose a reaction scheme for these processes (GLM stands for either glycopeptide BLM or TLM)

$$GLM + Fe(II) \rightleftharpoons GLM\ Fe(II) \qquad (1)$$

$$GLM\ Fe(II) + O_2 \longrightarrow GLM\ Fe(II).O_2 \qquad (2)$$

$$GLM\ Fe(II).O_2 \longrightarrow GLM\ Fe(III) + O_2^{\cdot -} \qquad (3)$$

$$GLM\ Fe(III) + NADPH \xrightarrow{-H^+} GLM\ Fe(II) + NADP \qquad (4)$$

$$GLM\ Fe(II) + O_2^{\cdot -} \xrightarrow{2H^+} GLM\ Fe(III) + H_2O_2 \qquad (5)$$

$$2\ O_2^{\cdot -} + 2H^+ \xrightarrow[\text{Dismutase}]{\text{Superoxide}} H_2O_2 + O_2 \qquad (6)$$

$$2\ H_2O_2\ \text{Catalase} \longrightarrow 2\ H_2O + C_2 \qquad (7)$$

$$GLM\ Fe(II) + H_2O_2 \longrightarrow GLM\ Fe(III) + OH^{\cdot} + OH^- \qquad (8)$$

$$OH^{\cdot} + DNA \longrightarrow \text{Strand breakage} \qquad (9)$$

HABER-WEISS REACTION

$$H_2O_2 + O_2^{\cdot -} \longrightarrow OH^{\cdot} + OH^- + O_2 \qquad (10)$$

The Haber-Weiss reaction (10) which is often invoked in *in vivo* systems is quite slow ($k < 0.30,\ M^{-1}\ sec^{-1}$ McClune and Fee, 1976; van Hemmen and Meuling, 1977; Halliwell, 1976) and is therefore unlikely to compete for $O_2^{\cdot -}$ compared with the very rapid steps 4 and 6.

Anthracycline Antitumour Antibiotics in which Oxygen Species Generation Correlates with Cardiotoxic Effects

A quite different example is provided by the anthracyclines. These represent a family of antibiotics characterised by a planar four ring chromophore and one or more sugar units of which the most important examples clinically are adriamycin and daunorubicin (Arcamone, 1978; DiMarco *et al.*, 1975). The results demonstrate that upon reductive activation the anthracyclines generate reactive oxygen species $O_2^{\cdot -}$, H_2O_2, and $OH^{\cdot}$ capable of cleaving DNA by a mechanism similar to the one proposed above for bleomycin and tallysomycin (Fig. 9).

The results in Table 2 also demonstrate that chemical modification of the aglycone (e.g. 5-iminodaunorubicin) leads to a reduction in this oxygen cycling which correlates with its observed lower cardiotoxic effects based on electrocardiogram tests in rats (Lown *et al.*, 1981). The rationale is that since anthracyclines accumulate in the heart (Arcamone, 1975) and since cardiac tissue is deficient in those

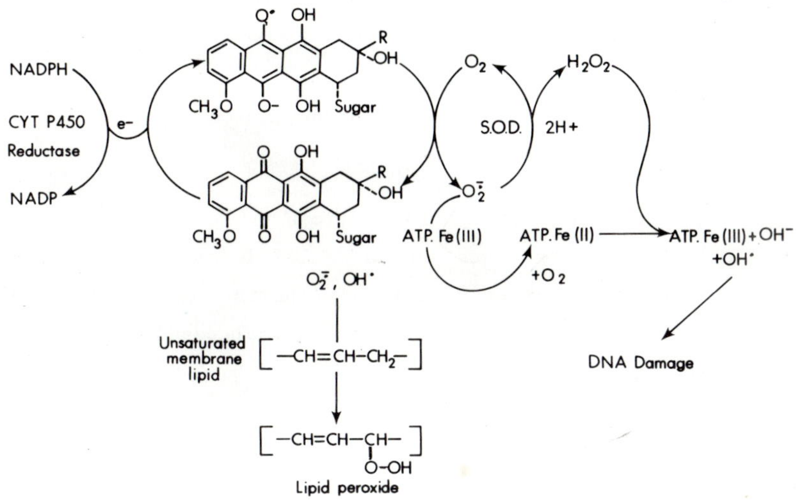

FIG. 9 Oxidative damage by bio-activated anthracyclines.

enzymes (Peskin *et al.*, 1977; Doroshow *et al.*, 1980) designed to protect the cell from oxidative lesions (i.e. superoxide dismutase, catalase, and glutathione peroxidase) factors which interfere with the oxygen cycling capacity of the drug lead to the alleviation of cardiotoxic effects by a factor of up to twenty. The agreement between the independent measurement of rat liver microsomal oxygen consumption and of superoxide generation is quite close. In addition the antileukaemic properties of the drugs are maintained. In conclusion it appears possible to separate the anti-tumour and cardiotoxicity effects of the anthracycline drugs by certain specific structural modifications, especially those that directly affect redox potential.

SUMMARY

A study has been made of the molecular mechanism of action of first, the glycopeptide antibiotics bleomycin and tallysomycin and second, the anthracyclines adriamycin, daunorubicin and their derivatives. In both cases bioreductive activation in the presence of oxygen leads to $O_2^{\bullet -}$, H_2O_2, and $OH^{\bullet}$ which may result in lipid peroxidation and DNA lesions. In the former examples this chemical mechanism correlates with the primary cytotoxic action, whereas in the latter examples, reactive oxygen species generation correlates with secondary cardiotoxic effects. This latter side-effect of the anthracyclines may be ameliorated by a factor of twenty by rational structural modification with no sacrifice in anti-leukaemic potency.

ACKNOWLEDGEMENTS

This research was supported by grants (to J.W. Lown) from the National Cancer Institute of Canada and the Natural Sciences and Engineering Council of Canada and the University of Alberta. We would like to thank Dr. J.A. Plambeck for the electrochemical results and Dr. E.M. Acton for the cardiotoxicity data.

REFERENCES

Arcamone, F. (1978). *In* "Topics in Antibiotic Chemistry" (Ed. P. Sammes) Vol. 2, pp.102-239, J. Wiley, New York.
Bachur, N.R., Gordon, S.L., Gee, M.V. and Kon, H. (1979). *Proc. Natl. Acad. Sci. USA* 76, 954-957.
Calvin, M. (1969). "Chemical Evolution" Oxford University Press, London.
Cone, R., Hasan, S.K., Lown, J.W. and Morgan, A.R. (1976). *Can. J. Biochem.* 54, 219-223.
Dabrowiak, J.C. and Santillo, F.S. (1979). *J. Electrochem. Soc.* 126, 2091-2095.
DiMarco, A., Arcamone, F. and Zunino, F. (1975). *In* "Antibiotics III. Mechanism of Action of Antimicrobial and Antitumour Agents" (Eds. J.W. Corcoran and F.E. Hahn), pp.101-128. Springer-Verlag, New York.
Dizdaroglu, M., von Sonntag, C. and Schulte-Frohlinde, D. (1975). *J. Am. Chem. Soc.* 97, 2277-2278.
Doroshow, J.H., Tonker, G.Y. and Myers, C.E. (1980). *J. Clin. Invest.* 65, 128-135.
Fridovich, I. (1972). *Acc. Chem. Res.* 5, 321-326.
Fridovich, I. (1974). *In* "Horizons in Biochemistry and Biophysics" Vol. 1, pp.1-38. Addison-Wesley, Reading MA.
Fridovich, I. (1977). *In* "Biochemical and Medical Aspects of Active Oxygen" (Eds. O. Hayaishi and K. Asada) pp.3-9. University Park Press, Baltimore.
Geran, R.I., Greenberg, N.H., MacDonald, M.H., Schumacher, A.M. and Abbot, B.J. (1972). *Cancer Chemother. Rep. Part 3* 3 (2), 9-112.
Goodman, J. and Hochstein, P. (1977). *Biochem. Biophys. Res. Commun.* 77, 797-803.
Gordon, G.R., Peters, J.H. and Acton, E.M. (1980). Second Chem. Congr. North Amer. Contient, Las Vegas, August 24-29, Abstract Bio 13.
Halliwell, B. (1976). *FEBS Lett.* 72, 8-10.
van Hemmen, J.J. and Meuling, W.J.S. (1977). *Arch. Biochem. Biophys.* 182, 743-748.

Kawaguchi, H., Tsukiura, H., Tomita, K., Konishi, M., Saito, K., Kobaru, S., Numata, K., Fujisawa, K., Miyaki, T., Hatori, M. and Koshiyama, H. (1977). *J. Antibiot. (Tokyo)* 30, 779-788.

Konishi, M., Saito, K., Numata, K., Tsuno, T., Asama, K., Tsukiura, H. Naito, T. and Kawaguchi, H. (1977). *J. Antibiot.* 30, 789-805.

Lown, J.W., Begleiter, A., Johnson, D. and Morgan, A.R. (1976). *Can. J. Biochem.* 54, 110-119.

Lown, J.W. and Sim, S.K. (1977). *Biochem. Biophys. Res. Commun.* 77, 1150-1157.

Lown, J.W., Sim, S.K., Majumdar, K.C. and Chang, R.Y. (1977). *Biochem. Biophys. Res. Commun.* 76, 705-710.

Lown, J.W., Sim, S.K. and Chen, H.H. (1978). *Can. J. Biochem.* 56, 1042-1047.

Lown, J.W., Chen, H.H., Plambeck, J.A. and Acton, E.M. (1979). *Biochem. Pharmacol.* 28, 2563-2568.

Lown, J.W. and Joshua, A.V. (1980). *Biochem. Pharmacol.* 29, 521-532.

Lown, J.W., Chen, H.H., Plambeck, J.A. and Acton, E.M. (1981). *Biochem. Pharmacol.* (in press).

McClune, G.T. and Fee, T.A. (1976). *FEBS Lett.* 67, 294-298.

McCord, T.M. (1974). *Science* 185, 529-531.

Morgan, A.R. and Pulleyblank, D.E. (1974). *Biochem. Biophys. Res. Commun.* 61, 396-403.

Overley, L.W. and Buettner, G.R. (1979). *Cancer Res.* 39, 1141-1149.

Peters, J.H. and Seymour, C.A. (1978). *Clin. Sci. Mol. Med.* 54, 549-563.

Peskin, A.V., Koen, Ya.M., Zbarsky, I.B. and Konstantinov, A.A. (1977). *FEBS Lett.* 78, 41-45.

Povirk, L.F., Hogan, M.S. and Dattagupta, N. (1979). *Biochemistry* 18, 96-101.

Povirk, L.F., Hogan, M., Dattagupta, N. and Buechners, M. (1981). *Biochemistry* 20, 665-671.

Rao, G.M., Lown, J.W. and Plambeck, J.A. (1978). *J. Electrochem. Soc.* 125, 534-539.

Rao, G.M., Begleiter, A., Lown, J.W. and Plambeck, J.A. (1977). *J. Electrochem. Soc.* 124, 199-202.

Sausville, E.A., Peisach, J. and Horwitz, S.B. (1976). *Biochem. Biophys. Res. Commun.* 71, 814-822.

Takeshita, M. and Grollman, A.P. (1979). *In* "Bleomycin, Chemical, Biochemical and Biological Aspects" (Ed. S.M. Hecht), pp.207-221. Springer-Verlag, New York.

Tomasz, M. (1976). *Chem. Biol. Interact.* 13, 89-97.

Tong, G.L., Lee, W.W., Black, D.R. and Henry, D.W. (1976). *J. Med. Chem.* 19, 395-398.

Tong, G.L., Wu, H.Y., Smith, T.H. and Henry, D.W. (1979a). *J. Med. Chem.* 22, 912-918.

Tong, G.L., Henry, D.W. and Acton, E.M. (1979b). *J. Med. Chem.* 22, 36-39.

Umezawa, H. (1975). *In* "Antibiotics III. Mechanism of Action of Antimicrobial and Antitumour Agents". (Eds. J.W. Corcoran and F.E. Hahn), pp.21-33, Springer-Verlag, New York.

Umezawa, H. (1976). *In* "Gann Monograph on Cancer Research No.19. Fundamental and Clinical Studies on Bleomycin". (Eds. S.K. Carter, T. Ichikawa, T. Mathé and H. Umezawa), pp.3-36, University Park Press, Baltimore.

White, H.L. and White, J.R. (1968). *Mol. Pharmacol.* 4, 549-565.
Zbinden, G., Bachmann, E. and Holdnegger, C. (1978). *Antibiotic Chemother. (Basel)* 23, 255-270.

DISCUSSION

Willson: With the quinones that you mentioned you have invoked metal ions in the generation of $OH^{\cdot}$. Do you know of any evidence for hydroxyl radical formation from the interaction of hydrogen peroxide with the semiquinone radical anion? It is known from old radiation studies that the $CO_2^{\cdot -}$ radical will react with hydrogen peroxide to give $OH^{\cdot}$.

Lown: Yes, that's quite possible. Thermodynamically I should say it is unlikely but possible. However, I know of no evidence to support that contention.

Willson: You didn't get rid of all the metal ions in your system then?

Lown: It's very difficult to remove the last traces of metals. Iron, even when chelated will react with hydrogen peroxide (Bielski, 1977).

Adams: I would like to ask you two general points regarding the $OH^{\cdot}$ radical. It is necessary to invoke some form of metal catalysis because of the very small rate constant of the $O_2^{\cdot}$ radical. One shouldn't overlook the fact that the rate constant of the protonated species, the $HO_2^{\cdot}$ radical, is several orders of magnitude greater. Since the pK_a of HO_2 is around 4.5 even though at biological pH, where only a very small proportion is in the HO_2 form, it could still predominate over O_2^- in its reaction. The $HO_2^{\cdot}$ radical is almost certain to be the reactive species, therefore, rather than O_2^-. The second point is that if the $OH^{\cdot}$ radical is generated and is responsible for the strand break, it is formed from some form of species which is presumably not reactive enough to prevent its diffusion. It will have a certain diffusion radius. It is known that reactivity of the $OH^{\cdot}$ radical is about 20 times greater with the bases than it is with the sugar residues. Base damage is much more likely to happen than the strand breakage, therefore.

Lown: Yes, that's right, but with bleomycin or tallysomycin the bases are released undamaged (Haidle *et al.*, 1972). For example, thymine is produced and is not attacked by $OH^{\cdot}$ whereas the sugar definitely is attacked giving dialdehyde fragments (Haidle, 1971). So evidently, the sugar is attacked preferentially. This may well have a stereochemical explanation.

Adams: It has to be, because, when in free solution, the rate constants are known precisely.

Lown: In that case it's a site specific radical generated close to the sugar and it's kept away from the base, otherwise there would be a kinetic preference for an attack on the base.

Symons: A question and a comment. The question is when you're generating $OH^{\bullet}$ radicals I take your point that it has to be site-specific in generating it near the sugar but in all these molecules have you got enormous reactivity towards OH in the unit itself?

Lown: Yes, in fact in the absence of DNA bleomycin destroys itself by generating $OH^{\bullet}$ radicals which attack succeptible sites (Hecht, 1979).

Symons: So it's the chance one that gets away that is doing the damage - is that right?

Lown: Yes. As soon as you activate bleomycin or tallysomycin by reduction in the presence of oxygen it starts degrading itself - a very curious suicidal activity.

Symons: The comment relates to Dr Willson's question concerning generating $OH^{\bullet}$ radicals from the semiquinone. I'm sure this is a truism but there is a very real difference between what ferrocyanin in a complex does and what a quinone anion would do. In the quinone anion reaction, as I would envisage it, there is a straightforward electron transfer to give you OH^{-} plus OH but in the reaction with iron I would imagine it is a coordination of hydrogen peroxide to the iron, followed by breaking of the O-O bond with the formation of an FeOH unit and and $OH^{\bullet}$ radical. Mechanistically, these are quite different things.

Ts'o: Lesko *et al.* (1980) using T7 DNA as a model showed you can put the DNA in hydrogen peroxide and superoxide radicals and get no chain breaks in the presence of metal chelators; so the conclusion of that paper is that the only reduced oxygen species that breaks DNA is the $OH^{\bullet}$ radical.

Lown: I'm glad to hear that. There's been a lot of controversy about this as you know, because many people wrongly implied that the superoxide radical can abstract an hydrogen atom from, for example, a sugar moiety. I don't think this is possible because it's from the same family as the semidiones or the semiquinones which are relatively stable.

Ts'o: With all the knowledge about binding specificity to the DNA conformation as well as information from the recent studies on polymorphism of DNA structure do you know whether this binding takes place with any preference for the A form of DNA or the Z form, etc.?

Lown: That's a very good question. I've just come from the Medicinal Chemistry Symposium in Buffalo and David Henry was there discussing bis intercalators. He presented evidence that he can make bis intercalators which will recognise the Z form preferentially so chemists are beginning to be concerned about this now. But whether or not this happens naturally I don't know. I think it's too early to tell, but certainly the conformation of DNA is very important in molecular recognition. What we are involved with now with bleomycin is to synthesise models or analogues designed to mimic the antibiotic action. We synthesised bis intercalators with an intercalative group bound through protein linkers to a capped porphyrin designed to bind to DNA and recognise different sequences from those that bleomycin recognises (Lown, J.W. and Joshua, A.V., unpublished results). One should thereby have a superoxide and hydroxyl generator in the capped porphyrin to nick the DNA at a sequence linked to the site. I think we're going to have to be concerned about the conformation of the DNA receptor in our future studies.

Ts'o: There is an hypothesis that when DNA is being transcribed by RNA polymerase it might switch into an A form because that is how RNA is made. In all your model building have you tried to fit your antibiotics into the A form of DNA?

Lown: No. It is tempting but I think it can be misleading to draw too many conclusions from CPK models. I think it's too soon to start drawing detailed conclusions about molecular recognition. We just don't know enought about it yet.

Swartz: Bill, in your scheme for bleomycin you had it picking up iron (II) and that raises an important question that seems to keep coming back: where does the iron (II) come from? It's a kind of article of faith, although it may be an erroneous one, that there is no ferrous iron in the cell available for something like bleomycin to pick up.

Lown: I didn't imply that it was free - the evidence suggests that the iron required is complexed to ATP or protein.

Swartz: I think there's a more general problem. Some people think that the critical event involves a reduction of ferric to ferrous iron and that this is really the triggering event in complex biological systems so that once you get the ferrous iron the damage is inevitable. Do you have any comments on how that ferrous iron might be generated within your scheme?

Lown: Well, as I mentioned before, the clinical grade bleomycin contains a small amount of iron already - about 0.02 atom % by atomic absorption (Lown and Sim, 1977). Perhaps that is sufficient when you inject it into the patient to allow the antibiotic to function. Because if you administer the one to one complex of bleomycin and iron, it's terribly toxic and, therefore, unsuitable clinically. Evidently, you need only a limited amount of iron. Perhaps bleomycin has enough as it is injected and since as we have seen, the antibiotic is degraded in the process, the trace of iron would be available for recycling? But you're right, the reduction step is clearly an important initial step in the activation of the antibiotic.

Connors: I like the concept of site specificity but then I was surprised with one of your results with tallysomycin. When you modify the tail of the molecule by spermine oxidase you found that you got very much reduced binding but the same amount of DNA scission. Surely the two should be related, reduced binding leading to less DNA scission?

Lown: Yes, but I think we were overloading the system in that case. The scission assay is very sensitive. One of its advantages is that you can use sub-micromolar concentrations of antibiotics but the disadvantage is that you can overload it very easily. So even at micromolar concentrations we were nicking all the DNA molecules at least once and I think that we were just using a little too much tallysomycin (Lown and Joshua, 1980).

Stier: Your concept could be tested by looking for the metabolites of the various antibiotics if there is self-destruction by $OH^{\bullet}$

radicals. You should have a great variety of products. Is anything known about this?

Lown: That takes us back to Professor Symons' question. Bleomycin is, in fact, extensively degraded by $OH^{\bullet}$ species generated and one obtains several fragments, e.g. the sugar moieties are released and degraded. Incidentally, I didn't mention it before but bleomycin has just been synthesised - quite an enormous task, which has been completed in Japan recently (Takita, T., personal communication). This is a significant step forward in synthetic chemistry and through their experience they were able to identify some of the metabolites which clearly come from oxidative damage.

Magee: You said that the gallium and cobalt complexes with bleomycin were used for tumour imaging. Does this mean that these are concentrated in the tumours?

Lown: That's correct, they are preferentially bound in neoplastic tissue (Hecht, 1979).

Magee: Is there any explanation why this is?

Lown: I don't know.

Connors: Gallium itself is concentrated, isn't it - is that the reason?

Lown: Yes, gallium is concentrated, and for that reason is used in cancer diagnosis.

Adams: The most common one is gallium citrate.

Magee: A second question. Is bleomycin by itself concentrated in the tumour?

Lown: It is activated preferentially because of the greater reducing environment in the tumour but as far as I know it doesn't concentrate in any organs like the anthracyclines (Hecht, 1979; Umezawa, 1975). It is, however, deactivated in the bone marrow owing to a greater concentration of bleomycin hydrolase (Umezawa, 1975).

Adams: You had an interesting slide where you compared the various anthracycline analogues with regard to their L1210 activity and superoxide anion production. You say the mechanism of action is mediated through the superoxide anion, both for the toxicity and anti-tumour activity. If you reduce the toxicity then you will reduce the activity.

Lown: I did not imply that. I mentioned at the beginning of that section that for the anthracyclines there are at least four different actions recognised in its cellular action (DiMarco *et al.*, 1975). It is difficult to pin-point which of these is the primary cause of the anti-cancer effect. My feeling is that the intercalative binding is necessary for anti-cancer activity but that the generation of superoxide, because it accumulates in the heart and, while it might be cytotoxic, is in this case deleterious, giving rise to cardiotoxicity. There is an apparent exception since, as you know, AD32 does not bind to DNA and yet it is quite active as an anti-cancer agent. This has been puzzling people for a long time but according to N.R. Bachur at the NIH (personal communication), AD32 is slowly hydrolysed and is in fact a pro-drug for adriamycin. That would tend to support the contention that the intercalative binding is a primary cause of anti-cancer activity. There may be a balance between the two mechanisms. We are trying to make drugs now that will shut off the superoxide generation completely in order to suppress the cardiotoxicity (Lown, J.W., Yen, S.F., Sondi, S., Acton, E.M. and Plambeck, J.A., unpublished results) as well, we just don't know yet.

Willson: Coming back to Harold Swartz's comment about scavenging iron. Iron may become ill-placed by the action of a drug. A neat method using bleomycin for estimating the amount of loosely bound, "free" or complexible iron in body fluids has recently been developed (Gutteridge *et al.*, 1981). When the iron-bleomycin complex interacts with DNA a malonaldehyde-like compound is produced which can be measured with thiobarbituric acid. This method has been used to measure the amount of "free" iron in synovial fluid of normal and arthritic patients.

Swartz: Did he have any information on the valence state of the iron?

Willson: I imagine it is probably Fe(II).

Mason: I have a comment on a paper of Professor Adams (Smith *et al.*, 1980) in which he reported that in Chinese hamster V79 cells the cytotoxicity of adriamycin is independent of oxygen concentration. He was looking for an oxygen effect in the radiobiology sense and there was none. I think that has profound implications for the role of free radicals in the cytotoxicity of the anthracyclines. If superoxide or some superoxide-derived species is the active species then hypoxia should protect. On the other hand, if the semiquinone is the reactive species, as others believe, then hypoxia should activate. But if hypoxia does neither, "the toxicity of adriamycin does not depend directly on the presence of O_2" one way or the other.

Lown: But clearly, oxygen is involved because you have the protective action of e.g. alphatocopherol *in vivo*. So with anti-oxidants you can suppress the cardiotoxicity of the anthracyclines (DiMarco *et al.*, 1975).

Adams: I think you both might be right. The work referred to was by a Ph.D. student of mine who was concerned with the effect of hypoxia in drug response *in vitro*. This is relevant to the problem of hypoxia in tumours. She examined the activity of adriamycin under oxic and hypoxic conditions. For short contact times in hypoxia there is no difference in sensitivity but if the cells remain hypoxic for a longer period before treatment one sees resistance developing and that resistance reaches a maximum when the cells have been in hypoxia for more than 8 h. The remarkable thing is that you can take these hypoxic cells and then make them oxic again. The resistance to adriamycin is retained and it takes 24 h before they lose it. A change of metabolic state arising from hypoxia can influence the subsequent response to adriamycin and some other drugs. But it is much more complicated than having oxygen there at the time of drug exposure.

Slater: I was going to make the point, perhaps a little naively, that anoxia is really a relative word in any biological system because it is virtually impossible to get all the oxygen out without killing the cells, whereas we know in experimental model systems one can work strictly anaerobically. In this paper that you mentioned, and which I did not know about, were the conditions genuinely anaerobic?

Adams: I would agree with that. One can achieve different levels of anoxia in mammalian cells. One can, for example, remove as much oxygen as possible in cells in glass vessels and then seal the vessel so that the cells can respire most of the remaining oxygen. The oxygen content in such conditions really becomes very low. Alternatively, one can equilibrate cells in suspension and equilibrate them with a nitrogen flow. The oxygen tension here is quite low too.

Again, one can achieve mild hypoxia by equilibrating the cells with nitrogen containing relatively low levels of oxygen, say 100 or 250 ppm. Interestingly, the severity of the hypoxia does not affect very much the so-called "anoxic" radiation response. In the drug experiments referred to the cells were equilibrated with N_2/CO_2 mixtures and the oxygen content was very low. Cells can be maintained in the hypoxic state (such that response to radiation or drugs can be affected) but this state of hypoxia alone does not kill the cells even though they are metabolically in a different condition. Restoration of oxygen will bring the cells into cycle. While it may be true that hypoxic cells do retain some oxygen, they can often behave like anaerobic bacteria in response to some agents, the nitroimidazoles for example.

Garner: I was just going to mention the work using the iron complex of adriamycin, it binds three iron atoms quite strongly.

Lown: Do you believe that? That's the Spanish work you are talking about?

Garner: Yes (Gosalvez *et al.*, 1978).

Lown: We looked at that and we could not reproduce their stoichiometry, perhaps you have been more successful than we have.

Garner: We did not check the stoichiometry. We were looking at it in the context of cytofluorimetry, trying to see whether the adriamycin was released again inside the cell, i.e. whether the iron was released from the adriamycin or not.

Lown: There are difficulties from the chemical point of view in seeing where the three irons would be sequestered.

Garner: It is probable that the binding constants vary for the three iron atoms, one is bound quite strongly, I believe.

Lown: Do they know where the iron atoms are bound?

Garner: I think it is tied up with the sugar amino group and the phenolic OH of the anthracycline.

Lown: What is the therapeutic story on this now, since several groups have been unable to reproduce the claims of the original authors (Brugarolas *et al.*, 1978)?

Garner: I'm not sure.

REFERENCES to Discussion

Bielski, B.H.J. (1977). *In* "Biochemical and Medical Aspects of Active Oxygen", p.7. University Park Press, Baltimore.

Brugarolas, A., Pachon, N., Gosalvez, M., Llanderal, A.P., Lacave, A.J., Buesa, J.N. and Marco, M.G. (1978). *Cancer Treat. Rep.* 62, 1527.

DiMarco, A., Arcamone, F. and Zunino, F. (1975). *In* "Antibiotics III - Mechanism of Action of Antimicrobial and Antitumor Agents" (Ed. J.W. Corcoran and F.E. Hahn), pp.101-128. Springer Verlag, New York.

Gosalvez, M., Blanco, M.F., Vivero, C. and Valles, F. (1978). *Eur. J. Cancer* 14, 1185-1190.

Gutteridge, J.M.C., Rowley, D.A. and Halliwell, B. (1981). *Biochem. J.* (in press).

Haidle, C.W. (1971). *Mol. Pharmacol.* 7, 645-652.

Haidle, C.W., Weiss, K.K. and Kuo, Mw.T. (1972). *Mol. Pharmacol.* 8, 531-537.

Hecht, S.M. (Ed.) (1979). "Bleomycin, Chemical, Biochemical and Biological Aspects", Springer Verlag, New York.

Lesko, S., Loventzen, R. and Ts'o, P. (1980). *Biochemistry* 19, 3023-3028.

Lown, J.W. and Joshua, A.V. (1980). *Biochem. Pharmacol.* 29, 521-532.

Lown, J.W. and Sim, S.K. (1977). *Biochem. Biophys. Res. Commun.* 77, 1150-1157.

Smith, E., Stratford, E.J. and Adams, G.E. (1980). *Br. J. Cancer* 41, 568-573.

Umezawa, H. (1975). *In* "Antibiotics III - Mechanism of Action of Antimicrobial and Antitumor Agents" (Ed. J.W. Corcoran and F.E. Hahn), pp.101-128. Springer Verlag, New York.

Radicals in Carcinogenesis by Aromatic Amines

A. STIER, R. CLAUSS, A. LÜCKE and I. REITZ

INTRODUCTION

DNA Adducts and Ultimate Carcinogens

Important questions related to the understanding of cancer, induced by aromatic amines, in terms of the somatic mutation theory, concern the quantity and pattern of distribution of carcinogen-DNA adducts within the chromatin which are necessary for tumour initiation. The number of those adducts may be much smaller than the number detected in experimental systems *in vivo* and *in vitro*. Furthermore, is the chemical structure of all adducts known? A reflection of these uncertainties is the number of reactive intermediates which have been suspected of being ultimate carcinogens (see Miller and Miller, 1977). This situation leaves free space for the search for alternatives.

COINCIDENCE OF RADICAL FORMATION AND CARCINOGENICITY

Radicals as possible metabolites of amines were first discussed by Heubner (1948) in relation to some toxic effects of these compounds. Table 1 gives the chronology of the detection of nitroxide radicals in toxicology and cancerology related to the present work (for recent reviews see Ts'o *et al.*, 1977 and Mason, 1979).

A recent development is the demonstration of nitroxide radical adducts to microsomal membrane constituents which will be of major concern in this review (Stier *et al.*, 1976; Floyd *et al.*, 1978; Stier *et al.*, 1980). Many carcinogenic aromatic N-containing compounds have been found to form nitroxide radicals under conditions of cytochrome P-450 dependent mixed function oxygenation in rabbit liver microsomal incubations (see Table 2). All these radicals are produced by reaction of primarily formed aromatic nitroxide radicals and/or other oxidation compounds with microsomal membrane constituents (see below for microsomal adduct radicals).

Of the 18 carcinogenic aromatic compounds which we have investigated, 14 produced radicals, of the 10 noncarcinogenic compounds only 2. Amongst the 4 exceptions in the group of carcinogenic compounds which did not form radicals are 2 nitrocompounds.

Some of the substances included in the group of carcinogenic compounds (1-aminonaphthalene, 6-aminochrysene, N-methylaniline) may be considered as marginally carcinogenic. Whereas 2-aminonaphthalene clearly produces bladder tumours in dogs, the 1- analogue does not, while with mice the 1-isomer has been found to produce lung tumours but to a much smaller extent than 2-aminonaphthalene. 6-Aminochrysene was found to produce tumours only in newborn, predominantly male mice, whereas in other animals it even inhibited polynuclear aromatic hydrocarbon-induced or spontaneous tumours (Arcos and Argus, 1974). Phenacetin is known to produce kidney tumours after excessively high and prolonged abuse in human beings (Bengtsson, 1974). The monocyclic amines aniline and N-methylaniline, are believed to be noncarcinogenic or only weak carcinogens. The carcinogenic potential of aniline is being reinvestigated (Ghess *et al.*, 1978). We know that the nitroxides of these compounds as well as the ones formed from some amines known to be only marginally carcinogenic are different with regard to their rate of formation and stability.

Of the aliphatic amines investigated only 2,2,6,6,-tetramethylpiperidine produces a nitroxide radical (which is well known as TEMPO, a spinlabel). The biochemical properties of this class of stable aliphatic nitroxides widely used in biophysical investigations of biological structures by ESR-spectroscopy will be referred to below in connection with their significance as a paradigm for aromatic amine induced carcinogenesis.

From an inspection of Table 2 a species variation in tissue specificity of tumour incidence is apparent. Admittedly, the data presented are highly selective. One thing to note is that the larger the number of animals investigated for a given compound, the larger is the number of different tissues observed to be involved in tumour development. This is only one example but it demonstrates the

TABLE 1 Chronology of aromatic nitroxide radicals in biochemical toxicology

Methemoglobinemia	Reactive intermediates formed from aromatic hydroxylamines involved in heme oxidation	Heubner (1948)
Methemoglobinemia	Autocatalytic cycle involving radical intermediates in aromatic amine and nitrocompound induced in heme oxidation	Kiese (1966)
Chemical carcinogenesis	Nitroxide radical formed by chemical oxidation from 4-hydroxylaminoquinoline-1-oxide detected by ESR-spectroscopy	Nagata *et al.* (1966)
Chemical carcinogenesis	Nitroxide radical formed by peroxidase from N-hydroxy-N-acetyl-2-aminofluorene, detected by ESR-spectroscopy	Bartsch and Hecker (1970)
Chemical carcinogenesis	Nitroxide radicals formed by mixed function oxygenation in microsomal incubations of different carcinogenic aromatic amines, detected by ESR-spectroscopy	Stier *et al.* (1972) Kimura *et al.* (1979)
Chemical carcinogenesis	Microsomal adduct radicals formed during mixed function oxygenation of aromatic amines	Stier *et al.* (1976) Stier *et al.* (1980)
Chemical carcinogenesis	Microsomal adduct radicals formed from nitrosofluorene	Floyd *et al.* (1978)

TABLE 2 Compounds tested by ESR spectroscopy for nitroxide radical formation in microsomal mixed function oxygenation and carcinogenicity[a]

Carcinogenic amines, amides and nitrocompounds	Radical detected by ESR	Experimental tumours formed in tissues[c]	in species[c]
2-aminofluorene	+	b	hu,d,h,mon
N-Acetyl-2-aminofluorene	+	li,b,i,s,mg,eg	r,mo,ra,h,d
N-Hydroxy-N-acetyl-2-aminofluorene	+	st,mg,li,i,eg,s	r,ra,mi,h,gp
2-Aminonaphthalene	+	b	hu,mon,ra,d,mo
1-Aminonaphthalene	0§	l	mo
3-Nitro-2-aminonaphthalene	0	mg,st,eg	r,mo
2-Aminoanthracene	+	li,b,mg,s	hu,mi
6-Aminochrysene	0§	li,l	mi
4-Aminostilbene	+	li,l,mg,i	r,mi
4,4'-Diaminostilbene	+	li	ra
4-Aminoazobenzene	+	li	r
N-Methylaniline	+§	k	r
N-Methyl-4-(phenylazo)aniline	+	li	r,mo
Benzidine	+	li,b,eg	r,d,mo
4-N,N-Dimethylaminodiphenyl	+	mg,eg,i	r
Phenacetin	+§	k	r
4-Nitroquinoline-1-oxide	+	l,s	mi,r,ra
1,2-Dichloro-3-nitronaphthalene	0		
Non-carcinogenic amines and Azo-compounds			
Azobenzene	0		
4-N,N-Diethylaminoazobenzene	0		
Aniline	+		
N-Acetylaniline	0		
N,N-Dimethyl-p-phenylendiamine	0		
1,2-Diaminoethane	0[b]		
2-Amino-2-methylpropane	0[b]		
Piperidine	0[b]		
2,2,6,6-Tetramethylpiperidine	+¶[b]		
9-Aminofluorene	0		

[a]Data on carcinogenicity are from Arcos and Argus (1974) and Schmähl (1970). [b]No data found on carcinogenicity. § Weak carcinogens. ¶ No adduct-nitroxide, from Stier and Reitz (1971). [c]Abbreviations used: b = bladder, li = liver, i = intestine, s = skin, mg = mammary gland, eg = earduct gland, st = stomach, l = lung, k = kidney, hu = human, d = dog, h = hamster, mon = monkey, r = rat, mo = mouse, ra = rabbit, mi = mice, gp = guinea pig.

difficulties in drawing generalised conclusions from those coincidences or correlations on the function of any particular chemical species in tumour initiation. Such hypotheses imply that a certain bioactivation step is limiting in the complex network of processes and reactions involved in tumour development. Moreover, within the frame of the somatic mutation theory of chemical cancer the more reactive the ultimate carcinogen is the nearer it must be formed to the localisation of the genetic material. Otherwise, unspecific cellular damage would preclude the development of cancer as is known for CCl_4 (Slater, 1979). A quite different interpretation may consider the radical forming capability as a peripheral expression of a basic molecular property which itself is causally related to carcinogenesis by another mechanism. Following this line of interpretation for instance the radical adduct formation in microsomes could be regarded as a chemical example for the formation of a DNA-adduct.

Nevertheless, the coincidence of radical formation and cancer induction presented in Table 2 is evidence supporting the theory that radicals may be involved in tumour initiation and/or promotion by carcinogenic aromatic N-containing compounds. The capacity of the liver to bioactivate carcinogens is greater than that of all other tissues. Moreover, the liver may be regarded as a prominent site for production of transport forms of ultimate carcinogens which may be distributed throughout the organism to reach the target organ where these transport forms promote the initiation process. Particular properties (longevity and redox properties) of radicals described later in this study allow for this possibility.

MICROSOMAL ADDUCTS: STABLE NITROXIDE RADICALS

The radicals formed from aromatic nitrogen compounds which are incubated with liver microsomes derived from phenobarbital stimulated rabbits under conditions of cytochrome P-450 dependent mixed function oxygenation have some remarkable attributes in common: (a) They display a striking longevity: hours in many cases of microsomal incubations and even days if kept in an organic solvent extract at room temperature. The radicals even survive chromatography. (b) All these radicals, surprisingly, show quite uniform shapes of the ESR-spectra taken after prolonged incubations (>20-30 min, for

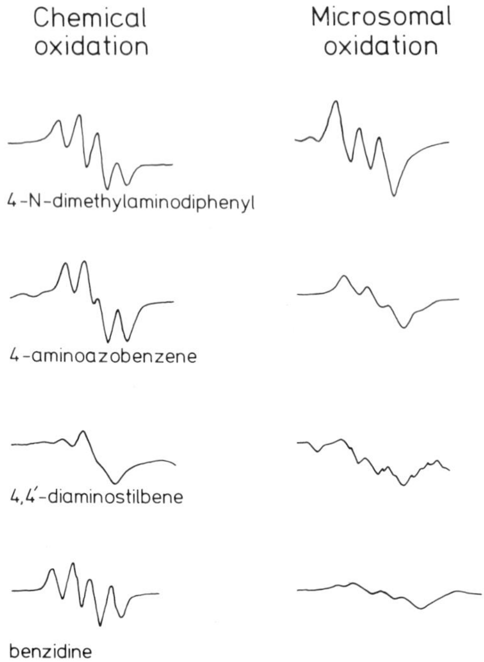

FIG. 1 Representative ESR-spectra of microsomal nitroxide adducts from various aromatic amines and spectra of corresponding arylnitroxides. ESR spectra of methanol-chloroform extracts of incubation mixtures of various amines with liver microsomes from phenobarbital-pretreated rabbits are compared with solutions of these amines to which 3-chloroperbenzoic acid was added. Modulation amplitude was 6.25 G. For details of experiments, see Stier *et al.*, 1980).

representative spectra see Fig. 1): a three band spectrum with a separation of the bands varying between 11 and 15 G due to hyperfine interaction with nitrogen. The position of the central band is the same among all compounds tested (Table 2) and nearly coincides with the central line of the spectrum recorded from the spin label TEMPO. These spectra, in all aromatic amines investigated, are clearly different from the spectra of the corresponding nitroxide radicals obtained by chemical oxidation of the amines (Fig. 1). This is a strong indication that the radicals are formed by a reaction of metabolites of the aromatic nitrogen compounds with membrane bound constituents. The adduct radicals remain bound to the microsomal membranes as they cosediment in ultracentrifugation. The microsomal

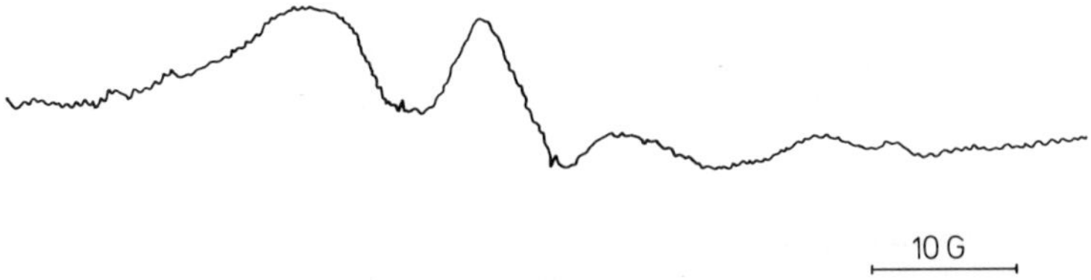

FIG. 2 ESR-spectra of microsomal incubations (microsomes from phenobarbital pretreated rabbits) of N-hydroxy-N-acetyl-2-aminofluorene. Modulation amplitude 6.25 G. Note the decrease in signal intensity from low to high field in the upper spectrum which is typical for anisotropic rotation of the molecule around the N-O-bond (Birrell *et al.*, 1972). (For experimental details see Stier *et al.*, 1980).

adduct radicals are immobilised within the microsomal membrane. For example, the adduct formed from N-hydroxy-N-acetyl-2-aminofluorene experiences restricted mobility in the microsomal membrane; the ESR spectrum obtained directly from the microsomal suspension (Fig. 2) is typical of an anisotropic rotation of the molecules around the N-O-bond (Birrell *et al.*, 1972). This anisotropy of motion points to the molecular shape of the microsomal component of the adduct being similar to that of a long chain fatty acid. Generally, radicals are much easier to detect in chloroform-methanol extracts from microsomal incubations since this removes the immobilisation within the membrane which causes the broadening of spectral shape. The adducts extracted into the solvent can freely rotate isotropically.

At least two species of adducts differing in the nature of the microsomal component can be formed (Stier *et al.*, 1980). Permeation chromatography on Sephadex LH-20, a hydrophobic gel, resolves the extracted radicals of phenylhydroxylamine into two fractions, the first eluting in a sharp band with phospholipids, and the second (40% total radical yield) migrating more slowly in a broad band containing many substances such as fatty acids, cholic acids, cholesterol and triglycerides. The ESR spectra of the two chromatographic fractions differ distinctly. In preparative thin layer chromatography (t.l.c.) on silica gel, only one fraction with an ESR signal was observed in the front region where fatty acids and cholesterol are found. This fraction gives an ESR spectrum similar to that of the first fraction eluting from the Sephadex LH-20 column. The radical eluting in the second fraction is apparently destroyed when chromatographed on silica gel. The more stable radical (representing about 60% of the total radical yield) behaves, on permeation chromatography, similarly to phospholipids but not on adsorption chromatography. In this typical experiment phenylhydroxylamine was used because arylhydroxylamines have been found to yield greater amounts of secondary nitroxides than any of the amines. This points to N-hydroxylation being the rate-limiting step of the whole reaction sequence for the formation of the adduct radical at physiological temperature (Fig. 3). Using 2-naphthylamine, however, microsomal adduct radicals with similar chromatographic behaviour is observed.

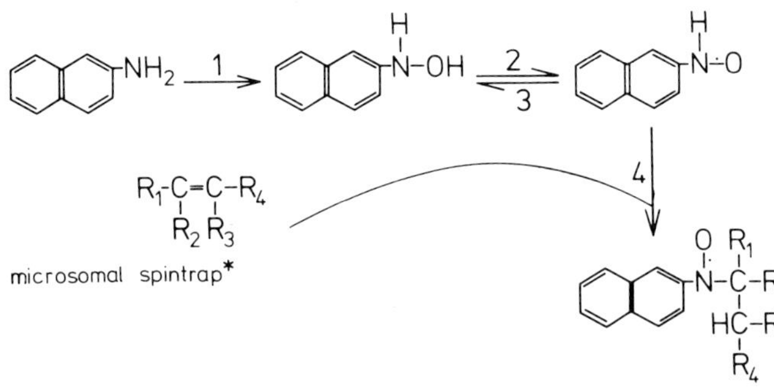

FIG. 3 Reaction scheme for formation of microsomal adduct nitroxides. Substituents $R_{1,4}$ are alkylgroups. Substituents $R_{2,3}$ may be hydrogen or alkylgroups.

The microsomal adducts are formed by addition of the aromatic nitroxides, originating in the course of mixed function oxygenation of aromatic amines, to double bonds of microsomal membrane constituents without involving the nitroxide radical group (Fig. 3). Evidence for this sort of spin trapping process (Janzen, 1979) stems mainly from changes in ESR signal observed during the microsomal incubation and chemical model reaction (Stier *et al.*, 1980).

In some cases (2-aminonaphthalene, 2-aminoanthracene, 4-aminoazobenzene and N-methylaniline) the inter-conversion of the intervening aromatic nitroxides to the adduct radical could be directly followed by ESR-spectroscopy. This transformation is best demonstrated by the microsomal incubation of 2-aminonaphthalene (Fig. 4). After 10 min incubation, two types of nitroxide radical spectra appear

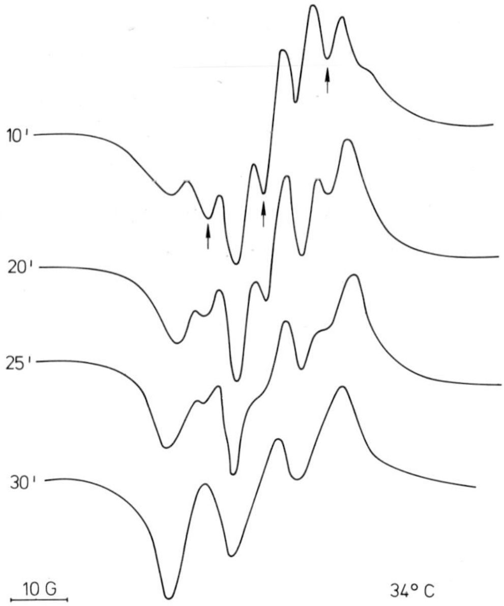

FIG. 4 ESR-spectra of microsomal solvent extracts after different times of incubation of 2-aminonaphthalene at 34°C with liver microsomes from phenobarbital stimulated rabbits. Modulation amplitude 2.5 G. Signals of the three band spectrum which resembles the spectra obtained from chemical oxidation of 2-aminonapthalene are indicated. Note the distinct shift by 5 G of the central band of this spectrum observed at the end of the incubation. (From Stier *et al.*, 1980).

superimposed, showing slightly different band separation and with considerable difference (5 G) in the position of the central band. The radical formed initially, which exhibits the spectral characteristics of the chemically-produced radical, is later transformed into a radical having the uniform spectral shape described above. In the other cases the interconversion is too fast for the aromatic nitroxide intermediates to be detectable. The reason for the slower interconversion of the aromatic nitroxides of the above mentioned amines might be because of their lower reactivity towards the microsomal spintrap as compared to the other nitroxides.

The addition reaction is analogous to spin-trapping (Janzen, 1979), has been observed in chemical systems (Banks *et al.*, 1971), and is substantiated by model reactions using substances relevant to the microsomal spintraps. 2-Naphthylamine oxidised by 3-chloroperbenzoic acid in the presence of egg lecithin forms a radical which displays an ESR spectrum similar to that of secondary radicals formed in microsomal oxidations, different from that of radicals formed in the absence of egg lecithin, or in the presence of dipalmitoyl lecithin - a lipid lacking fatty acid double bonds. Similarly, phenylhydroxylamine oxidised in the presence of oleic acid gives a spectrum similar to that obtained in an extract from microsomal oxidation, and different from that obtained without addition of oleic acid.

Arylnitroxides strongly disproportionate to hydroxylamines and nitroso compounds (Bowman *et al.*, 1971). As an alternative mechanism of microsomal adduct formation an "ene"-reaction of the arylnitroso compounds with the fatty acid double bonds giving the nitroxide through subsequent oxidation may be considered and has been proposed for the case of nitrosofluorene (Floyd *et al.*, 1978). This mechanism implies (a) the accumulation of considerable amounts of nitroso derivatives (several orders of magnitude greater than the nitroxides) of the amines giving the ESR signals, and (b) that the similarity of time course of formation of the adduct and of the disappearance of the aromatic nitroxide (Fig. 4) is purely accidental, the latter reaction being geared to an independent reaction which consumes large amounts of the nitroso compound. On the other hand, the bimolecular disproportionation may be retarded in the liquid crystalline lipid phase of the membrane to the extent that the radical double bond addition reaction can compete with it.

The yield of the microsomal adduct radical is low. Under optimum conditions in the case of phenylhydroxylamine, adduct nitroxides are formed to the extent of 0.2% of substrate, or e.g. 0.2 - 0.3% of the total microsomal phospholipids present in the incubation mixture. In view of this low yield of adduct radicals, microsomal spin-traps represent only a minor constituent of the microsomal membrane, presumably not phospholipids. The results presented indicate that the microsomal constituents which act as spin traps may be membrane-bound strongly lipophilic compounds, which contain reactive double bonds sterically accessible to the primary aromatic nitroxide. Substituent R_2 on the adduct nitroxide (Fig. 3) may represent a β-proton.

This was indeed observed in the nitroxide produced from phenylhydroxylamine in the presence of oleic acid. An adduct nitroxide possessing no β-protons may be formed from spin-trapping by compounds like dolichol or retinol. Secondary nitroxides with β-protons would be more susceptible to oxidation and this may be important in connection with the persistence of the redox cycle (see below).

The structure of a mixed type nitroxide assigned to the adduct radical (Fig. 3) explains the remarkable chemical stability, due to stabilisation of the nitroxide group by delocalisation of the radical electron in the aromatic moiety on the one side and by the secondary (in the presence of a β-proton) or tertiary carbon on the other. The latter group is the structural element responsible for stabilisation of the spin-label class of nitroxides. Thus, the adduct nitroxides resemble spin-label compounds with regard to their chemical reactivity and structure.

NITROXIDE ADDUCT RADICALS: CARRIER FORMS OF ULTIMATE CARCINOGENS?

The nitroxide-hydroxylamine redox couple-produces oxygen free radicals

The microsomal adduct radical can be reduced by NADPH (Stier *et al.*, 1980) and regained by chemical oxidation (Floyd *et al.*, 1978). As the adduct nitroxide is similar in structure to spin labels we may infer more about this redox behaviour from the known biochemistry of these compounds.

For instance 2,2,6,6-tetramethylpiperidine (TMP) has been found to be oxidised by rat and rabbit liver microsomes to TEMPO in a reaction requiring O_2 and NADPH (Stier and Reitz, 1971). An oxidation sequence (Fig. 5) leads from TMP via the corresponding hydroxylamine TMPOH (step 1) to TEMPO (step 2) which is further oxidised to an unknown product (step 5). TEMPO is reduced via TMPOH (step 3) to TMP (step 4). Cytochrome P-450-reductase is involved in steps 3, 4, 5 and, together with cytochrome P-450, in steps 1, 2. Cytochrome P-450 and/or the aminoxidase described by Ziegler and Mitchell (1972) may contribute to step 1. Step 1 is rate-limiting since reaction 2 proceeds at a considerably faster rate. A nonenzymic oxidation also contributes to step 2 to the extent of 10%. At oxygen concentrations as low as 10^{-5} M TMPOH is readily reoxidised. This nonenzymic oxidation yields $O_2^{\cdot -}$ while a haemoprotein and cytochrome P-450

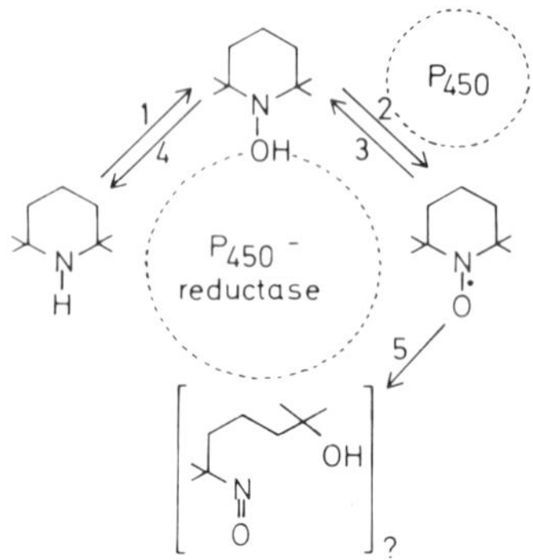

FIG. 5 Scheme of reactions involved in formation of the spin label TEMPO and its reduction in microsomal incubations (see text).

catalysed oxidation produces H_2O_2. From these oxygen species the powerful $OH^{\bullet}$ radical may originate (for mechanism see Willson, 1979). On the other hand, since the nitroxides are good electron acceptors, they may initiate a redox cycle (Fig. 6), which may become highly effective in production of active oxygen species. One-electron oxidations by O_2 are involved in this cycle. Their possible significance to cancer and cancer therapy is discussed in this volume also by Lesko *et al.* (1982) and by Lown *et al.* (1982).

Thus, the microsomal adduct nitroxides may serve as catalysts for promotion of oxygen free radicals. The nature of the microsomal component may confer to the molecules a specific carrier function resulting in a selective intracellular and tissue distribution.

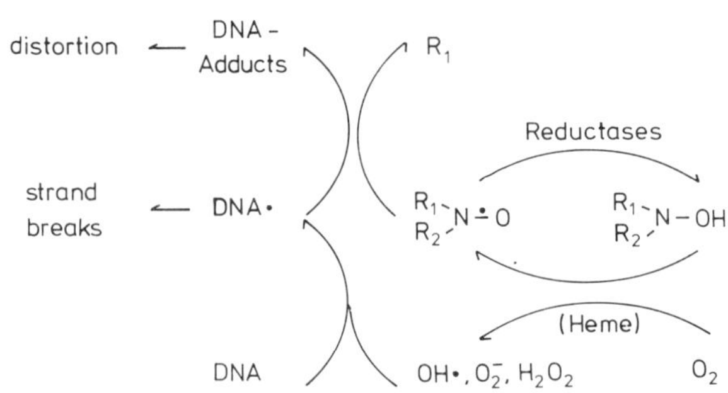

FIG. 6 Scheme of the proposed redox cycle of the microsomal adduct carrier and the concerted reaction of the carrier and reactive oxygen species with DNA.

DNA may be Modified by a Concerted Action of Nitroxide and Oxygen Free Radicals

If the reduced transport form of the carcinogen (microsomal adduct carrier) bound to the target is reoxidised reactive oxygen species would be generated *in situ*. $OH^{\bullet}$ radicals may initiate a radical chain by reaction with DNA. The resulting change in the heteroaromatic bases would be translated into strand breaks (see Adams and Wardman, 1977). Also hydrogen peroxide is known to break DNA strands (Lesko *et al.*, 1980). The DNA radicals can also recombine with the carrier to yield DNA adducts resulting in distortion of DNA. During adduct formation the mixed nitroxide representing the carrier may be split. If the leaving group is the aromatic residue, originally radioactively labelled, the DNA adduct (of the endogenous constituent of the carrier) will remain undetected by the analytical techniques usually applied. In an experiment relevant to this reaction the spin label 2,2,6,6-tetramethylpiperidine-4-one nitroxide was bound covalently to DNA when irradiated with X rays (Brustad *et al.*, 1973). The chemical structure of this adduct is not known.

Another branch of a radical chain would be opened by reaction of the DNA radical with the hydroxylamine form of the carrier to give the nitroxide radical. A third radical chain would start with hydrogen abstraction from a reducing agent (e.g. from a thiol) by the carrier nitroxide leaving a carbon centred radical. These suppositions are based on results obtained from reactions of nitroxides in chemical systems (see Kochi, 1973; Brustad *et al.*, 1973).

CONCLUSIONS

If the concept of a nitroxide carrier functioning *in situ* as a redox couple producing reactive oxygen species is valid this means that the ultimate carcinogens should have additional properties favouring a more selective interaction with the targets for tumour initiation. The electrophilicity of ultimate carcinogens is not, itself, a property sufficiently specific to permit a high degree of selectivity of interaction. This reactivity would come into play in an earlier step of the sequence of initiation which may be distant, in time and space, from the target. Therefore, this concept does not lead to the expectation of a good correlation between covalent binding to DNA and carcinogenicity and/or mutagenicity. The longevity of the carrier nitroxides and the ubiquity of conditions favouring the redox reactions of the carrier allows for a wide distribution of their oxygen radical producing function within the organism. It means that damage to DNA could be independent of the presence of special activating enzymes in target tissues. The distribution of the carrier within cells and in the organism depends mainly on the nature of its endogenous component. Furthermore, the carrier may be able to bring its nitroxide group into a distinct position and steric orientation at the target DNA.

The present concept increases the multiplicity of targets attacked by ultimate carcinogens, namely DNA, RNA, proteins and lipophilic constituents of microsomal membranes. Furthermore, the critical step for tumour initiation (namely, adduct formation in the endoplasmic reticulum) might be modulated by hormonal or dietary factors which modify the composition of this membrane. In addition, parameters altering membrane structure, which may influence the probability of encounters between the primary aromatic nitroxide and the spin traps, may become important. The idea of ultimate carcinogen acting as a mediator of oxygen toxicity links tumour initiation with the system protecting against oxygen toxicity, namely, superoxide dismutase and catalase, and predicts the radiosensitising action of carcinogenic amines.

All these considerations are made only within the frame of the somatic mutation theory of chemical carcinogenesis and totally neglecting any epigenetic aspects whatever their importance might be.

ACKNOWLEDGEMENT

This work was supported by the "Fond der Chemie".

REFERENCES

Adams, G.E. and Wardman, P. (1977). *In* "Free Radicals in Biology" (Ed. W.A. Pryor) Vol. III, pp.53-95. Academic Press, New York.

Arcos, J.C. and Argus, M.F. (1974). "Chemical Induction of Cancer". Academic Press, New York.

Banks, R.E., Haszeldine, R.N. and Justin, B. (1971). *J. Chem. Soc. (Chem. Commun.)*, 2777-2785.

Bartsch, H. and Hecker, E. (1970). *Biochim. Biophys. Acta* 237, 567-578.

Bengtsson, U. (1974). *Clin. Nephrol.* 2, 123-126.
Birrell, G.B., Van, S.P. and Griffith, O.H. (1972). *J. Am. Chem. Soc.* 95, 2451-2458.
Bowman, D.F., Brokenshire, J.L., Gillian, T. and Ingold, K.U. (1971). *J. Am. Chem. Soc.* 93, 6651-6655.
Brustad, T., Jones, W.B.G. and Wold, E. (1973). *Int. J. Radiat. Biol.* 24, 33-44.
Floyd, R.A., Soong, L.M., Stuart, M.A. and Reigh, D.L. (1978). *Arch. Biochem. Biophys.* 185, 450-457.
Ghess, M.J., Bartsch, H., Huff, J.E. and Tomatis, L. (1978). "Information Bulletin on the Survey of Chemicals Being Tested For Carcinogenesis Nr. 7", International Agency for Research on Cancer, Lyon.
Heubner, W. (1948). *Naunyn-Schmiedeberg's Arch. Exp. Pathol. Pharmakol.* 205, 310.
Janzen, E.G. (1979). *In* "Free Radicals in Biology" (Ed. W.A. Pryor) Vol. IV, pp.115-154. Academic Press, New York.
Kiese, M. (1966). *Pharmacol. Rev.* 18, 1091-1161.
Kimura, T., Kodama, M. and Nagata, C. (1978). *Biochem. Pharmacol.* 28, 557-560.
Kochi, J.K. (1973). "Free Radicals", John Wiley, New York.
Lesko, S.A., Lorentzen, R.J. and Ts'o, P.O.P. (1980). *Biochemistry* 19, 3023-3028.
Lesko, S.A., Ts'o, P.O.P., Yang, S.-U. and Zheng, R. (1982). This volume.
Lown, J.W., Joshua, A.V. and Chen, H.-H. (1982). This volume.
Mason, R.P. (1979). *Rev. Biochem. Toxicol.* 1, 151-200.
Miller, J.A. and Miller, E.C. (1977). *In* "Origins of Human Cancer, Book B, Mechanisms of Carcinogenesis" (Eds. H.H. Hiatt, J.D. Watson and J.A. Winsten) Vol. 4, pp.605-627. Cold Spring Harbor Laboratory.
Nagata, C., Kataoka, N., Imamura, A., Kawazoe, Y. and Chihara, G. (1966). *GANN* 57, 323-335.
Schmähl, D. (1970). "Entstehung, Wachstum und Chemotherapie maligner Tumoren", Editio Cantor KG, Aulendorf in Württ.
Slater, T.F. (1979). *In* "Submolecular Biology and Cancer" (Ciba Foundation Symposium 65), pp.301-328. Excerpta Medica, Amsterdam.
Stier, A. and Reitz, I. (1971). *Xenobiotica* 1, 499-500.
Stier, A., Reitz, I. and Sackmann, E. (1972). *Naunyn-Schmiedeberg's Arch. Pharmakol.* 274, 189-191.
Stier, A.,Clauss, R., Lücke, A., Rösen, R. and Rosenberg, P. (1976). *Panminerva Med.* 18, 449-453.
Stier, A., Clauss, R., Lücke, A. and Reitz, I. (1980). *Xenobiotica* 10, 661-673.
Ts'o, P.O.P., Caspary, W.J. and Lorentzen, R.J. (1977). *In* "Free Radicals in Biology" (Ed. W.A. Pryor) Vol. III, pp.251-303. Academic Press, New York.
Willson, R.L. (1979). *In* "Oxygen Free Radicals and Tissue Damage" (Ciba Foundation Symposium 65), pp.19-42. Excerpta Medica, Amsterdam.
Ziegler, D.M. and Mitchell, C.H. (1972). *Arch. Biochem. Biophys.* 150, 116-125.

DISCUSSION

Magee: I will ask you two questions: one is that you've shown some experiments you have done with 2-naphthylamine - have you done any work with 1-naphthylamine?

Stier: Yes.

Magee: Does it give the same answer or not?

Stier: No it doesn't. It doesn't give an ESR signal.

Magee: The second question is, as everybody knows, a lot of work has been done on the metabolic activation of drugs and carcinogens in the nucleus and isolated nuclei. I wondered if you had been able to do these sorts of experiments, where the reactant wouldn't be so remote from the DNA, as it would be after formation in the cytoplasm.

Stier: That would be a good suggestion to do these experiments.

Lohmann: It is well-known that the ESR triplet signal of a spin label changes characteristically when attached to phospholipids. The high field signal is changed first in spin concentration and line width, finally the splitting parameter of the triplet has reached its optimal value.

Stier: You are talking about the immobilised signal?

Lohmann: Yes.

Stier: When I said that it might rotate anisotropically around the N-O bond I referred to the decrease of the triplet signal with field strength.

Lohmann: Then I have two questions. You are talking about the spin concentration as obtained from the height of a particular signal despite the fact that other signals or even triplets might overlap this particular one. This might result in a considerable error of the spin concentration. Furthermore, how can you explain the two different triplets?

Stier: Unfortunately, I did not go too much into experimental details. With regard to your second question: Generally the ESR spectra have been recorded in chloroform-methanol extracts of microsomal incubations because line broadening, due to immobilisation, renders weak signals undetectable from ESR spectra measured directly in microsomal suspension. Only in cases of compounds which gave strong signals - for example, in the case of N-hydroxy-N-acetyl-2-aminofluorene - can we detect the ESR signal directly in microsomal incubations.

Lohmann: And how about spin concentration?

Stier: You are talking about the superposition of two triplet signals in the case of the early incubation period of 2-amino-naphthalene. I agree that this is only a qualitative description of interconversion of of naphthalene-2-nitroxide to the microsomal adduct nitroxide. I would like to add that this interconversion is strongly dependent on temperature. It is quite slow at temperatures below around 30°C. This suggests that the microsomal spin trap is too immobile below this temperature to be able to react sufficiently well with the aromatic nitroxide. I do not think that this spin trap is a phospholipid. Under optimum conditions we may titrate out the microsomal spin trap. For this purpose we use phenylhydroxylamine. By this choice we circumvent the first slow rate limiting step in the whole reaction sequence. Only 0.2% of the total substrate was found to be converted to a stable nitroxide. If this stable nitroxide is a phospholipid adduct, only two out of a thousand microsomal phospholipid molecules are acting as spin traps. So we don't think that the microsomal spin traps are phospholipids even if the adduct nitroxides behave in one of the chromatographic procedures like phospholipids. We could imagine that dolichols or retinals may act as spin traps. These compounds could provide a tertiary carbon to which the nitroxide binds, which would explain the high stability of the adduct radical. Unsaturated fatty acids would not provide a tertiary carbon near the nitrogen. Perhaps the difference in stability we observe between the two chromatographic fractions may be explained by the presence or absence of a β-proton near the nitroxide.

Lohmann: Might it be due to the different degree of unsaturation as R. Floyd has suggested?

Stier: Yes, Floyd has no other evidence as we have which may indicate a possible importance of the degree of unsaturation (see Floyd *et al.* 1978).

Dianzani: This is just a short comment to the second question of Professor Magee. He asked if isolated nuclei could metabolise carcinogenic amines. I would expect a positive answer. Nuclear membranes are derived from the endoplasmic reticulum and have been shown to metabolise carbon tetrachloride by the Castro group. So I would expect some metabolism in the case of the carcinogenic amines. Now a short question to Professor Stier. Is there any change in lipid peroxidation in your system?

Stier: We do not know about that. It's a very good question whether lipid peroxidation occurs in microsomal suspensions in the presence of carcinogenic amines.

Adams: On your final overhead projection you described a general concept. You related cytotoxicity, carcinogenicity and radio-sensitisation. I think you said that this would predict that the amino-aromatics would be radio-sensitisers.

Stier: Yes.

Adams: They are not.

Stier: This is interesting.

Adams: Yes, it is interesting because the fully oxidised nitro compounds are very powerful radio-sensitisers and so are the nitroxyls too. When the compounds are reduced to the amino derivatives radio-sensitising action is lost.

Stier: Well, what you are saying is that aromatic amines are not radio-sensitisers, but what we propose is that the nitroxides are.

Adams: Yes they are. The nitroxyls are very efficient radio-sensitisers. Are you saying that you can put the amino-aromatics in there and expect to develop sensitising ability by oxidation to a nitroxyl derivative?

Stier: I expect them to be radio-sensitisers because they form nitroxides and the nitroxides could reach the DNA, particularly the stable nitroxide carrier form.

Adams: If one treats cells with amino-aromatics and heterocyclics and then leaves them a long time, one sees no sensitisation. But if one treats cells with nitroxides, even under conditions where the contact time is extremely short, sensitisation occurs.

Stier: But you must treat cells that are able to form this type of nitroxide. You must treat, for example, liver cells or other cells which are able to oxidise amines to the N-hydroxy and to the nitroxide compounds, and contain molecules like the microsomal spin traps described here. That would be the right system to be tested.

At this point I would like to make a general comment. All these predictions and suppositions are corollaries of a general concept, the concept of redox couples as ultimate carcinogens creating reactive oxygen species, applied to the special case of aromatic amines. Other corollaries of these concepts applied to the case of benzpyrene carcinogenesis and bleomycin carcinostatic action are given in this volume by Professor Ts'o and Professor Lown. The only further modification of this concept specific for the case of aromatic amines is the formation of a stable nitroxide adduct radical to which we may assign a carrier function. As long as we do not know the exact chemical nature of the microsomal constituent of this carrier we may speculate that the microsomal parts provide for the means of a specific transport of the carrier within cells to the nucleus or within the organism to a specific organ. The redox properties of the carrier, necessary for the production of reactive oxygen species, have been mainly extrapolated from experimental results with spin labels which are nitroxides possessing chemical properties quite similar to the microsomal adduct nitroxides. Thus, the scheme given in Fig. 6 of my presentation is mere speculation.

Asmus: You showed several samples where you had hydroxylamine type species reacting with oxygen to give the nitroxide radical and the $O_2^{\cdot -}$ radical. Now, on the other hand, it is known that nitroxide radicals can be reduced by other radicals, alcohol radicals for instance (Asmus *et al.*, 1976), which would be a kind of reverse process. This poses a question about the redox potential of the hydroxylamines. Do you know them?

Stier: The adduct nitroxide can be reduced by NADPH and reoxidised by oxygen. More information we have from the redox behaviour of spin labels, e.g. tetramethylpiperidinehydroxylamine is easily oxidised by oxygen to the spin label TEMPO. Heme compounds like microsomal cytochrome P_{450} greatly increased the rate of oxidation.

Asmus: My other question would be: is it a straightforward reaction, i.e. irreversible, or do you have signs for the reversibility of this reaction?

Stier: We have signs for reversibility: if we enzymatically reduce nitroxide spin labels by NADPH or NADH in microsomal systems (see for example Stier and Sackmann, 1973), there are difficulties to measure clearly the reduction rate, because even oxygen concentrations as low as 10^{-5} M are sufficient to reoxidise part of the reduced spin labels (Bosterling, B and Stier, A., unpublished).

Esterbauer: I was wondering very much about the high stability of the radical, which you can extract with chloroform, purify and so on. Did I understand you right that this radical was a constituent of the membrane or is it derived from the amine only?

Stier: The ESR spectrum indicates that it must be a nitroxide radical. The reaction scheme given in Fig. 3 explains the observed high chemical stability. Addition of the aromatic nitroxide to a double-bond of a microsomal constituent yields an adduct radical whose nitroxide is bound on the one side to a tertiary carbon. On the other side delocalisation of the radical electron in the aromatic system contributes to the stability. Thus two structural features, aromatic ring delocalisation and the tertiary carbon explain a high stability of the microsomal adduct nitroxide radical.

Esterbauer: So it is a radical from the amine compound?

Stier: Yes, it is a radical derived from the aromatic nitroxide in a sort of spin trapping reaction with a double-bond of a microsomal constituent.

Ts'o: Two comments and one simple question. Tomorrow I will describe some of the redox cycles of the quinone-hydroquinone of benzo(a)pyrene. These are already practically established. As to the question of the nucleus pointed out by Professor Magee we also have investigated this rather carefully using benzo(a)pyrene with the purified nucleus (Lesko *et al.*, 1978). You can still get about 1% of microsomal-like activities from the purified nucleus. The question is, is it due to microsomal contamination? The products profile we got from the nucleus was different from microsomes, and, therefore, at first, we were very confident that this could not be due to microsomal contamination. It was pointed out later, however, that it could still be a partial or specific contamination of certain microsomal components. This argument could be readily refuted and thus we will never be able to know whether these enzymic activities came totally from the nucleus. With the best method we know, and by microscopic examination, these preparations contained clean nuclei and had 1% microsomal-like activity. Now the question I want to raise is whether the major issue in establishing the biological function of these redox cycles can be based on the variable toxicity exhibited in the treated cells as a function of the oxygen tension. Have you done those experiments carefully?

Stier: We have not done any experiments with nuclei. With regard to microsomal contamination of nuclei one should not forget that the endoplasmic reticulum membrane is continuous with the external nuclear membrane and perhaps the cytochrome P_{450}-system diffuses into the membrane. I think a careful study has shown that nuclei indeed contain a cytochrome P_{450}-system.

Mason: This could be a difficult experiment but you might hope to get some idea of the rate of redox cycling either by observing oxygen uptake over periods of time necessary to form the nitroxide, or by adding purified nitroxide to the microsomal incubation, and monitoring the stimulated oxygen consumption. Have you done any experiments of that kind?

Stier: No. What we have done is we found that nitroxides can be enzymatically reduced in microsomal suspensions and hydroxylamines can be oxidised. The redox cycle may not be perfect. Something we cannot explain at the moment came up in the case of phenobarbital stimulated rabbit liver microsomes. We see an additional signal, a 5-band spectrum appears which is quite similar to the spectra observed with dinitroxide spin labels. From this we may speculate that the spin label TEMPO may be further oxidised and subsequently two oxidised nitroxides may dimerise to a dinitroxide. A curious feature of this reaction is that we can totally suppress the appearance of the additional signal if we do the reaction in the presence of glycerol.

Slater: I think the comments of Professor Stier on the stabilised radical takes my memory back to some work we did a number of years ago, probably about 12 years ago I think, with isolated perfused rat livers in rats with external biliary canulae and we were interested in changing the redox state of the liver using a compound called phenazine methosulphate. Phenazine methosulphate is an interesting compound biochemically because it very rapidly and non-enzymatically oxidises reduced nicotinamide adenine dinucleotides. We wanted, in the intact liver, in the intact animal, to oxidise NADPH and NADH and look for the effects on drug metabolism. In fact, we weren't able to do this because the compound turned out to be extremely toxic, and to get a large dose into the animal results in very rapid death, but if you inject a small dose which, of course, is not sufficient to change the $NADH/NAD^+$ and the $NADPH/NADP^+$ ratio the interesting thing that you observe is that this compound forms a very stable free radical. The observation we made (Lott and Slater, 1973) was that when this compound was injected into animals the bile colour changed to a very brilliant red. Our first thought was that the rats were bleeding into the biliary canulus, but it turned out not to be blood, but a highly stabilised free radical. The stability of the radical was remarkable because you can leave it on the bench, as we did in fact, for days and days and days. We were very surprised by the stability, it seems to be secreted in the bile in lipid micelles and is attached in some way to a lipid component, and it seems to me to have some relevance to the type of radicals that you have described, and it raises the question: is phenazine methosulphate carcinogenic, for example. Has anyone any information about its carcinogenicity? It is widely used of course in cycling procedures, I may say, for estimating NAD^+ and $NADP^+$.

Stier: Can I ask a question of Professor Lown? What is known about carcinogenicity of bleomycin and these other antibiotics?

Lown: Well, most of them are carcinogenic and it often depends on the dose level. Nitrosoureas, for instance, are quite carcinogenic (Fishbein *et al.*, 1970), but at the same time they exhibit an anti-tumour effect (Wheeler, 1976). I am not aware if anyone has done a systematic study of the carcinogenicity of anti-tumour agents, it is certainly something one needs to be concerned about.

Adams: I think people are very much concerned with this now. Because of some sucess in treating some childhood leukaemias one is now beginning to observe second primaries in patients who have been in remission for many years. There is much current interest in the carcinogenicity of the common anti-cancer drugs. The International Agency will publish a booklet very soon which surveys all the literature on bleomycin, adriamycin, the vinca alkaloids, nitrosoureas and the alkylating agents and all the evidence for their carcinogenicity. That is epidemiological studies in man and both animal tests and short term tests.

REFERENCES to Discussion

Asmus, K.D., Nigam, S. and Willson, R.L. (1976). *Int. J. Radiat. Biol.* 29, 211-219.

Fishbein, L., Flamm, W.G. and Folk, H.L. (1970). "Chemical Mutagens", Academic Press, New York.

Floyd, R.A., Soong, L.M., Stuart, M.A. and Reigh, D.L. (1978). *Arch. Biochem. Biophys.* 185, 450-457.

Lesko, S., Lorentzen, R. and Ts'o, P. (1978). *In* "Polycyclic Hydrocarbons and Cancer", Vol. 1, pp.261-269. Academic Press, New York.

Lott, K.A.K. and Slater, T.F. (1973). *Biochem. Soc. Trans.* 1, 926.

Stier, A. and Sackmann, E. (1973). *Biochim. Biophys. Acta* 311, 400-408.

Wheeler, G.P. (1976). *In* "Cancer Chemotherapy". Am. Chem. Soc. Symp. Series 30, pp.87-119, Am. Chem. Soc.

Interaction of Activated Intermediates of Chemical Carcinogens with Cellular DNA and its Possible Prevention

P.N. MAGEE

INTRODUCTION

A number of chemical carcinogens has been shown to require metabolic activation to yield biologically active products which are chemically reactive nucleophiles (Miller and Miller, 1966; Miller, 1970; Miller, 1978; Magee, 1974). The terms precarcinogen, proximate carcinogen and ultimate carcinogen were introduced by Miller and Miller (1966) to describe, respectively, the parent carcinogen, metabolites on the metabolic pathway leading to the active form and this product which is the ultimate carcinogen. All ultimate carcinogens studied so far have proved also to be mutagens (Miller and Miller, 1971; Ames *et al.*, 1973). The most extensively studied classes of precarcinogens include polycyclic aromatic hydrocarbons, aromatic amines, aromatic azo dyes, nitrosamines, various alkyl hydrazine derivatives, aflatoxins, nitrofurans and 4-nitroquinoline 1-oxide.

Most, but not all, precarcinogens are activated in the body by enzymes known variously as drug-metabolising enzymes, microsomal hydroxylases and microsomal mixed function oxidases (see reviews by Conney, 1967; Cooper and Rosenthal, 1975; Lu and West, 1980). The metabolic activation of chemical carcinogens has been recently reviewed by Sims (1980). The microsomal mixed function oxidases comprise a membrane-bound multi-component enzyme system containing cytochrome P_{450}, cytochrome b_5, NADH- and NADPH-cytochrome reductases and various lipid and other components. The system hydroxylates and otherwise modifies steroids, fatty acids and various foreign compounds including drugs, insecticides and carcinogens. The enzymes occur mainly in the liver but also in other organs in varying amounts and they are induced by phenobarbitone, polycyclic hydrocarbons, pesticides, polychlorinated biphenyls and dioxins. Activation of chemical carcinogens occurs by various processes (see Sims, 1980) including: epoxidation of polycyclic hydrocarbons, aflatoxins and some chlorinated aliphatic compounds; N-hydroxylation of aromatic amines, such as N-acetylaminofluorene; free radical formation, for example polycyclic hydrocarbons (Ts'o *et al.*, 1976) and carbon tetrachloride (Slater, 1972) and N-dealkylation with formation of an alkylating intermediate as shown by nitrosamines, other N-nitroso compounds, dialkyl hydrazines, and aliphatic azoxy and azo compounds (Magee *et al.*, 1975; Sims, 1980).

It is currently thought that those carcinogens that are metabolically activated to nucleophiles exert their carcinogenic potency by interaction of the latter with a cellular constituent, probably macromolecular (Miller and Miller, 1966; Magee, 1974). Although the evidence is not conclusive, it appears increasingly probable that the crucial intracellular target for ultimate carcinogens is DNA, the genetic material of the cell, and the term genotoxic carcinogen has been proposed for such agents (Williams, 1980). For the remainder of this discussion it will be assumed that DNA is the crucial target for activated chemical carcinogens and consideration of the interaction of activated intermediates in chemical carcinogenesis will be limited to the carcinogenic N-nitroso compounds, in part because the author is most familiar with these agents and also because they have clear advantages for studies involving the intact animal.

N-NITROSO COMPOUNDS

Biological Actions and Metabolic Activation

The N-nitroso compounds have a variety of biological actions including cytotoxicity, carcinogenesis, mutagenesis and teratogenesis and several are finding extensive use in cancer chemotherapy. The toxic actions of the nitroso compounds depend on whether they require metabolic activation or not (see below). The nitrosamines are usually acutely hepatoxic with less damaging effects on other organs while the directly acting compounds, such as the nitrosamides tend to show varying degrees of local tissue injury at the site of application, and to damage

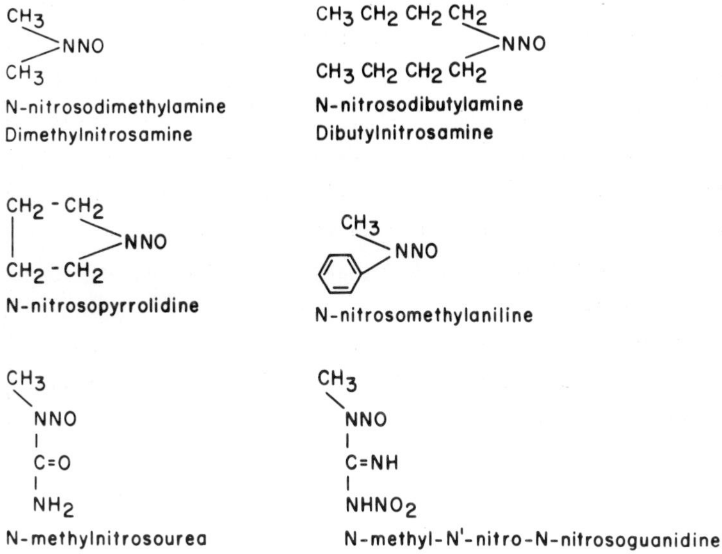

FIG. 1 Some carcinogenic N-nitroso compounds. Chemical structures.

organs with rapid cell turnover such as the small intestine, the bone marrow and the lymphoid tissues (see Magee and Swann, 1969). The mutagenic (Neale, 1976), carcinogenic (Druckrey *et al.*, 1967; Magee and Barnes, 1967; Magee *et al.*, 1976), teratogenic (Druckrey, 1973) and chemotherapeutic (Ludlum, 1977) actions of the nitroso compounds have all been reviewed in detail and only a brief introduction to their actions will be provided here.

The chemical structures of some carcinogenic nitroso compounds are shown in Fig. 1. The four nitrosamines all require metabolic activation by enzymes while the two compounds on the lowest line of the figure, N-methyl-nitrosourea and N-methyl-N'-nitro-N-nitrosoguanidine do not. Thus both of the latter compounds react directly with DNA in buffer solutions under physiolological conditions (i.e., pH 7.4 and a temperature of 37°C) while the four upper compounds, which are nitrosamines, are inactive under these conditions but can become active in the presence of a rodent liver enzyme preparation with appropriate cofactors, as will be described below. The nitroso compounds show remarkable organ specificity which varies with their chemical structures. For example, phenylmethylnitrosamine induces tumours only in the oesophagus of rodents, even after repeated subcutaneous injection.

A similar degree of organ specificity is shown by (4-hydroxybutyl)-butylnitrosamine for the rodent urinary bladder. There are several factors involved in the organ specificity of the nitrosamines (Magee, 1979) including the capacity for the organ or tissue to activate the compound. This capacity is a necessary but not sufficient condition for carcinogenesis by nitrosamines. Nearly all the organs of the body have been shown to be sensitive to the action of one or more of the compounds. A very wide range of species is known to be susceptible to nitrosamine carcinogenesis. This area has recently been reviewed by Bogovski and Bogovski (1981) who report that tumours have been induced in 39 species belonging to 25 families, 17 orders and 5 classes of animals. The species comprise fish, amphibia, birds and mammals, including monkeys. There is no direct evidence that human beings are susceptible to nitrosamine carcinogenesis but it seems unlikely that man is resistant since there is evidence that he can activate dimethylnitrosamine to yield a methylating intermediate that reacts with DNA to give a similar pattern of products as is produced by rodent activating enzyme systems both *in vitro* and *in vivo* (Montesano and Magee, 1970; Herron and Shank, 1980).

There is considerable evidence that the metabolic activation of the dialkyl and cyclic nitrosamines is initiated by α-hydroxylation of the carbon adjacent to the amino nitrogen followed by release of the aldehyde and formation of the alkyldiazohydroxide which spontaneously decomposes to give the alkyl diazonium cation which releases molecular nitrogen and the alkylating species. The earlier work on which this metabolic scheme is based was done mainly with the simple methylating compounds N-nitrosodimethylamine (dimethylnitrosamine) and N-methyl-nitrosourea and the postulated metabolic pathways are shown in Fig. 2. Much subsequent work, reviewed by Lai and Arcos (1980) has confirmed that a similar process of α-hydroxylation is involved in the activation of longer chain dialkylnitrosamines and of cyclic nitrosamines.

The formation of hydroxymethylnitrosamine has been omitted from Fig. 2 because, until very recently, its existence had not been demonstrated. There is, however, strong circumstantial evidence for the transient formation of the hydroxymethyl derivative because acetoxymethylmethylnitrosamine and higher acetoxyalkylalkylnitrosamines have

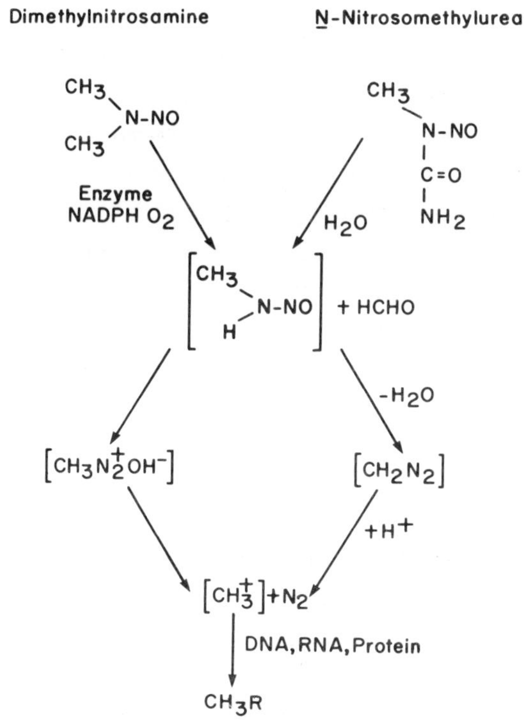

FIG. 2 Proposed metabolic pathways of dimethylnitrosamine (N-nitrosodimethylamine) and N-methylnitrosourea.

been prepared and shown to have the biological properties expected of a stabilised hydroxyalkylalkylnitrosamine which is decomposed in the body by non-specific esterases (Joshi *et al.*, 1977; Kleihues *et al.*, 1979; Frank *et al.*, 1980; Okada, 1976). Moreover, the isolation and characterisation of N-alkyl-N-(hydroxymethyl)nitrosamines from (hydroperoxymethyl)-nitrosamines by peroxidation has been reported from the laboratory of Okada (Mochizuki *et al.*, 1980). These authors demonstrated that both N-butyl- and N-methyl-N-(hydroxymethyl)nitrosamine decompose under physiological conditions to yield the aldehydes and a methylating agent thus substantiating the postulated metabolic activation pathway of carcinogenic dialkylnitrosamines.

Microsomal Metabolism of Dimethylnitrosamine

Metabolism of dimethylnitrosamine *in vitro* was first reported by Magee and Vandekar (1958) who showed that rat liver slices and post-mitochondrial fractions of rat liver could catalyse the decomposition of the compound. Metabolism by this post-mitochondrial fraction was shown to require reduced pyridine nucleotides and oxygen. Similar results were obtained by Brouwers and Emmelot (1960) who reported that formaldehyde was a metabolic product of dimethylnitrosamine *in vitro*. Since then, formaldehyde production has been widely used as a measure of metabolism of dimethylnitrosamine (see recent reviews: Lai and Arcos, 1980; Magee, 1980; Lotlikar, 1981).

Methylation of DNA incubated *in vitro* with DNA and liver microsomal preparations has been reported by Chin and Bosman (1976) and subsequently methylation on the 7-position of guanine was detected (Grilli *et al.*, 1977; Chin and Bosman, 1980). The author and his colleagues also detected methylation on the O^6-position of guanine under similar *in vitro* conditions (Jensen *et al.*, 1979). Some discrepancies arose, however, between *in vivo* effects of agents affecting the rate of dimethylnitrosamine metabolism and the effects on metabolism of the compound by microsomal preparations *in vitro*, raising the question of the validity of formaldehyde production as a measure of dimethylnitrosamine metabolism *in vitro* (Chin and Bosman, 1976). Recently published work by Jensen *et al.* (1981) has provided some clarification of this question. Using a microsomal fraction prepared from hamster liver, calf thymus DNA was incubated with [^{14}C]dimethylnitrosamine in the presence of necessary cofactors and the extents of methylation of the DNA and of production of formaldehyde were measured. The yield of radiolabelled formaldehyde was determined by precipitation of the dimedone derivative, formaldemethone and the major methylated purines released by mild and hydrolysis were measured by cation exchange high pressure liquid chromatography (Fig. 3). 7-Methylguanine, 3-methyladenine and O^6-methylguanine were found in the hydrolysates in the same relative proportions as found in similar hydrolysates of DNA treated with methylnitrosourea *in vitro* and in DNA isolated from the livers of rats shortly after treatment with [^{14}C]dimethylnitrosamine *in vivo*. The rate of DNA

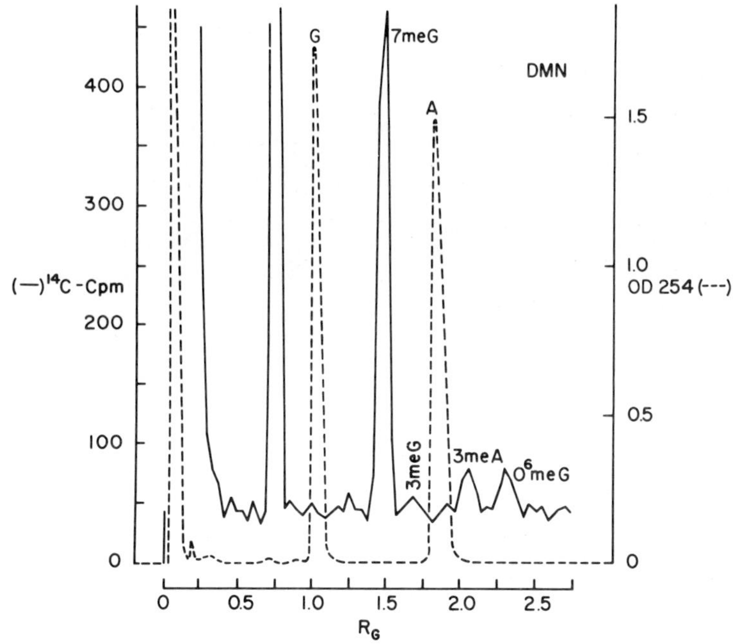

FIG. 3 Cation exchange high pressure liquid chromatogram of the purine residues released by mild acid hydrolysis of DNA incubated with [^{14}C]-DMN in the presence of hamster liver microsomes *in vitro* (Jensen *et al.*, 1981).

methylation correlated well with the rate of formaldehyde formation although the extents of DNA methylation were considerably lower than the amounts of formaldehyde formed. Both processes were dependent on NADPH and were inhibited by carbon monoxide, which is consistent with an involvement of cytochrome P_{450}. Agents reported to interfere with the metabolism of dimethylnitrosamine *in vivo* affected DNA methylation and formaldehyde production to the same extents. These findings suggest that the enzymic activity in the isolated microsomal system that is responsible for the metabolic activation of dimethylnitrosamine to yield a methylating agent is very similar, if not identical, with the system responsible for DNA methylation in the intact animal *in vivo*.

Metabolic Production of Molecular Nitrogen (N_2) from Dimethylnitrosamine

The metabolic pathways shown in Fig. 2 indicate that the postulated common product, methyldiazohydroxide, decomposes to yield molecular nitrogen and the methylating intermediate. The equations require that for every molecule of N_2 released a molecular equivalent of the methylating species must be formed. Clearly further confirmatory evidence for the postulated metabolic pathways of the nitrosamines would be obtained if the metabolic formation of molecular nitrogen from N-nitroso compounds *in vivo* and *in vitro* could be obtained. Several workers have reported experiments designed to demonstrate and quantify this metabolic production of N_2 with strongly conflicting results. Cottrell *et al.* (1977) studied the metabolism of dimethylnitrosamine labelled in both nitrogens with ^{15}N([$^{15}N^{15}N$]dimethylnitrosamine) by post-mitochondrial rat liver homogenates (S-9 fraction) and reported that less than 5% of the ^{15}N in the added nitrosamine was released as $^{15}N_2$. In sharp contrast Milstein and Guttenplan (1979), using unlabelled dimethylnitrosamine and liver microsomes, reported near quantitative production of molecular nitrogen. In recent studies aimed at elucidation of these contrary findings Kroege-Koepke and her colleagues (1981) have studied the *in vitro* metabolism of [$^{15}N^{15}N$]-dimethylnitrosamine and [$^{15}N^{15}N$]methylaniline by rat liver S-9 fractions and found that approximately 34% of the nitrogen from the dimethylnitrosamine and approximately 19% of that from that nitrosomethylaniline were released. Under the same conditions, [$^{15}N^{15}N$]-methylnitrosourea, studied as a positive control yielded 96% of the labelled nitrogen. Beyond noting the markedly different experimental conditions for those used by Cottrell *et al.* (1977) and by Milstein and Guttenplan (1979) it is difficult to offer an explanation for the variations in the quantitative findings of the different laboratories.

Some work on the metabolic production of molecular nitrogen from carcinogenic N-nitroso compounds by intact rats *in vivo* that is currently in progress in the laboratory of the author will now be described. This work has been carried out by Cecilia Chu in collaboration with Marilyn Kroege-Koepke, Steven Koepke, Gary McClusky and Christopher Michejda of the Frederick Cancer Research Center,

Frederick, Maryland, using a special metabolism chamber designed and developed in the United Kingdom by John Hollsman of the Courtauld Institute of Biochemistry at the Middlesex Hospital Medical School, London and David Halliday of the MRC Clinical Research Centre, Harrow, Middlesex. In these experiments rats have been given doubly ^{15}N-labelled dimethylnitrosamine, N-nitrosomethylaniline and N-methylnitrosourea by intraperitoneal injection and placed in the metabolism chamber breathing an atmosphere of 50% oxygen and 50% sulphurhexafluoride for a period of time sufficient for completion of the metabolism of the compound. Sulphurhexafluoride is known to be a safe replacement for atmospheric nitrogen and has the advantage that it can be condensed and thus removed from the system. At the end of the experimental period the animals were killed by injection of chloroform into the chamber and the contained gases were passed through a series of traps to remove oxygen, CO_2, unchanged dimethylnitrosamine and sulphurhexafluoride, the latter being condensed out in a trap immersed in liquid nitrogen. The small quantity of residual gases was collected in vials by a mercury-manometer system and analysed by mass spectrometry. A known quantity of neon was admitted to the system before exhaustion to serve as a quantitative internal standard for recovery of the $^{15}N_2$. The results of experiments on the metabolism of [^{15}N^{15}N]dimethylnitrosamine, [^{15}N^{15}N]nitrosomethylaniline and [^{15}N^{15}N]methylnitrosourea are shown in Table 1. The high recovery

TABLE 1 Metabolism of ^{15}N-labelled nitrosamines by rats *in vivo*

	Dose (mg/kg)	No. rats	$^{15}N_2$ expired (% injected dose, mean ± SD)
N-methylnitrosourea	24	4	88.0 ± 2.6
Dimethylnitrosamine	20	5	67.1 ± 11.1
Phenylmethylnitrosamine	37	4	52.3 ± 10.9

Male rats (120-150 g body wt.) received equimolar doses of nitrosamines i.p. and were killed 6 h after injection.

recovery of N_2 (88% of the injected dose) from methylnitrosourea, together with the use of neon as an internal standard, suggests that the apparatus was functioning satisfactorily and that the quantitative results with the other nitroso compounds are reasonably reliable. The recovery of 67% of the injected nitrogen in dimethylnitrosamine indicates that the metabolic pathway depicted in Fig. 2 probably does occur in the intact animal *in vivo* and that it is quantitatively the major one. Recovery of less than 100% of the N_2 from dimethylnitrosamine is not unexpected since Heath and Dutton (1958) showed that some of the nitrogen from $[^{15}N^{15}N]$dimethylnitrosamine appeared in the urinary urea after administration to rats.

This finding of incorporation of isotope into urinary urea has been confirmed in the laboratory of the author and found also to occur in germ-free rats (Holsman, Halliday and Magee, unpublished). There appears to be no recorded example of nitrogen fixation by mammalian cells, therefore any incorporation of ^{15}N into cellular constituents or products must indicate metabolism of the nitrosamine by pathways other than the one shown in Fig. 2. Metabolic denitrosation of N-nitrosomorpholine by liver microsomes has recently been reported (Appel *et al.*, 1980). It is possible that dimethylnitrosamine also is denitrosated in the body to yield products that could be further metabolised to urea. The finding that about half of the $[^{15}N^{15}N]$-phenylmethylnitrosamine was exhaled is interesting since relatively little is known about the metabolism of this oesophagus-specific carcinogen. Clearly the compound could be decomposing to yield either the phenyl or the methyl diazo intermediates or both, but there is no indication of their relative proportions. These results give strong support to the hypothesis that the carcinogenic nitroso compounds act by alkylation (arylation) of a cellular component.

POSSIBILITIES FOR PREVENTION OF INTERACTION OF ULTIMATE CARCINOGENS WITH CELLULAR DNA *IN VIVO*

Since many chemical carcinogens require metabolic activation it is clear that any factor that reduces the extent of their metabolism to their ultimate carcinogenic form will reduce the extent of the interaction of the latter with cellular constituents, including DNA.

There is ample evidence that this is, in fact, the case, and the induction of cancer in animals has been inhibited by substances that inhibit activation of chemical carcinogens of all the major classes (Wattenberg *et al.*, 1977). Clearly, also, any scavenging agent that can react with the ultimate carcinogen to a sufficient extent would be expected to reduce cancer induction, as with free radical scavengers in protection against radiation injury (Bacq, 1967).

An attempt to prevent some of the damaging effects of dimethylnitrosamine on rat liver *in vivo* was made by Kleihues *et al.* (1975) who showed that pretreatment of the animals with the radioprotective agent cystamine (Bacq, 1967) prevented the inhibition of hepatic protein synthesis induced by the nitrosamine and greatly reduced the *in vivo* methylation of hepatic DNA. These authors discuss the possibility that cystamine reacts with carbonium ions, presumed to be the active products of the nitrosamine, and thus reduce their interactions with the cell, but admit that the possibility that the cystamine might also inhibit the metabolism of dimethylnitrosamine and thus reduce the intracellular concentration of the methylating intermediate. The latter possibility has recently been investigated in the laboratory of the author by Julia Zubroff. Rats were treated with cystamine and dimethylnitrosamine under similar conditions to those of Kleihues and his colleagues (1975) and the inhibitory effect on hepatic DNA methylation was confirmed. The effect of cystamine on the metabolism of dimethylnitrosamine was then studied under the same conditions of dosage, with measurement of $^{14}CO_2$ exhalation after administration of the labelled compound. Labelled CO_2 production has been shown to be a valid measure of the metabolism of dimethylnitrosamine *in vivo* (Heath, 1962). As shown in Fig. 4, the metabolism of the nitrosamine was powerfully inhibited, strongly suggesting that the observed protective effect of the cystamine was largely due to this inhibitory action on nitrosamine metabolism rather than as a scavenger of the methylating intermediate.

Although protective effects against chemical carcinogenesis by nitrosamines and other chemical carcinogens by agents that effect the microsomal mixed function oxidases have been recorded, the use of such agents in any attempt to block carcinogenesis in human subjects could

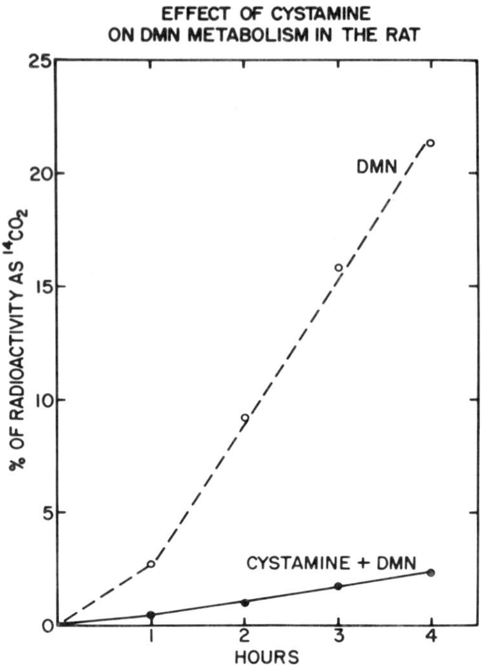

FIG. 4 Female Wistar rats (180 g body wt.) were given cystamine (600 mg/kg body wt.) i.p. followed 2 h later by [^{14}C]dimethylnitrosamine (30 mg/kg body wt.) and $^{14}CO_2$ exhalation was monitored for 4 h. Control animals did not receive cystamine.

be hazardous because of unknown and unforseen effects on the many functions of the mixed function oxidases other than the metabolism of xenobiotics. It would, therefore, be very desirable to find an agent that would serve as a trap for alkylating and other reactive carcinogenic intermediates, and would thus reduce the extent of interaction with the DNA on the cell. Such a material, ideally, would have very low mammalian toxicity and would be cheap. Ascorbic acid, which meets some of the above criteria, has been proposed as a blocking agent for dimethylnitrosamine by Edgar (1974) who drew attention to the ability of this compound to react with alkylating agents. At physiological pH ascorbic acid (pK_a 4.2) is largely in the anionic form and is therefore particularly susceptible to alkylation *in vivo*. The compound ascorbigen is formed very rapidly in plants by alkylation of the ascorbic acid anion by indole-3-methanol and Edgar pointed out that ascorbic acid might become alkylated in mammalian cells by the alkylating intermediates produced by nitrosamines, and thus function as a scavenger or trap (Edgar, 1974). This possibility has been investigated in the laboratory of the author by Julia Zubroff and David Jensen, in collaboration with Alan Conney and Wolf Koenzig of the Department of Biochemistry and Drug Metabolism, Hoffmann-LaRoche, Inc., Nutley, New Jersey.

The feasibility of prevention of DNA methylation by the methylating intermediate of dimethylnitrosamine was investigated by incubation of [^{14}C-methyl]-N-methyl-N-nitrosourea with calf thymus DNA in phosphate buffer at pH 7.4 in the presence of varying concentrations of sodium ascorbate. As shown in Table 2 some inhibition of DNA methylation

TABLE 2 *In vitro* methylation of DNA by N-methylnitrosourea as a function of sodium ascorbate concentration

Sodium ascorbate (mM)	$7meG/_{10^5G}$	$3meA/_{7meG}$	$O^6meG/_{7meG}$
0	482	0.11	0.10
5	479	0.11	0.10
10	391	0.11	0.10
15	339	0.11	0.13
20	309	0.11	0.10

Calf thymus DNA (5.76 mM) was incubated with 0.48 μM [^{14}C]methylnitrosourea (16.7 mCi/mmole) in 50 mM K_2HPO_4, 0.1 mM Na_2EDTA, pH 7.4, 5% dimethylsulphoxide at 23^oC for 2 h. DNA isolated by a Sephacryl-centrifugation procedure and analysed by HPLC after mild acid hydrolysis. Methylation of DNA is expressed as a ratio of 7-methylguanine to guanine, i.e., 7meG/10^5G.

did occur which increased with increasing concentrations of ascorbate in the range from 5 mM to 20 mM. These results suggested a similar inhibitory action might occur in the intact animal *in vivo* and this was investigated by Julia Zubroff in collaboration with Alan Conney and Wolf Koenzig of Hoffman LaRoche, Inc. The guinea pig was chosen because like the human being, but unlike other common laboratory rodents, this species lacks the capacity for biosynthesis of ascorbic acid. Furthermore, guinea pigs can be maintained on varying dietary regimes such that their body load of ascorbic acid varies over a substantial range. The experimental plan was to administer dimethylnitrosamine to groups of guinea pigs with high and low body levels of ascorbic acid and to compare the resulting methylation of the liver DNA. The doses of dimethylnitrosamine given were very low for two reasons. Obviously the lower the concentration of the methylating intermediate, the better the chance that the ascorbic acid anion could compete with the other nucleophilic sites in the cell. Also very low doses would be more comparable to the conditions apparently present in human beings where the occurrence of very small concentrations of dimethylnitrosamine in the circulating blood has been reported (Fine *et al.*, 1977; Lakritz *et al.*, 1980). Previous work had shown that methylation of rat liver DNA could be detected and measured (in terms of 7-methylguanine) after single doses of dimethylnitrosamine as low as 1 μg per kg body wt. and that the methylation declined proportionately with the dose of the nitrosamine (Diaz-Gomez *et al.*, 1977; Pegg and Perry, 1981). The extent of methylation of DNA, as 7-methylguanine, at decreasing dose levels of dimethylnitrosamine from 50 μg/kg body wt. down to 0.1 μg/kg body wt. in the guinea pigs with high and low body levels of ascorbic acid are shown in Table 3. The production

TABLE 3 Methylation of liver DNA by [^{14}C] or [^{3}H]dimethylnitrosamine in guinea pigs with high and low body levels of ascorbic acid

Dose of dimethyl-nitrosamine (μg/kg body wt)	Ascorbic acid in the liver (mg/100g wet wt)	$^{14}CO_2$ production (% of injected radioactivity)	Methylation of DNA (7meG as % of G × 10^4
50 [^{14}C]	4.3	48	6.9
50 "	27.7	45	6.8
10 [^{14}C]	4.0,3.7	39,40	1.2,-
10 "	41.1,41.1	42,41	1.3,1.2
0.1 [^{3}H]	5.5,3.7,-	-	0.020,0.019,0.018
0.1 "	37.0,32.2,-	-	0.019,0.019,0.017

Male Hartley guinea pigs (320-400 g body wt.) were fed semi-synthetic diets containing 0.01% and 3.3% ascorbic acid respectively for 3-4 weeks. The animals received the labelled nitrosamine i.p. and were killed 15 min later.

of $^{14}CO_2$ from those animals receiving [^{14}C]dimethylnitrosamine is also shown. It is clear that there is no difference in the rat of $^{14}CO_2$ production between the two groups, indicating that the differing body levels of ascorbic acid had no influence on the rate of metabolism of the nitrosamine and also that there is no difference between the groups in the extent of DNA methylation. These findings indicate, therefore, that under these conditions ascorbic acid did not affect the level of interaction of the carcinogen with the hepatic DNA by acting as a trap for the methylating intermediate or by any other mechanism.

SUMMARY

The metabolic activation of the main types of chemical carcinogens is briefly discussed indicating that the cytochrome P_{450}-dependent microsomal mixed function oxidase enzyme systems are frequently involved and that the activated product, or ultimate carcinogen, is an electrophile which reacts with various macromolecular and other nucleophilic receptors in the cell. Although not conclusively established the crucial cellular target for ultimate carcinogens is widely thought to be DNA. A short overview of the metabolism of carcinogenic N-nitroso compounds is given and some recent experimental findings are presented. Methylation of DNA by dimethylnitrosamine activated by subcellular preparations of hamster liver *in vitro*, as shown by formation of 7-methylguanine, 3-methyladenine and 0^6-methylguanine, is described and evidence presented that this methylation reaction is closely coupled to the formation *in vitro* of formaldehyde from the nitrosamine. The pattern of methylated purines was identical to that observed in calf thymus DNA incubated with N-methylnitrosourea *in vitro* and with that found in liver DNA extracted from rats treated with dimethylnitrosamine *in vivo*. The metabolic formation of molecular nitrogen (N_2) from doubly ^{15}N-labelled dimethylnitrosamine, phenylmethylnitrosamine and N-methylnitrosourea by intact rats *in vivo* is reported. Inhibition by ascorbic acid of methylation of calf thymus DNA by N-methylnitrosourea *in vitro* was demonstrated but no inhibitory action of the vitamin on the methylation by dimethylnitrosamine of liver DNA in guinea pigs *in vivo* was found even at the lowest dose of the carcinogen administered (0.1 μg per kg body wt.).

ACKNOWLEDGEMENTS

The author wishes to acknowledge support from NIH Research Grants CA 12227 and CA 23451 from the National Cancer Institute, and from the Samuel S. Fels Fund of Philadelphia.

REFERENCES

Ames, B.N., Durston, W., Yamasaki, E. and Lee, F. (1973). *Proc. Natl. Acad. Sci. USA* 70, 2281-2285.

Appel, K.E., Schrenk, D., Schwarz, M., Mahr, B. and Kunz, W. (1980). *Cancer Lett.* 9, 13-20.

Bacq, Z.M. (1967). "Chemical Protection Against Ionizing Radiation" Charles C. Thomas, Springfield.

Bogovski, P. and Bogovski, S. (1981). *Int. J. Cancer* 27, 471-474.

Brouwers, J.A.J. and Emmelot, P. (1960). *Exp. Cell Res.* 19, 467-474.

Chin, A.E. and Bosmann, H.B. (1976). *Biochem. Pharmacol.* 25, 1921-1926.

Chin, A.E. and Bosman, H.B. (1980). *Toxicol. Appl. Pharmacol.* 54, 76-89.

Conney, A.H. (1967). *Pharmacol. Rev.* 19, 317-366.

Cooper, D.Y. and Rosenthal, O. (Eds.) (1975). *In* "Cytochromes P_{450} and b_5, Structure, Function and Interaction", p.554. Plenum Press, New York.

Cottrell, R.C., Lake, B.G., Phillips, J.C. and Gangolli, S.C. (1977). *Biochem. Pharmacol.* 26, 809-813.

Diaz-Gomez, M.I., Swann, P.F. and Magee, P.N. (1977). *Biochem. J.* 164, 497-500.

Druckrey, H. (1973). *Xenobiotica* 3, 271-303.

Druckrey, H., Preussmann, R., Ivankovic, S. and Schmahl, D. (1967). *Z. Krebsforsch.* 69, 103-201.

Edgar, J.A. (1974). *Nature (London)* 248, 136-137.

Fine, D.H., Ross, R., Rounbehler, D.P., Silvergleid, A. and Song, L. (1977). *Nature (London)* 265, 753-755.

Frank, N., Janzowski, C. and Wiessler, M. (1980). *Biochem. Pharmacol.* 29, 383-387.

Grilli, S., Bragaglia, R.B. and Prodi, G. (1977). *Gann* 68, 129-137.

Heath, D.F. (1962). *Biochem. J.* 85, 72-91.

Heath, D.F. and Dutton, A. (1958). *Biochem. J.* 70, 619-626.

Herron, D.C. and Shank, R.C. (1980). *Cancer Res.* 40, 3116-3117.

Jensen, D.E., Lotlikar, P.D. and Magee, P.N. (1979). *Proc. Am. Assoc. Cancer Res.* 20, 121.

Jensen, D.E., Lotlikar, P.D. and Magee, P.N. (1981). *Carcinogenesis* 2, 349-354.

Joshi, S.R., Rice, J.M., Wenk, M.L., Roller, P.P. and Keefer, L.K. (1977). *J. Nat. Cancer Inst.* 58, 1531-1535.

Kleihues, P., Doerjer, G., Keefer, L.K., Rice, J.M., Roller, P.P. and Hodgson, R.M. (1979). *Cancer Res.* 39, 5136-5140.

Kleihues, P., Margison, J.M. and Margison, G.P. (1975). *Cancer Res.* 35, 3667-3672.

Kroege-Koepke, M.B., Koepke, S.R., McClusky, G.A., Magee, P.N. and Michejda, C.J. (1981). *Proc. Natl. Acad. Sci. USA* (in press).

Lai, D.Y. and Arcos, J.C. (1980). *Life Sci.* 27, 2149-2165.

Lakritz, L., Simenhoff, M.L., Dunn, S.R. and Fiddler, W. (1980). *Food Cosmet. Toxicol.* 18, 77-79.
Lotlikar, P.D. (1981). *J. Cancer Res. Clin. Oncol.* 99, 125-136.
Lu, A.Y.H. and West, S.B. (1980). *Pharmacol. Rev.* 31, 277-295.
Ludlum, D.B. (1977). *In* "Cancer, a Comprehensive Treatise" (Ed. F. Becker), Vol.5, pp.285-307. Plenum Press, New York.
Magee, P.N. (1974). *In* "Essays in Biochemistry" (Eds. P.N. Campbell and F. Dickens), Vol.10, pp.105-136. Academic Press, London.
Magee, P.M. (1979). *In* "Advances in Medical Oncology, Research and Education" (Ed. G.P. Margison), Vol.1, pp.213-221. Pergamon Press, Oxford.
Magee, P.N. (1980). *In* "Microsomes, Drug Oxidations and Chemical Carcinogenesis" (Eds. M.J. Coon *et al.*), pp.1081-1092. Academic Press, New York.
Magee, P.N. and Barnes, J.M. (1967). *Adv. Cancer Res.* 10, 163-246.
Magee, P.N., Montesano, R. and Preussmann, R. (1976). *In* "Chemical Carcinogens, A.C.S. Monograph 173" (Ed. C.E. Searle), pp.491-625. American Chemical Society, Washington, D.C.
Magee, P.M., Pegg, A.E. and Swann, P.F. (1975). *In* "Handbuch der Allegmeinen Pathologic Sechster Band, Tumors II" (Ed. E. Grundmann) pp.329-419. Springer, Berlin.
Magee, P.M. and Swann, P.F. (1969). *Br. Med. Bull.* 25, 240-244.
Magee, P.N. and Vandekar, M. (1958). *Biochem. J.* 70, 500-605.
Miller, E.C. (1978). *Cancer Res.* 38, 1479-1496.
Miller, E.C. and Miller, J.A. (1966). *Pharmacol. Rev.* 18, 805-838.
Miller, E.C. and Miller, J.A. (1971). *In* "Chemical Mutagens: Principles and Methods for their Detection" (Ed. A. Hollaender) Vol.1, pp.83-119. Plenum Press, New York.
Miller, J.A. (1970). *Cancer Res.* 30, 559-576.
Milstein, S. and Guttenplan, J.B. (1979). *Biochem. Biophys. Res. Commun.* 87, 337-342.
Mochizuki, M., Anjo, T. and Okada, M. (1980). *Tetrahedron Lett.* 21, 3693-3696.
Montesano, R. and Magee, P.N. (1970). *Nature (London)* 228, 173-174.
Neale, S. (1976). *Mutat. Res.* 32, 229-266.
Okada, M. (1976). *In* "Fundamentals in Cancer Prevention" (Ed. P.N. Magee *et al.)* pp.251-266. Univ. of Tokyo Press, Tokyo/Univ. Park Press, Baltimore.
Pegg, A.E. and Perry, W. (1981). *Cancer Res.* 41, 3128-3132.
Sims, P. (1980). *Br. Med. Bull.* 36, 11-18.
Slater, T.F. (1972). "Free Radical Mechanisms in Tissue Injury" Pion, London.
Ts'o, P.O.P., Barrett, J.C., Caspary, W.J., Lesko, S.A., Lorentzen, R.J. and Schechtman, L.M. (1976). *In* "Aging, Carcinogenesis, and Radiation Biology" (Ed. K.C. Smith) pp.373-398. Plenum Press, New York.
Wattenberg, L.W., Lam, L.K.T., Speier, J.L., Loub, W.D. and Borchert, P. (1977). *In* "Origins of Human Cancer" (Eds. H.H. Hiatt, J.D. Watson and J.A. Winsten) Vol.4, pp.785-799. Cold Spring Harbor, New York.
Williams, G.M. (1980). *Ann. N.Y. Acad. Sci.* 349, 273-282.

DISCUSSION

Connors: We showed that compounds such as cysteine and thiourea could protect against the toxicity of the alkylating agents. The trouble is that if the drug forms a methyl carbonium ion, the moment it's formed, it will react with what it's closest to. So if you form it close to DNA you'll find it very difficult to protect, won't you?

Magee: That is correct. However, it seems quite certain that there are other intermediates, the methyl diazo hydroxide and so on, and it seems fairly well established that there is a finite time between the first decomposition of the DMN and the final formation of the carbonium ion. I don't think you could trap an intermediate there, but one hopes that you might be able to get somewhere in between, possibly. The ascorbic acid, of course, should be in the nucleus too - it's uniformly distributed I believe. But it didn't work so I take your point.

Willson: You mentioned the Millers' work and the activation to electrophilic intermediates. You described your own work and the suggested role of the carbonium ion. You said there was some concern about the lifetime of this particular species and suggested that another species might be present. I assume this species is also electrophilic. You had cystamine on the slide. Should this have been cysteamine (the reduced form) because this is a better nucleophile and is more likely to trap an electrophilic species.

Magee: No, we used cystamine, following Kleihues and his colleagues, as I indicated.

Willson: Do you then envisage that cystamine, once you give it, increases the cysteamine levels, or do you think the cystamine is actually trapping the electrophilic species?

Magee: Well, we did this based on Kleihues' findings you see. He showed you get this remarkable reduction in the methylation of the liver DNA of rats treated with dimethylnitrosamine. I should say we confirmed Kleihues absolutely; there is this substantial 90% reduction in the methylation of the DNA but there's also a 90% inhibition of the metabolic activation of the dimethylnitrosamine so the cystamine is probably working that way and not as a trap.

Adams: On the S-S/SH point again, I think that cysteamine itself is metabolically fairly unstable but there are other SH compounds which are much more stable. Methylcysteine is one and lipoic acid is another which you might be able to try.

Magee: Well, I think Conney has tried, or is trying now, methylcysteine. I am not sure what his results are.

Slater: Another thiol perhaps to consider is mercapto propionyl glycine. I don't know if any work's been done on that in relation to your studies. Because it's reasonably non-toxic you can use relatively high concentrations *in vivo*; it's under clinical trial as a protector against liver damage in a number of centres now. I think you can get higher tissue concentrations with this substance than with the older SH-containing substances.

Perhaps I could change the line a little bit. You mentioned right at the beginning the hepatoxic action of DMN. I aways try to remember what my friends tell me (of course I don't always succeed), but a very, very long time ago you told me, maybe 20 years ago now, that DMN produces a much more hemorrhagic necrosis than CCl_4. Do you know why?

Magee: Well, I can suggest a reason why. I would suggest it's probably because the intermediate must have a longer life than the carbon tetrachloride intermediates, and I think it gets far enough outside the hepatocyte to attack the blood vessels.

Slater: But do you think it's the primary intermediate or some secondary intermediate?

Magee: Well, that's what I was trying to stress. One of the intermediates between the hydroxymethyl and the methyl carbonium must be relatively stable because, for example, dimethylnitrosamine works in the host-mediated assay system of Legator where bacteria are put into the peritoneal cavity and carcinogens are injected systemically. Therefore, the activated species has to get out into the peritoneal cavity. I would therefore suggest that in the case of carbon tetrachloride, if it is the CCl_3 radical that's important, it has such a short life that it would never get to the vascular cells of the blood vessels. With 1,2-dimethylhydrazine, for example, vascular cells have been separated from the hepatocytes and the vascular cells were found to be methylated. I think that is probably the reason for the difference between dimethylnitrosamine and carbon tetrachloride, simply that the active intermediates of the nitrosamine have a longer duration.

Symons: If there were any tendency to get CH_3^+ by an S_N1 process it would immediately react with water by diffusion-controlled process to form methanol. So you would have to have a system that was water-free in order to get methylation of anything else by such a process. I would think that it's incredibly unlikely that you would get CH_3^+. However, if one goes along with that formulation, the tendency to form $CH_3N_2^+$ would be strongly acid-catalysed and base inhibited. Is there any evidence for a pH dependence?

Magee: Well, insofar as one is talking about work in the intact animal, one is only concerned with pH. Concerning methanol there is experimental evidence that methanol is produced, there's no doubt about that. In terms of CH_3^+, many of my chemist friends have told me it reacts very quickly. Presumably, therefore, one of those intermediates I put up on the slide, like methyl diazo hydroxide, has got somewhat greater stability. Okada has recently reported the isolation of hydroxymethylmethyl nitrosamine so some of those intermediates must have a long enough life to be able to get far enough to methylate DNA and protein.

Symons: If we think of CH_3N^+ as a potential intermediate (which I would be quite happy with) this of course is going to be very susceptible to nucleophilic attack so that overcomes the need to call in the carbonium ion.

Magee: Should I then re-do my slides and remove the carbonium ion? It's only hypothetical.

Symons: Well, you did, in fact, say in your talk it was only hypothetical but from the discussion it seemed that some people considered that this was a serious postulate. It's fine as a mechanistic device but I think in terms of real chemistry it is unlikely.

Magee: Well, as far as we are concerned that's fine too, because we only want to explain the final methylation.

Slater: Is there any evidence that the formaldehyde could produce the methanol because it must be a very small amount of methanol that's produced?

Magee: Well, I suppose there is, but I don't see how one can distinguish between the two pathways. These were *in vitro* experiments. The people at BIBRA have shown methanol formation and my colleague, Dr S. Kim, also.

Slater: Yes, I was just wondering if you could use that for evidence for the CH_3^+ production by Professor Symons' reaction because it could come from formaldehyde.

Connors: If it is $CH_3N_2^+$ should Peter be looking for a different sort of protector?

Symons: Well, water would attack $CH_3N_2^+$, again to form methanol plus nitrogen, because water isn't a bad nucleophilic reagent. However, a better nucleophile might compete effectively.

Connors: But Peter has been trying ascorbic acid and ionised thiols; if it's $CH_3N_2^+$ is there something that might be more selective?

Symons: Well, certainly RS^- would be good.

Adams: Then you have the problem that penetrability of the cell could be affected in the ionised state.

Symons: And the problem with a "hard" nucleophile is that it will protonate in water and then it's no longer a good nucleophile. One needs to play this game rather carefully.

Magee: Of course some of these reactions are occurring not in water at all, but in a membrane.

Willson: In what part of the body, tissue or even cell, are you envisaging this electrophilic species to be?

Magee: Well, I think we're pretty confident about this. We think that it's formed primarily within the liver cell and that it can get a little way out but we do not believe it gets very far in the bloodstream for various reasons. One of the main reasons is that dimethylnitrosamine has no obvious effects on the bone marrow. If the reactive intermediate was getting into the bloodstream one would expect it to do that.

Willson: But you do get tumours in other parts of the body, other than the liver, do you not?

Magee: It depends which nitrosamine we're talking about. The kidney tumour I showed was induced by dimethylnitrosamine. But the kidney has got the enzymes to activate it, you see.

Adams: What about the oesophagus then?

Magee: This is one of the questions nobody knows the answer to. We have just started a programme of work on the pig in collaboration with the University of Illinois. One of the main purposes is to be able to get enough oesophageal tissue to work with. We assume that nitrosamines are activated in the oesophagus too.

Ts'o: I really enjoyed your talk. Congratulations. You've pushed really far now on these studies, but I think there is a real puzzle there; this question of the methylation of the DNA has come back to a full cycle. The emphasis started with Peter Alexander in methylation on phosphates, it went to N-7 with Peter Brookes and Lawley, and now to O-6. As we know, right now there's a lot of methylation on the phosphates, and it is a predominant product though it doesn't necessarily produce the kind of ultimate product postulated earlier. The discussion has so far indicated that no matter what the species is the species must be really very active. If there's a lot of water and a lot of phosphates and a lot of everything which can be reacted with, how do you expect ascorbic acid to compete with all the other so-called receptors for the reactive species - unless the ascorbic acid gets in to interfere with the metabolism, as you earlier inferred. But once you get the reactive species, there are already many substances which can react with the reactive species. It seems to be very difficult for the ascorbic acid to be more effective, and it is particularly difficult to see how the reactive species can be blocked by ascorbic acid so that it will not react with O-6 of guanine located deep inside the DNA.

Magee: Well, I wasn't very optimistic about it but I thought it was worth trying. The idea was put forward by Edgar, but the reason why I thought it was worth trying was first because Dave Jensen in our laboratory got the small *in vitro* effect, and second because ascorbic acid is very non-toxic; it's known that people can take very large amounts of it with no problem and it's very cheap. So if there had been any blocking effect that's exactly the sort of compound we want. I wasn't too optimistic that it would work and I wasn't too surprised it didn't, but what I hoped was it might have a chance to work at very low doses of dimethylnitrosamine (0.1 μg/kg body wt.), but it didn't.

Ts'o: Recently there was a report on ascorbic acid by Will Benedict (Benedict *et al.*, 1980) which suggests that it can block neoplastic transformation. So ascorbic acid is a very interesting agent. But trying to use it to block a highly activated methyl group is another matter.

Magee: Well, you're right - we couldn't do it.

Cheeseman: You mentioned the group at BIBRA (British Industrial Biological Research Association). As I understand it they see a role for amine oxidase rather than cytochrome P_{450} in dimethylnitrosamine metabolism. What is the current situation?

Magee: Well, I honestly don't know the answer there. I've discussed this with them and they say "this is what we find". I think it could well be that two enzymes are involved. I certainly think there is a cytochrome P_{450} component because my colleague, Dr Prabhaker Lotlikar, got inhibition with CO but part of the metabolism may well be with amine oxidase.

Connors: Just to follow on from that question because the group from BIBRA think DMN is metabolised mainly be amine oxidase. Everybody else tells me the major pathway is microsomal. Someone has got to be wrong, if one group claims the vast majority is metabolised by amine oxidase and the other group says it's microsomal. What is the answer to the problem?

Magee: Well, I don't know how to answer it. They have their results and other people have theirs. But one thing I do know and have known from when we first studied the enzymes that metabolise dimethylnitrosamine - it's not a typical cytochrome P_{450} enzyme system. It differs in many ways from the one that metabolises, for instance, aminopyrene. I've always known that. But on the other hand, it does have some of the properties of the P_{450} enzymes.

Slater: Does the amine oxidase come down with the peroxisomal fraction, do you know Tom? Because if so, then it would certainly sediment together with the microsomes?

Connors: No, they can clearly separate what they call an amine oxidase fraction and a microsomal fraction, but what they show with the microsomal fraction is that they don't get any nitrogen evolved.

Magee: Well, that I can't explain. Some work I didn't mention is that Christopher Michejuda has a paper, of which I am a co-author, accepted in, I think, PNAS, where we show that about 40% of the nitrogen from dimethylnitrosamine is released on incubation with liver microsomes. Why our results are different from their's I can't explain. We certainly do have the neon internal marker in the system so we feel confident that nitrogen *is* produced in the proportion I indicated.

REFERENCE to Discussion

Benedict, W., Wheatley, W. and Jones, P. (1980). *Cancer Res.* 40, 2796-2801.

Free Radical Metabolites of Chemical Carcinogens

R.P. MASON, W.G. HARRELSON, B. KALYANARAMAN, C. MOTTLEY, F.J. PETERSON and J.L. HOLTZMAN

INTRODUCTION

Interest in free radical metabolites of xenobiotics as possible toxic intermediates or ultimate carcinogens dates to the early 1940s. These early speculations were based primarily on the chemical reactivity of almost all free radicals (Swartz, 1972). Support for this type of speculation was found in the fact that some physical carcinogenic processes such as ionising radiation and UV light produce free radicals. Tobacco smoke was also discovered to contain large numbers of free radicals.

Before free radical metabolism can clearly be implicated in the origin of chemical carcinogenicity, at least three conditions must be met. First, the free radical metabolite must be demonstrated to exist. The only general method of detecting free radicals in biological systems is electron spin resonance. Second, if the carcinogenicity of free radicals is the result of purely chemical reactions of these reactive species, a knowledge of the radicals' chemistry under physiological conditions is also necessary. Note that free radicals are not usually substrates for enzymes, but react spontaneously. The third connection is that the location of the tumour must be consistent with the known enzymatic and non-enzymatic free radical reactions of the given chemical carcinogen. For example, a highly reactive free radical formed in the kidney cannot react with DNA in the bladder.

Many classes of free radicals are known to form during the metabolism of aromatic chemical carcinogens (Mason, 1979). In most cases, direct unambiguous ESR evidence has been obtained for at least one member of these classes of free radical metabolites, but the significance of the free radical metabolite to chemical carcinogenicity is generally unknown. Free radical metabolites of azo dyes, quinone anti-cancer drugs, and gentian violet are given as examples of the free radical metabolism of chemical carcinogens.

RESULTS

Azoaromatic Radical Anion

Red dye No. 2 was banned recently as a food dye by the US Food and Drug Administration. This food colouring is a weak carcinogen, and its high consumption (about 19 mg per person per day) necessitated its removal from our diet. The reductive metabolism of azo compounds such as red dye No. 2 by a wide variety of biological systems has long been known. Sulfonazo III is a diazonaphthol compound which is used in the titrimetric determination of sulphates and organic sulphur. Sulfonazo III is structurally related to the monoazo food dyes such as red dye No. 2.

We recently observed the electron spin resonance spectrum of a free radical metabolite of sulfonazo III in anaerobic rat hepatic microsomal incubations containing the azo dye and NADPH (Fig. 1).

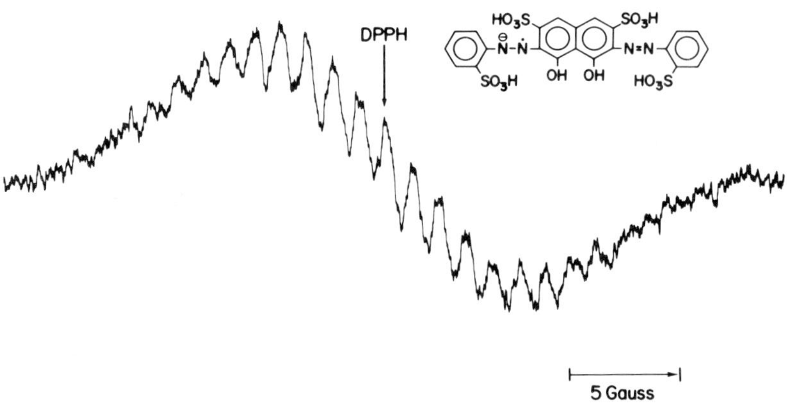

FIG. 1 The ESR spectrum of the sulfonazo III radical anion metabolite seen in an anaerobic hepatic microsomal incubation containing an NADPH-generating system. The *g*-value of 2,2-diphenyl-1-picrylhydrazyl (DPPH) is indicated by the arrow. The assignment of the unpaired electron to one of the azo groups is made for the sake of convenience (from Mason *et al.*, 1978, with permission).

NADPH is the ultimate source of the extra electron in this biological system (Mason *et al.*, 1977). This spectrum is characterised by a partially resolved 17-line hyperfine pattern and a *g*-value of the centre line equal to 2.0034. The 8 lines up field and 8 lines down field of the centre line indicate that the unpaired electron is delocalised onto at least one of the aromatic rings and probably onto both azo groups. The *g*-value of sulfonazo III metabolite is indistinguishable from the *g*-values of the azobenzene anion free radical or the chemically related 2,2-diphenyl-1-picrylhydrazyl. This result suggests that the sulfonazo III radical metabolite is in fact an azo anion free radical.

Next we studied the effect of dissolved gases on the steady-state ESR signal (Table 1) and on the rate of sulfonazo III dye disappearance in rat hepatic microsomal incubations (Table 2). The reduction of an azo compound to a hydrazine destroys the conjugation between the aromatic rings, causing a loss of the azo colour.

$$R\text{-}N{=}N\text{-}R \xrightarrow{e^-} R\text{-}\dot{N}\text{-}\overset{\ominus}{N}\text{-}R \xrightarrow[2H^+]{e^-} R\text{-}NH\text{-}NH\text{-}R$$

In air, the initial ESR steady-state signal is only 7% of that seen in a nitrogen atmosphere. Similarly, dye disappearance is inhibited markedly by oxygen. If the incubation system is left closed to the atmosphere, the steady-state ESR signal and the rate of dye disappearance increase in 2.5 min to reach activity similar to that seen in the deoxygenated samples. Carbon monoxide has a minimal effect on both the ESR signal and the rate of dye disappearance. This indicates that the reduction of the dye is not mediated through cytochrome P_{450}. When microsomes are omitted, or heated to 57°C for 15 min, one observes a loss of the ESR signal and a marked decrease in dye disappearance.

Our postulated mechanism for the formation of the azo anion free radical metabolite is shown in Fig. 2. Hernandez *et al.* (1967) have shown that NADPH-cytochrome c(P_{450}) reductase is the primary azo reductase in rat hepatic microsomes. In addition, Iyanagi and Makino (1980) have proposed that the one-electron donation to cytochrome P_{450} occurs by a shuttle between an O_2-stable flavin semiquinone and an O_2-unstable flavin semiquinone. With this in mind, it is natural

TABLE 1 The effects of atmospheric gases and heat denaturation on the steady-state ESR signal of the sulfonazo anion free radical metabolite in rat hepatic microsomal incubations*

Atmosphere	Relative amplitudes
N_2	100.0 ± 0.1
Air	7.3 ± 5.2
Air (after 2.5 min)	98.2 ± 1.0
CO	96.0 ± 0.9
N_2 (microsomes heated 57° for 15 min)	1.0 ± 0.2
N_2 (no microsomes)	0.0 ± 0.6
N_2 (no microsomes x 10 generating system	0.5 ± 0.1

* From Mason *et al.* (1977) with permission

TABLE 2 The effect of atmospheric gases on the disappearance of sulfonazo III in rat hepatic microsomal incubations*

Atmosphere	Dye disappearance (nmoles/min-mg protein)	Relative activity
N_2	58.5 ± 1.0	100.0
Air	1.7 ± 0.1	2.9
CO	51.1 ± 0.8	87.4
N_2 (microsomes-heated)	1.7 ± 0.1	2.9
N_2 (no microsomes)	1.4 ± 0.1	2.4

*From Mason *et al.* (1977) with permission

for us to propose that azo compounds can, like cytochrome P_{450}, accept a single electron to form the azo anion free radical.

Ultimately the enzymatic formation of the reactive azo anion free radical metabolites may cause toxicity. Three chemical reactions of azo free radicals could be of importance in the toxicity of azo

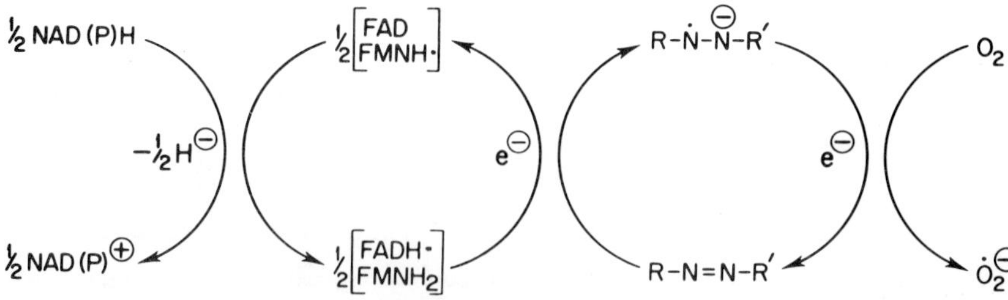

FIG. 2 The proposed mechanism of azo radical anion formation. The exact scheme of electron donation by NADPH-cytochrome c(P_{450}) reductase to sulfonazo III is unknown, but may be the same as the mechanism of electron donation to cytochrome P_{450} as proposed by Iyanagi and Makino (1980).

compounds. The first is the reaction of the free radical with itself, that is, disproportionation. This could be either a detoxification reaction, because the free radical destroys itself, or an activation step, if the hydrazine product is on the pathway to the ultimate carcinogen.

$$2\ R\text{-}\dot{\underline{N}}\text{-}\overset{\ominus}{\underline{N}}\text{-}R + 2\ H^{+} \longrightarrow R\text{-}N{=}N\text{-}R + R\text{-}\underline{N}H\text{-}\underline{N}H\text{-}R$$

A second possibly important reaction is hydrogen abstraction by the free radical metabolite. 2-2-Diphenyl-1-picrylhydrazyl, which is chemically related to the azo anion free radicals, is known to abstract hydrogen from tocopherol, cysteine (Blois, 1958) and other amino acids (Dearden and Odusina, 1973).

$$R\text{-}\dot{\underline{N}}\text{-}\overset{\ominus}{\underline{N}}\text{-}R + R'H + H^{+} \longrightarrow R\text{-}\underline{N}H\text{-}\underline{N}H\text{-}R + R'^{\bullet}$$

The third reaction, the air oxidation of azo anion free radicals, will be shown to be the dominant reaction in the presence of oxygen.

$$R\text{-}\dot{\underline{N}}\text{-}\overset{\ominus}{\underline{N}}\text{-}R + O_2 \longrightarrow R\text{-}N{=}N\text{-}R + O_2^{\bullet -}$$

Free radicals are not usually substrates for enzymes, but react spontaneously, so these chemical reactions should be important in the context of the reduction of sulfonazo III.

Our suggested mechanism of oxygen inhibition of sulfonazo III reduction is also shown in Fig. 2. The rapid air oxidation of the azo anion radical is the pivotal event. In such a scheme, there would be no net reduction of the azo compound since the parent compound would be reformed. Thus, sulfonazo III would catalyse the production of superoxide anion radical. Superoxide formation has been shown to be toxic to microbes, and superoxide is thought to be toxic to mammals, including man. Unfortunately, superoxide anion radical does not have a detectable electron spin resonance spectrum at 37°C. Although the azo anion radical formation is inhibited by oxygen, it is possible that oxygen merely inhibits the enzymatic formation of the radical by acting as a competitive electron acceptor. This would result in lower azo anion radical concentrations.

On the other hand, studies on the uptake of oxygen should give different results depending on the mechanism of oxygen inhibition of the microsomal azo-reductase. If the inhibition is due to a direct reaction between oxygen and the azo anion radical, then there will be a significant concentration of the superoxide and hydrogen peroxide produced, whereas if the radical is not formed, no production of superoxide is expected. In view of these considerations, observations on the stimulation of oxygen uptake by sulfonazo III and the reversal of this stimulation by superoxide dismutase and catalase would be a useful way to determine whether the azo anion radical is also formed in the presence of oxygen. We examined the effect of 50 μM sulfonazo III on the NADPH-supported oxygen consumption by hepatic microsomes; the oxygen uptake was increased 10-fold over basal levels and this stimulation was partially reversed by superoxide dismutase (Table 3). The presence of superoxide anion radical strongly suggested that the sulfonazo III anion free radical is formed by microsomal azo reductase under aerobic conditions (Mason *et al.*, 1978). This oxygen uptake rate is over five times greater than that observed for cytochrome P_{450}-catalysed reactions, and is the largest rate of oxygen consumption ever observed for rat hepatic microsomes. As expected, the disproportionation of hydrogen peroxide by catalase also decreased the sulfonazo III-stimulated uptake of oxygen. The rate of dye disappearance in this incubation is less than 2% of the rate of oxygen consumption. This implies that the consumption of oxygen is indeed catalytic, as is consistent with Fig. 2. The oxidation of NADPH by

TABLE 3 Effect of superoxide dismutase and catalase on sulfonazo III stimulation of oxygen uptake by rat hepatic microsomal incubations*

Sulfonazo III (50 μM)	Superoxide dismutase (40 μg/ml)	Catalase (67 μg/ml)	O_2 uptake (nmoles/min/mg protein)
–	–	–	12.2 ± 0.2
+	–	–	122.6 ± 1.2
+	+	–	111.2 ± 0.6
+	–	+	83.1 ± 1.9
+	+	+	79.3 ± 1.9

* From Mason *et al.* (1978) with permission.

microsomal incubations is also increased greatly by sulfonazo III, but it is not influenced by superoxide dismutase or catalase. This result implies that if superoxide, hydrogen peroxide, or a related species, such as the hydroxyl radical, participates in the microsomal oxidation of NADPH, the rate of these reactions must be much less than the rate of the futile azo reduction (Mason *et al.*, 1978).

The key prediction of our mechanism of oxygen inhibition of microsomal azo reductase is that superoxide anion will be generated. The conversion of epinephrine to adrenochrome is inhibited by superoxide dismutase and has been used by many workers to indicate the formation of the superoxide anion free radical in microsomal incubations. The initial rate of adrenochrome formation was 8-fold greater in the presence of 50 μM sulfonazo III than the basal level (Mason *et al.*, 1978), and both basal and stimulated rates were completely inhibited by superoxide dismutase.

One final point is that sulfonazo III anion radical formation in the presence of oxygen will not lead to the formation of the ultimate products of azo reduction, anilines and/or hydrazines, unless the oxygen concentration is very low. The absence of these reductive metabolites *in vitro* or *in vivo* does not imply that azo reduction to the anion radical has not occurred. Therefore, better known methods of detecting drug metabolites such as thin layer chromatography, which can not detect unstable free radicals, may lead to erroneous conclusions concerning the extent of reductive drug metabolism. For instance, our oxygen uptake results imply that each molecule of sulfonazo III in the incubation was reduced to the anion radical every 9 seconds, but the nearly quantitative air oxidation of the azo anion radical results in little net disappearance of the sulfonazo III until all of the oxygen is consumed. Because this futile metabolism is characteristic of many classes of phantom free radicals, many *in vitro* and whole animal studies, which show no net formation of products, may be totally misleading in ascertaining the importance of free radical intermediates, and, therefore, the true extent of metabolism.

In contrast to the reduction of sulfonazo III, the reduction of red dye No.2 is completely CO-sensitive, suggesting that this reaction is catalysed by cytochrome P_{450}. Although cytochrome P_{450} reduces red dye No.2 by an oxygen-sensitive mechanism, only a very weak ESR spectrum has been obtained from microsomal incubations. Since the oxygen inhibition of this azo reduction may be due to the air oxidation of the reduced cytochrome P_{450}, the formation of an azo anion free radical metabolite by cytochrome P_{450} is an open question.

Mitomycin C Semiquinone

Mitomycin C is an antineoplastic N-heterocyclic quinone natural product. It is carcinogenic in rodents, mutagenic in the *Salmonella* test, and induces dominant lethal mutations, chromosome abberations, micronuclei, sister-chromatid exchanges and spermhead abnormalities (Cole *et al.*, 1981). Activation of mitomycin C to cytotoxic metabolites occurs preferentially in hypoxic cells, which implies reductive activation (Kennedy *et al.*, 1980). This metabolic activation occurs by a widely distributed NADPH-dependent quinone reductase, to form alkylating derivatives. These metabolites damage DNA by alkylation of guanine, and by forming cross links between DNA bases.

Detection of the mitomycin C semiquinone free radical was expected to be somewhat difficult. Although this free radical has been observed with ESR in chemical systems, this species has not been observed in biological systems. Recently, a broad spectrum was observed in rat liver microsomal incubations, which disappeared within 4 min (Fig. 3). The transient nature of this spectrum is, presumably, the reason why many other workers have been unable to detect this

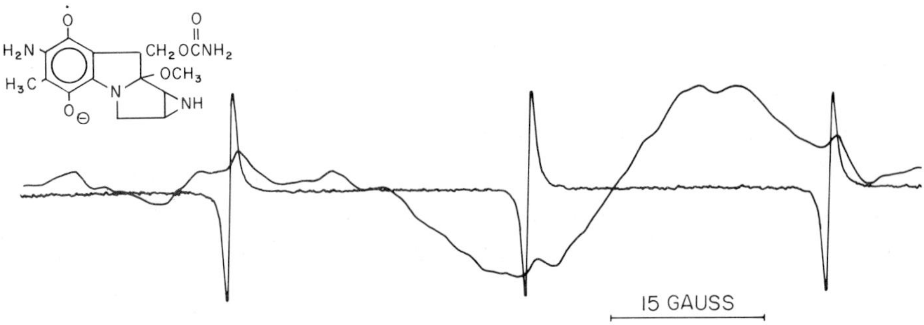

FIG. 3 The simultaneous ESR spectrum of the semiquinone metabolite of mitomycin C and the Fremy's salt *g*-standard obtained with a dual sample cavity and a dual recorder. The microsomal incubation (4 mg/ml) contained 1 mM mitomycin C and an NADPH-generating system (from Kalyanaraman *et al.*, 1980, with permission).

free radical (Kalyanaraman *et al.*, 1980). The spectrum was completely dependent upon the presence of the NADPH-generating system, microsomes and mitomycin C. The *g*-value for the free radical metabolite of mitomycin C was determined with a Fremy's salt *g*-standard and a dual sample cavity. The *g*-value of 2.0035 agrees with the value reported for the chemically-generated mitomycin C semiquinone in an aqueous medium, but we could not distinguish this *g*-value from that of the other NADPH-dependent paramagnetic species within microsomes, such as the NADPH-cytochrome c (P_{450}) reductase flavin semiquinone, which has a *g*-value of 2.00. Fortunately, the peak-to-peak width of the mitomycin C semiquinone spectrum is 9 G, whereas the NADPH-cytochrome c reductase flavin semiquinone is much broader with a peak-to-peak width of about 20 G. An earlier spectrum of the mitomycin C semiquinone in NADPH-cytochrome c reductase incubations shows a peak-to-peak line width of 20 G and is apparently due to the flavin semiquinone. In addition, the microsomal reduction of mitomycin C is 95% inhibited by CO (Kennedy *et al.*, 1980), implying that cytochrome P_{450}, not its reductase, is the primary one-electron donor.

Adriamycin and Daunomycin Semiquinone

Adriamycin, also called doxorubicin, and daunomycin, also called daunorubicin, are anthracycline anticancer drugs noted for their carcinogenicity, mutagenicity and cardiotoxicity (Benedict *et al.*,

1977). These anthracycline anticancer drugs have both quinone and hydroquinone structures and include a sugar moiety which confers water solubility. Microsomal NADPH-cytochrome c (P_{450}) reductase reduces the quinone functional group to form anthracycline semiquinones in a manner entirely analogous to the reduction of nitro compounds (Mason, 1979) or sulfonazo III.

The first evidence of enzymatic semiquinone formation from a quinone anticancer drug was indirect. Handa and Sato (1975) demonstrated that daunorubicin and adriamycin mediated the formation of superoxide in microsomal incubations containing NADPH. Later, they also demonstrated that these compounds stimulated aerobic NADPH oxidation in the absence of any net reduction of these antitumour compounds (Handa and Sato, 1976). The presence of semiquinone metabolites of anthracyclines has been demonstrated more recently with electron spin resonance in anaerobic incubations containing microsomes (Sato *et al.*, 1977; Bachur *et al.*, 1977) or the purified NADPH-cytochrome P_{450} reductase (Bachur *et al.*, 1979) and even in incubations of Ehrlich ascites tumour cells (Sato *et al.*, 1977). Once formed, the semiquinone and/or superoxide-derived species may damage DNA. Reductive activation of adriamycin and daunorubicin by microsomes and NADPH results in covalent drug binding to DNA (Sinha, 1980), which also occurs *in vivo* (Sinha and Sik, 1980).

The one-line spectrum in Fig. 4 is that of the semiquinone metabolite of daunorubicin in an anaerobic incubation containing rat liver microsomes and NADPH. Our g-value for the semiquinone metabolite of daunorubicin (g=2.0036) is in agreement with the literature value (Sato *et al.*, 1977; g=2.004). The long duration of this signal is probably due to the well known disproportionation-comproportionation equilibrium which continually destroys and reforms the semiquinone free radical. Sato *et al.* (1977) found that the ESR spectra of the adriamycin and daunorubicin semiquinones in aerobic microsomal incubations appear only after a time lag. They proposed that the ESR signal appeared only after the dissolved O_2 had been consumed by the semiquinone autoxidation. Under our conditions an induction period of about 10 min was found. This lag period was approximately five times longer in incubations which had been initially saturated with

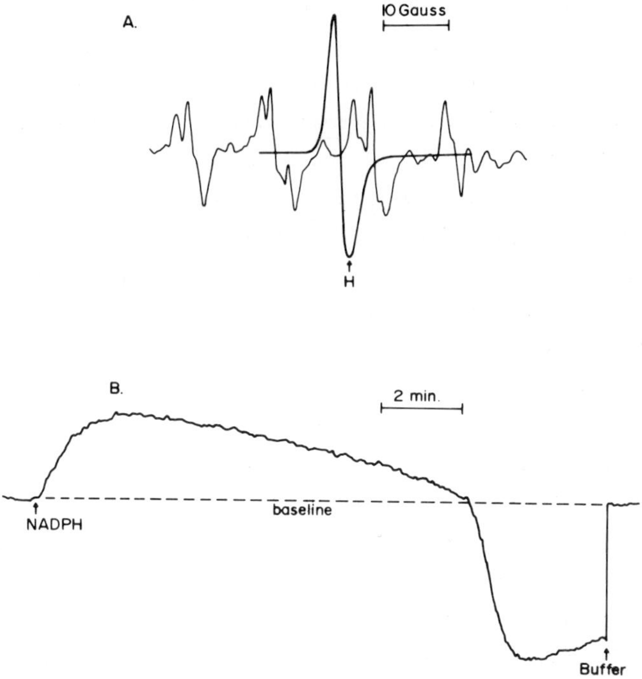

FIG. 4 (A) ESR spectra of the semiquinone metabolite of daunorubicin and the DMPO-superoxide radical adduct. (B) Changes in the ESR signal amplitudes of the DMPO-superoxide radical adduct and the daunorubicin semiquinone with time in a microsomal incubation (1 mg/ml) containing 1.0 mM daunorubicin, 80 mM DMPO, and an NADPH-generating system (from Kalyanaraman *et al.*, 1980, with permission).

oxygen, implying that the lag period does indeed reflect depletion of dissolved oxygen as proposed by Sato *et al.* (1977).

We have used the spin trap 5,5'-dimethyl-1-pyrroline-1-oxide (DMPO), which reacts with superoxide to give a DMPO-superoxide nitroxide adduct, to detect superoxide in these microsomal incubations (Fig. 4). This 12-line spectrum can be suppressed totally by superoxide dismutase. The DMPO-superoxide adduct was observed only during the induction period and remained until the appearance of the semiquinone spectrum, at which time the DMPO-superoxide spectrum disappeared (Kalyanaraman *et al.*, 1980).

This result was obtained in the following manner (Fig. 4). The magnetic field was fixed at the field position indicated by the arrow.

At this point, the DMPO-superoxide spectrum gives a positive deflection and the daunorubicin semiquinone gives a negative deflection. The reaction was initiated by the addition of NADPH. The signal amplitude increased due to the formation of the DMPO-superoxide radical adduct. After reaching a maximum, the concentration of the DMPO-superoxide radical adduct slowly decreased until 10.5 min had passed. At this time it was rapidly replaced by the semiquinone spectrum, as shown by the negative amplitude.

At least three factors could contribute to this phenomenon (Kalyanaraman *et al.*, 1980). First, the DMPO-superoxide adduct has a half-life of 45 s at pH 7.4, and, once the molecular oxygen is depleted, the formation of the DMPO-superoxide adduct must cease. Secondly, the nitroxide group of the spin adduct may be reduced enzymatically, as are other nitroxide free radicals. The third possibility is that once all of the oxygen has been reduced to superoxide, the anthracycline semiquinones may then reduce the DMPO-superoxide adduct. Although there is already evidence for the reduction of nitroxides by semiquinones in a purely chemical system, the inherent instability of the DMPO-superoxide adduct is sufficient to explain our observations.

When calf thymus DNA was preincubated with daunorubicin, the semiquinone free radical signal was greatly diminished under anaerobic conditions. A small residual signal may be due to free drug. This result is in agreement with Sato *et al.* (1977), who concluded that intercalated anthracyclines are much poorer substrates for enzymatic reduction. Furthermore, intercalated daunorubicin does not mediate the production of superoxide under aerobic conditions, which supports the idea that autoxidation of the semiquinones is responsible for superoxide generation (Kalyanaraman *et al.*, 1980). This result is in contrast to the reported chemical reduction of intercalated anthracyclines by $NaBH_4$ (Lown *et al.*, 1977).

At present, two general free radical mechanisms for the anticancer properties of many quinone compounds have been proposed (Kalyanaraman *et al.*, 1980 and references therein). One mechanism postulates that the semiquinones of these antitumour compounds are sufficiently stable to enter the nucleus, where they may intercalate and/or react with

DNA and/or with other macromolecules. The second mechanism of antitumour activity focuses instead on the quinone-catalysed superoxide-derived species, such as the hydroxyl radical. The hydroxyl radical has been implicated in the DNA scission caused by both chemically-reduced (Lown *et al.*, 1977) and enzymatically-reduced (Berlin and Haseltine, 1981) quinone anticancer drugs.

It should be emphasised that these two mechanisms cannot be operating simultaneously, because superoxide generation necessarily destroys the semiquinone (Fig. 5). In fact, the known rates of reactions between bi- or polycyclic semiquinones and oxygen at pH 7 are

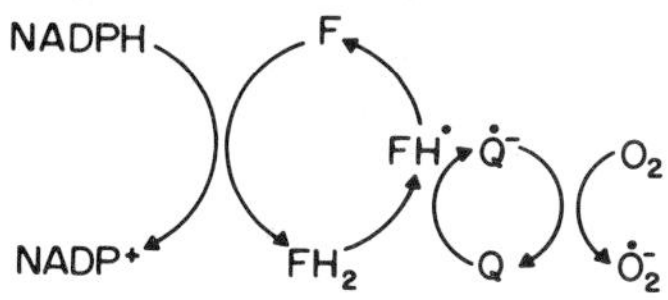

FIG. 5 The proposed mechanism of the quinone-catalysed superoxide anion radical generation by NADPH-cytochrome c reductase according to Iyanagi and Yamazaki (1969) and Handa and Sato (1976). The exact scheme of electron donation by the flavoprotein is unknown (from Kalyanaraman *et al.*, 1980, with permission).

greater than 10^8 M^{-1} s^{-1}. Although this reaction is reversible, the reverse reaction is one to two orders of magnitude slower. Assuming an oxygen concentration of 1 μM, which is less than 0.5% of the oxygen concentration found in air-saturated water, and assuming pseudo-first-order irreversible decay (*i.e.* $O_2 >> \dot{O}^-$), the half-life for the semiquinone radical can be estimated to be less than $\ln 2/k[O_2]$ or 6 millisec (Kalyanaraman *et al.*, 1980). If the O_2 concentration is greater than 1 μM, the half-life for the semiquinone radical will be correspondingly shorter. Consequently, semiquinone metabolites normally cannot be expected to be stable *in vivo*, and any reactions of semiquinones with macromolecules must be very rapid if a reaction is to occur. With the exception of simple electron transfer reactions, such as the reduction of methemoglobin or cytochrome c by semiquinones, most chemical reactions will be too slow to compete with electron transfer to O_2 at most *in vivo* oxygen concentrations.

Poorly perfused hypoxic tumours or the intestinal flora are possibly important exceptions to this argument, because these environments will have much lower levels of intracellular oxygen. The mitochondrion contains both cytochrome oxidase and quinone reductase, and therefore is the organelle most likely to become hypoxic. The mitochondrial quinone reductase will support the anthracycline-catalysed reduction of oxygen to superoxide, which, in conjunction with cytochrome oxidase, may cause the mitochondria to become essentially devoid of oxygen, thereby greatly extending the life time of these semiquinone metabolites.

In contrast to mitomycin C, adriamycin is less toxic to hypoxic sarcoma cells than to aerobic cells (Martin and McNally, 1980). This result would appear to rule out the possibility of anthracycline semiquinone radicals damaging the cell by reacting with DNA or other macromolecules. Although semiquinone-derived superoxide formation would still appear to be a viable mechanism for cellular toxicity, it should be noted that intercalated anthracyclines are not substrates for enzymatic reduction. Therefore, intercalated anthracyclines cannot catalyse either superoxide formation (Kalyanaraman *et al.*, 1980) or superoxide-mediated DNA strand scission (Berlin and Haseltine, 1981). In fact, the cytotoxicity of adriamycin to Chinese hamster V79 cells does not appear to depend *directly* on the presence of oxygen (Smith *et al.*, 1980). The mechanism of adriamycin cytotoxicity may depend upon the cell line because hypoxic EMT6 mammary tumour cells have been described as more susceptible than aerobic cells in one report, but as not in another (Teicher *et al.*, 1981).

Our major contribution to this area is the observation that the anthracycline semiquinone spectrum changes shape within minutes of the initiation of the radical formation to become asymmetric (Kalyanaraman *et al.*, 1980). Over a period of two to three h, the spectrum of the daunorubicin semiquinone (Fig. 6A) acquires the features of a strongly immobilised, axially symmetric g-tensor (Fig. 6E), characterised by g-perpendicular = 2.0046 and g-parallel = 2.0021. The final spectrum (Fig. 6E) is also a semiquinone as evidenced by the fact that the average g-value (trace of the g-tensor) is unchanged from the initial spectrum. In the initial spectrum molecular motion has averaged g-perpendicular and g-parallel to give the average g-value (g=2.0036), whereas, in the final spectrum, molecular motion has not averaged g-perpendicular and g-parallel,

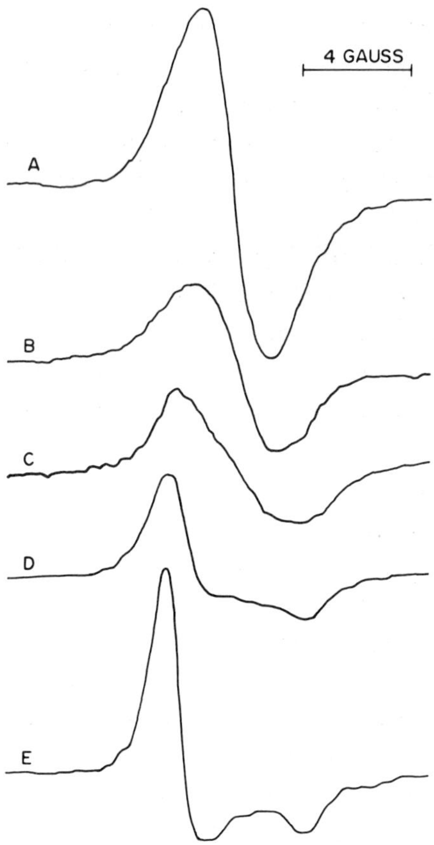

FIG. 6 The ESR time-profile of the daunorubicin semiquinone radical showing the progressive change of the symmetric motionally-narrowed spectrum into a completely immobilised spectrum (from Kalyanaraman *et al.*, 1980, with permission).

necessitating arithmetic averaging to obtain the average g-value, g=(2g-perpendicular + g-parallel)/3.

These spectra indicate that, initially, this free radical metabolite is rotating in solution; by the time the last spectrum of Fig. 6 is observed, the free radical has stopped moving on the ESR time scale. It can be shown that, in order to observe such a spectrum, the semiquinone metabolite must be rotating at a rate much less than 12 megahertz (Kalyanaraman *et al.*, 1980), which is the reciprocal of the ESR time scale. This motion is too slow for a small molecule in solution. Therefore, the semiquinone must be firmly associated with the microsomes, which are relatively large vesicles. Under the same conditions, daunorubicin metabolites become covalently attached to microsomal protein (Sinha, 1980). The binding of the daunorubicin semiquinone to the microsomes may be part of the answer, but this alone cannot explain the progressive immobilisation of the semiquinone metabolite. This sequence of spectra must imply either a change in the microsomes, or a transformation of the semiquinone radical. Under anaerobic conditions, microsomal incubations of daunorubicin are known to form deoxyaglycone products, which do not have the attached sugar moiety that gives water solubility to the compound. A semiquinone of this metabolite would be more lipophilic and more tightly bound to the microsomes, and could, perhaps, account for the final spectrum. Another possibility is that a semiquinone polymerisation product of daunorubicin and microsomal protein is responsible for the final immobilised spectrum (that is, a melanin-like polymer). Melanin, of course, has ESR spectra with less *g*-anisotropy. In any case, the progressive immobilisation of the daunorubicin-derived semiquinone in the microsomal membrane is of considerable interest, and requires further investigation.

Triarylmethyl Radical

Benzyl violet 4B, light green SF and related triarylmethane dyes are used as biological stains, to dye wool and silk, as food dyes and in cosmetics. Gentian violet is used as a biological stain and is used extensively in human and veterinary medicine. It is given internally to children and adults for pinworm, and is applied topically for fungus infections such as thrush. Gentian violet is mutagenic in the Rosenkranz assay and causes DNA strand breaks in Chinese hamster cells (Au *et al.*, 1979). Ingestion of guinea green B by the rat significantly increases the frequency of hepatic carcinomas (Hansen *et al.*, 1966). Ingested benzyl violet 4B causes squamous cell carcinomas and mammary carcinomas in the rat (Ikeda *et al.*, 1974).

When these compounds are metabolised under a nitrogen atmosphere by rat hepatic microsomes supplemented with NADPH, a single-line electron spin resonance spectrum is obtained (Fig. 7).

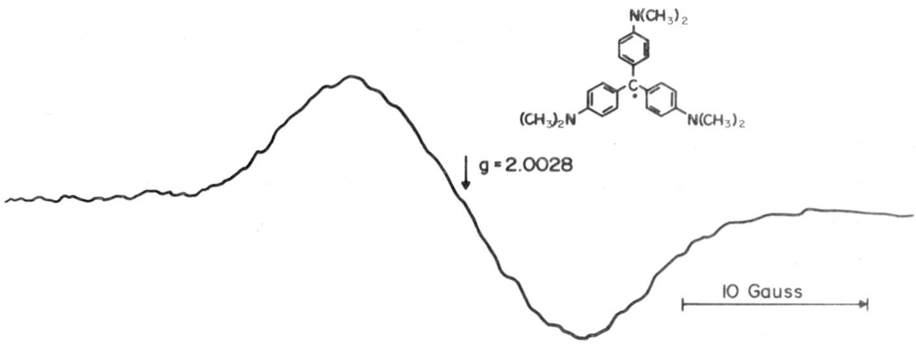

FIG. 7 The ESR spectrum of the tri-N,N-dimethyl-anisyl methyl radical observed on incubation of 1 mM gentian violet with 2 mg/ml of rat hepatic microsomes and an NADPH-generating system.

The one electron reduction of gentian violet forms the tri-N,N-dimethyl-anisyl methyl radical, which is characterised by g = 2.0028 (Leaver, 1972). Apparently, this free radical forms (at least in part) by a one-electron transfer from reduced cytochrome P_{450}, as indicated by the CO sensitivity (Fig. 8).

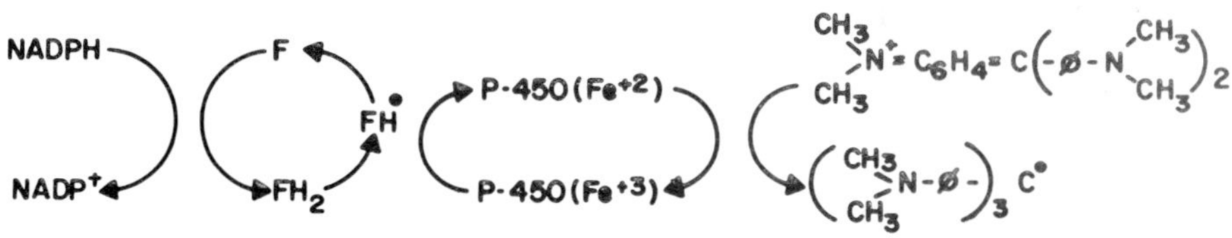

FIG. 8 The proposed mechanism of carbon-centred free radical formation by the rat hepatic microsomal reduction of gentian violet. The exact scheme of cytochrome P_{450} reduction by NADPH-cytochrome P_{450} reductase is unknown (Iyanagi and Makino, 1980), but reduced cytochrome P_{450} can donate only one electron at a time to gentian violet, and the carbon-centred free radical so formed is presumably the species detected with electron spin resonance.

The known chemistry of the triphenylmethyl free radical suggests that the reactions of the tri-N,N-dimethyl-anisyl methyl radical may be of toxicological significance. Like most carbon-centred free radicals, the triphenylmethyl radical reacts with oxygen to form a very reactive peroxyl free radical, which should initiate lipid peroxidation. Instead of forming a peroxy free radical, the tri-N,N-dimethyl-anisyl methyl radical may air oxidise to form superoxide. In addition, the triphenylmethyl free radical can add across conjugated double bonds (Forrester *et al.*, 1968).

Although we have chosen to discuss free radical metabolites of carcinogens, it should be noted that free radicals can, in principle, be generated from almost any aromatic organic chemical, carcinogen or noncarcinogen (Mason, 1979). Most biochemicals are not aromatic, and, therefore, are not easily metabolised through free radical intermediates. In contrast, many synthetic aromatic organic compounds and closely related natural products are readily metabolised to reactive free radicals. In fact, the enzymatic formation of free radical metabolites of synthetic aromatic compounds is the rule and not the exception. The generality of the free radical metabolism of aromatic compounds precludes any simple relationship between free radical formation and carcinogenicity. The aromaticity of a chemical facilitates both free radical formation and its intercalation between DNA bases, but, as has been noted, the intercalation of the free radical precursor inhibits the enzymatic formation of free radicals, which further complicates the relationship. The involvement of yet other free radical metabolites in chemical carcinogenesis has been reviewed (Ts'o *et al.*, 1977).

REFERENCES

Au, W., Butler, M.A., Bloom, S.E. and Matney, T.S. (1979). *Mutat. Res.* 66, 103-112.

Bachur, N.R., Gordon, S.L. and Gee, M.V. (1977). *Mol. Pharmacol.* 13, 901-910.

Bachur, N.R., Gordon, S.L., Gee, M.V. and Kon, H. (1979). *Proc. Nat. Acad. Sci. USA* 76, 954-957.

Benedict, W.F., Baker, M.S., Haroun, L., Choi, E. and Ames, B.N. (1977). *Cancer Res.* 37, 2209-2213.

Berlin, V. and Haseltine, W.A. (1981). *J. Biol. Chem.* 256, 4747-4756.

Blois, M.S. (1958). *Nature (London)* 181, 1199-1200.

Cole, R.J., Taylor, N., Cole, J. and Arlett, C.F. (1981). *Mutat. Res.* 80, 141-157.

Dearden, J.C. and Odusina, A.O. (1973). *Mech. Ageing Dev.* 2, 309-314.

Forrester, A.R., Hay, J.M. and Thomson, R.H. (1968). *In* "Organic Chemistry of Stable Free Radicals", pp.69-71, Academic Press, New York.

Handa, K. and Sato, S. (1975). *Gann* 66, 43-47.

Handa, K. and Sato, S. (1976). *Gann* 67, 523-528.

Hansen, W.H., Long, E.L., Davis, K.J., Nelson, A.A. and Fitzhugh, O.G. (1966). *Food, Cosmet. Toxicol.* 4, 389-410.

Hernandez, P.H., Gillette, J.R. and Mazel, P. (1967). *Biochem. Pharmacol.* 16, 1859-1875.
Ikeda, Y., Horiuchi, S., Imoto, A., Kodama, Y., Aida, Y. and Kobayashi, K. (1974). *Toxicology* 2, 275-284.
Iyanagi, T. and Yamazaki, I. (1969). *Biochim. Biophys. Acta* 172, 370-381.
Iyanagi, T. and Makino, R. (1980). *In* "Microsomes, Drug Oxidations and Chemical Carcinogens" (Eds. M.J. Coon, A.H. Conney, R.W. Estabrook, H.V. Gelboin, J.R. Gillette and P.J. O'Brien) Vol. I, pp.407-410. Academic Press, New York.
Kalyanaraman, B., Perez-Reyes, E. and Mason, R.P. (1980). *Biochim. Biophys. Acta* 630, 119-130.
Kennedy, K.A., Rockwell, S. and Sartorelli, A.C. (1980). *Cancer Res.* 40, 2356-2360.
Leaver, I.H. (1972). *Photochem. Photobiol.* 16, 189-196.
Lown, J.W., Sim, S.-K., Majumdar, K.C. and Chang, R.-Y. (1977). *Biochem. Biophys. Res. Commun.* 76, 705-710.
Martin, W.M.C. and McNally, N.J. (1980). *Br. J. Cancer* 42, 881-889.
Mason, R.P., Peterson, F.J. and Holtzman, J.L. (1977). *Biochem. Biophys. Res. Commun.* 75, 532-540.
Mason, R.P., Peterson, F.J. and Holtzman, J.L. (1978). *Mol. Pharmacol.* 14, 665-671.
Mason, R.P. (1979). *In* "Reviews in Biochemical Toxicology" (Eds. E. Hodgson, J.R. Bend and R.M. Philpot) Vol. I, pp.151-200. Elsevier North Holland, Inc., New York.
Sato, S., Iwaizumi, M., Handa, K. and Tamura, Y. (1977). *Gann* 68, 603-608.
Sinha, B.K. (1980). *Chem.-Biol. Interact.* 30, 67-77.
Sinha, B.K. and Sik, R.H. (1980). *Biochem. Pharmacol.* 29, 1867-1868.
Smith, E., Stratford, I.J. and Adams, G.E. (1980). *Br. J. Cancer* 41, 568-573.
Swartz, H.M. (1972). *Adv. Cancer Res.* 15, 227-252.
Teicher, B.A., Lazo, J.S. and Sartorelli, A.C. (1981). *Cancer Res.* 41, 73-81.
Ts'o, P.O.P., Caspary, W.J. and Lorentzen, R.J. (1977). *In* "Free Radicals in Biology" (Ed. W.A. Pryor) Vol. III, pp.251-303. Academic Press, New York.

DISCUSSION

Swartz: In adriamycin one has this tempting looking quinone/hydroquinone on the same molecule. The mechanisms you discussed were bimolecular mechanisms, that is you had two adriamycins for your redox pair. Is it possible that you are getting an internal disproportionation/conproportionation in those adriamycin derivatives where there are adjacent quinone/hydroquinone pairs?

Mason: We have a quinone, semiquinone/hydroquinone couple. Benzoquinone is a 2-electron oxidation product of hydroquinone, so if we add an electron to a quinone, that forms a semiquinone. If you wanted to make the semiquinone ring into a hydroquinone ring and vice versa, that would just be a resonance structure and you are quite welcome to do that, but that is not a different species. It's just another valence bond structure. The hydroquinone is already fully reduced, so if it was oxidised by the semiquinone that would just swap the position of the semiquinone and hydroquinone, but that is just a valence bond structure. So what you are aluding to does occur but it's just another valence structure of the radical. It is an appropriate representation of the radical, but it is not a different species. One possibility that you do have in the anthracyclines, which I am interested in, is that a peroxidase could oxidise the hydroquinone moiety. Now this would form a different entity. Pietronigro *et al.* (1973) have reported oxidising the hydroquinone moiety of adriamycin. I think they were observing the semiquinone formed by reduction, but there is a lot of room for confusion there.

Willson: I think what Professor Swartz was referring to was your slide where you had a quinone and hydroquinone together, and you said you got dismutation of these two to give a semiquinone. In this case wouldn't the structure be a bi-radical, a bi-semiquinone? Both rings would be semiquinones and you could envisage a compound with two free electrons.

Mason: O.K. A bi-radical is yet another possibility.

Willson: But would such a bi-radical be stable?

Mason: Yes, that is at the same redox state as the parent anthracycline, and that is another resonance structure. Anthracyclines do not have room temperature ESR signals, but that proves nothing because it is not easy to detect triplet signals in solution at room temperature. Anyway, the bi-radical is just another resonance structure.

Adams: But how important are the rings on either side? It's not an homogeneous structure so your contribution of the bi-radical will be correspondingly lower. The contribution of the bi-radical to the total structure I would imagine to be rather small.

Mason: I would think so too, but it might be fun to look for a $\Delta M = 2$ transition at half field at liquid nitrogen temperature - you never know.

Symons: I enjoyed your talk. It seems to me one of the essential points you are bringing out is the catalytic formation of superoxide and consequences thereof. I wonder if you could expound a bit on that and the question of why putting in one of these redox dye systems should catalyse the formation of superoxide. I do not understand why that should be.

Mason: It is not generally understood. The arguments are the following. These redox enzymes are usually cytochrome reductases, which normally reduce iron. They have the thermodynamic potential to reduce oxygen to superoxide, but they have been designed through the eons not to do that, so even though thermodynamically they have more than enough potential to reduce oxygen to superoxide the structure of the enzyme prevents that in some kinetic way. If you add a redox dye (a nitro compound, azo compound or quinone) this kinetic barrier is somehow overcome and the enzyme will donate an electron to this foreign compound, not knowing any better presumably, and the thermodynamics take over. Why reductases are not oxidases is a question that has no answer as far as I know.

Stier: What you measure is an increased oxygen consumption and an increased NADPH consumption in the presence of the dye substrate. Perfluororinated hydrocarbons have the same effect. How do you exclude a possibility like this, a decoupling of the microsomal electron transfer chain? Did you do experiments for instance with a purified reductase or did you measure the reduction of the dye substrate?

Mason: Many of these redox dyes have been looked at with the purified NADPH-cytochrome c (P_{450}) reductase. The quinones have been extensively studied by Iyanagi and Yamazaki (1969) and Bachur *et al.* (1979). Your question is a good one though. I think the biggest difference between the sulfonazo III stimulation or the nitrofurantoin stimulation is the magnitude. Shunting electrons from the reductase you can obtain stimulations of microsomal oxygen uptake of ten-fold to a rate of 123 nmole/min mg protein (Table 3), and this is at least five times greater than any cytochrome P_{450}-mediated phenomenon known. The cytochrome P_{450} catalysed reactions are exceedingly slow in comparison with the reductase-mediated reactions. The perfluoro-*n*-hexane stimulation of NADPH-supported O_2-uptake is only three-fold with a final consumption of 6.4 nmole/min mg protein (Staudt *et al.*, 1974).

Stier: Yes, but that is not the decoupling reaction. The oxygen consumption and NADPH consumption are not to be compared with mixed function oxidation product formation.

Mason: Agreed. The fundamental difference is - I know I have metabolism here, because I can detect the azo anion radical metabolite.

Stier: That does not give you the stoichiometry of the reaction; the ESR signal you see may only represent a very minor amount. I think the only experiment that would give unequivocal results would be with the purified cytochrome P_{450} reductase.

Mason: Well, these stimulations of oxygen consumption are insensitive to P_{450} inhibitors - maybe that would convince you. They are insensitive to CO, for instance, if you use an O_2/CO atmosphere. The parallel between the two phenomena is striking, though, and I have often wondered if perfluoro-*n*-hexane or CCl_4 itself is reduced to an anion radical by the microsomal system, and then they would be identical. But the redox phenomenon is better understood than the uncoupling phenomenon, so I'll stand behind my mechanism.

Adams: There are a number of examples of catalysed electron transfer. Dr Willson referred to this yesterday regarding some pulse radiolysis systems where electron transfer from one molecule A to molecule C can be accelerated by putting in molecule B. It seems to me that you could use a model pulse radiolysis system to show that one can obtain catalysis by these agents.

Mason: It is known with both the semiquinone anion radicals (Svingen and Powis, 1981) and the nitro anion radicals (Wardman and Clarke, 1976) that the rate constant for the reaction of oxygen with the anion radicals is very rapid. I think the other thing that tends to support the scheme that superoxide formation is the result of anion radical metabolite formation is the experiment with DMPO and the semiquinone (Fig. 4). Sealy *et al.* (1978) have performed similar experiments with nitro compounds and DMPO. What you see is initially the DMPO-superoxide adduct, and, when it disappears, it is immediately replaced by the respective anion radical metabolite. The sequence of events is very convincing evidence that one is the result of the other.

Adams: You referred to the hypothesis of the action of anthracyclines in which the semiquinone attacks the DNA. When I ask what is meant by this I am told this involves electron transfer to the DNA. This is impossible on energetic grounds. There are lots of examples where one can show electron transfer *from* DNA or from nucleotides to quinones using pulse radiolysis, but not in the reverse direction.

Slater: Perhaps we can come back to that one in general discussion. Professor Ts'o has something to say with relevance to that in his lecture. On several of your slides you had NADPH going to reduce the flavine coenzyme of the flavoprotein to form the flavone semiquinone. Is there any evidence to show which component is so reduced in your system? Is it the high potential or the low potential coenzyme? In other words is it the FAD or the FMN of the NADPH P_{450} reductase?

Mason: This question has only been studied in the context of cytochrome P_{450} reduction by NADPH-cytochrome P_{450}(c) reductase. I refer to the work of Iyanagi and Makino (1980) and earlier work with H.S. Mason on how electrons are shuttled into the flavoprotein from NADPH and how they are shuttled out. As you mentioned, there are two flavins, FMN and FAD. At present their scheme is incomplete, but they propose that the air-stable redox state of the semiquinone is a flavin semiquinone, FAD/FMNH$^{\bullet}$. They propose that the flavoprotein is reduced by a hydride transfer from NADPH forming $FADH_2$/FMNH$^{\bullet}$, which transfers the electron from one flavin to the other forming FADH$^{\bullet}$/$FMNH_2$ which is the actual electron donor to cytochrome P_{450} (Vermilion *et al.*, 1981). For lack of any other evidence I assume that cytochrome c and these redox dyes accept electrons in a manner totally analogous to cytochrome P_{450}, whatever that may be.

Slater: There is evidence from Coon's group for example that different dyes will accept electrons from either FMN or FAD. I wondered if you had evidence with your particular substances that there is really a different pathway of electron transport. On your early work you had NADH as a reducing source, NADH with P in brackets. I wonder if you could comment on that method of reduction, because as far as I know NADH reductase doesn't go through a semiquinone stage, it is a 2-electron reduction.

Mason: The parentheses are in there to remind me that when NADH is added to a microsomal incubation you observe the same free radicals. Electron transfer is presumably catalysed by the NADH-cytochrome b_5

reductase, but I have not in any way attempted to understand the NADH-dependent "black box" that donates electrons.

Slater: Of course, you know in that case with NADH that the cytochrome c is reduced from the cytochrome b_5 rather than the flavoprotein, so it is a different route from that with the NADPH/cytochrome c reductase where the electron comes direct from the flavoprotein.

Mason: Yes. The reconstituted systems are very interesting and I would greatly profit from that sort of work but it is exceedingly labour intensive and I find it a more economical use of my time to search for different types of free radical metabolites. I believe the mechanism of electron donation from the flavoproteins is better studied by a biochemist.

Slater: If there is a pathway of reduction by NADH *in vivo* then it should be favoured by chronic alcohol intoxication. Is there any evidence that the toxicity of these drugs is increased in such persons because that disturbs the $NADH/NAD^+$ ratio?

Mason: I don't believe so.

Slater: That is encouraging!

Mason: A nitroimidazole, Flagyl R is an "antabuse" drug, but it is thought that the mechanism is due to inhibition of aldehyde oxidase as in the case of disulfiram (Antabuse R). I know of no other report of a relationship.

REFERENCES to Discussion

Bachur, N.R., Gordon, S.L., Gee, M.V. and Kon, H. (1979). *Proc. Natl. Acad. Sci. USA* 76, 954-957.

Iyanagi, T. and Yamazaki, I. (1969). *Biochim. Biophys. Acta* 172, 370-381.

Iyanagi, T. and Makino, R. (1980). *In* "Microsomes, Drug Oxidations and Chemical Carcinogenesis" (Eds. M.J. Coon, A.H. Conney, R.W. Estabrook, H.V. Gelboin, J.R. Gillette and P.J. O'Brien), Vol. I,pp. 407-410. Academic Press, New York.

Pietronigro, D.D., McGinness, J.E., Koren, M.J., Crippa, R., Seligman, M.L. and Demopoulos, H.P. (1979). *Physiol. Chem. Phys.* 11, 405-414.

Sealy, R.C., Swartz, H.M. and Olive, P.L. (1978). *Biochem. Biophys. Res. Commun.* 82, 680-684.

Staudt, H., Lichtenberger, F. and Ullrich, V. (1974). *Eur. J. Biochem.* 46, 99-106.

Svingen, B.A. and Powis, G. (1981). *Arch. Biochem. Biophys.* 209, 119-126.

Vermilion, J.L., Ballou, D.P., Massey, V. and Coon, M.J. (1981). *J. Biol. Chem.* 256, 266-277.

Wardman, P. and Clarke, E.D. (1976). *Biochem. Biophys. Res. Commun.* 69, 942-949.

Benzo(a)pyrene Radicals and Oxygen Radical Involvement in DNA Damage, Cellular Toxicity and Carcinogenesis

S.A. LESKO, P.O.P. TS'O, S.-U. YANG and R. ZHENG

INTRODUCTION

Most of the identifiable metabolites of chemical carcinogens are formed by two-electron oxidation reactions. However, an ever-increasing body of evidence indicates that one-electron oxidation also takes place in metabolic processes. These one-electron oxidations produce organic free radicals, and if the oxidant is molecular oxygen, the autoxidation process can produce reactive, reduced oxygen species such as superoxide radical anion, hydrogen peroxide and hydroxyl radicals. Both the organic free radicals and the reduced oxygen species can react with important cellular macromolecules in a variety of ways, including hydrogen abstraction, which can readily lead to DNA strand scission or crosslinking.

Oxygen is also reduced univalently by all aerobic cells during normal metabolic processes. Oxygen toxicity probably results from the action of one or more of these species that arise by partial reduction. This is attested to by the ubiquitous distribution of protective enzymes, viz., superoxide dismutase, catalase and glutathione peroxidase in aerobes. An enormous amount of oxygen must be reduced to meet daily energy requirements. Thus, only a miniscule amount of reduced oxygen species needs to escape the cellular oxygen defence system to have a low steady state rate of radical reaction occurring with critical cellular macromolecules. Such damage could be the initiating event leading to senescence, somatic mutation or neoplastic transformation and thus represents a risk that all aerobic cells must bear.

This chapter will focus firstly on one-electron oxidation of chemical carcinogens (mostly benzo(a)pyrene) and then on the involvement of organic radicals and reduced oxygen species in DNA damage and cellular toxicity.

RADICALS FROM BENZO(A)PYRENE AND OTHER POLYCYCLIC HYDROCARBONS

Mild chemical oxidation. Electron paramagnetic resonance (EPR) studies in our laboratory have shown the presence of benzo(a)pyrene [B(a)P] radicals induced by I_2 at 25°C and measured in frozen solutions of benzene, methanol, and cyclohexane (Caspary *et al.*, 1973). The steady-state concentration of B(a)P radicals in benzene was reached within 1 min upon addition of I_2 and remained constant for at least 2 h. The maintenance of constant steady-state radical concentrations was also observed with other hydrocarbons in this system. The highest steady-state concentration of radicals found in solutions of B(a)P was about 10% and the formation of these radicals was critically dependent on I_2 concentration.

The steady-state radical concentration of the B(a)P radicals in benzene was not reduced by the introduction of methanol, isopropanol, acetaldehyde, and water, or by bubbling nitrogen gas through the system. The B(a)P radical concentration, however, was drastically reduced upon introduction of substituted adenosine or guanosine. Many nitrogenous compounds, such as imidazole, purine, pyrimidine, aniline, and nucleosides could quench the B(a)P radical signal in methanol.

The steady-state radical concentration of 14 hydrocarbons formed in the presence of I_2 have been investigated by EPR. In general, the carcinogenic compounds such as B(a)P, 7,12-dimethyl-benz(a)anthracene, 3-methylcholanthrene, and dibenzo(a,h)pyrene had a much higher concentration of radicals than the noncarcinogenic compounds, such as B(e)P, benz(a)anthracene, pyrene, anthracene, picene, dibenz(a,c)-anthracene, naphthalene, and naphthacene. The steady-state radical concentrations of these compounds did not correlate well with their ionisation potentials since the radical concentration is govenered by potentially complex pathways with variable rates of formation and decay. If the initiation process in hydrocarbon carcinogenesis is related to the production of these radicals, then the combination of a high steady-state concentration and the ability to react with biologically important macromolecules might be related to carcinogenic activity.

The chemical nature of the iodine-induced B(a)P radical remains uncertain since its EPR signal lacks the hyperfine structure needed for its identification. The formation of 6,6'-B(a)P dimers and the 6-B(a)P pyridinium salt has been reported upon exposure of the hydrocarbon to I_2 vapour in the presence of pyridine (Rochlitz, 1967). He interpreted this as an indication of the formation of a radical cation of B(a)P with a high charge localisation at position six. The data of Wilk and Girke (1969, 1972) and Jeftic and Adams (1970) also support this hypothesis.

Covalent binding of B(a)P to DNA has been induced with three oxidation systems (Hoffmann *et al.*, 1970; Lesko *et al.*, 1969) viz. iodine, H_2O_2/Fe^{++} and ascorbic acid hydroxylating system of Udenfriend *et al.* (1954). Considerable DNA degradation occurs with the latter two systems which are known to produce hydroxyl or perhydroxyl radicals (Rhaese and Freese, 1968; Massie *et al.*, 1972). DNA interstrand crosslinking was observed in the iodine-induced reaction (Maher *et al.*, 1971).

The chemical mechanism for the activation of B(a)P in the H_2O_2/Fe^{++} system is not the same as the I_2 system since a product other than the 6-B(a)P pyridinium salt was found (Hoffmann *et al.*, 1969). Ioki *et al.* (1974) reported that the 6-oxo-B(a)P radical is formed upon oxidation of B(a)P with H_2O_2/Fe^{++}.

ENZYMIC FORMATION OF THE 6-OXO-B(A)P RADICAL

There is no direct evidence for the formation of the B(a)P radical cation in metabolising systems. The six position B(a)P is chemically more reactive than the other sites on the hydrocarbon (Cavalieri and Calvin, 1971; Jeftic and Adams, 1970) but 6-OH-B(a)P often is not reported as a metabolite although its formation has been implied by the detection of the 6-OH-B(a)P glucuronide *in vivo* (Falk *et al.*, 1962). Nagata *et al.* (1968, 1974) demonstrated that 6-OH-B(a)P can be detected in the metabolism of B(a)P in rat liver homogenate, as well as in mouse and rat skin homogenates, *via* its phenoxy radical, 6-oxo-B(a)P. This observation was confirmed and extended by Lesko *et al.* (1975). The same EPR signal could be extracted from rat liver homogenates after incubation with B(a)P or synthetic 6-OH-B(a)P. The signal has been identified as that of the 6-oxo-B(a)P radical by its hyperfine structure. The only products detected after 6-OH-B(a)P was incubated for 40 min in a rat liver homogenate were three stable isomeric B(a)P diones (1,6-; 3,6-; 6,12-).

The percentage of B(a)P metabolism proceeding through the 6-OH-B(a)P pathway was determined to be about 20% using female rate liver homogenates. This value agrees reasonably well with the proportion of B(a)P diones produced from B(a)P metabolism by rat liver microsomes (Kinoshita *et al.*, 1973). Thus, 6-OH-B(a)P appears to be the precursor of most of the B(a)P diones formed during metabolism of B(a)P.

AUTOXIDATION OF 6-OH-B(A)P

In aqueous buffer ethanol solutions, 6-OH-B(a)P is autoxidised to the same three stable B(a)P diones detected with rat liver homogenates (Lorentzen *et al.*, 1975). The 6-oxo-B(a)P radical is also produced during the autoxidation. In the reaction, molecular oxygen is reduced as evidenced by the appearance of H_2O_2. The paramagnetic nature of ground-state molecular oxygen virtually ensures that the autoxidation proceeds by one-electron steps. This is supported by the formation of the 6-oxo-B(a)P. Thus any H_2O_2 must arise from the spontaneous dismutation of superoxide, the initial species produced upon univalent reduction of oxygen. The kinetics of formation and decay of the 6-oxo-B(a)P radical indicate that it is an obligatory intermediate in the autoxidation of 6-OH-B(a)P to B(a)P diones (Lesko *et al.*, 1975; Lorentzen *et al.*, 1975). In fact, the isolated radical is autoxidised in aqueous buffer-ethanol solutions and yields products identical to those observed with 6-OH-B(a)P (Lorentzen *et al.*, 1975).

When synthetic [^{3}H]-6-OH-B(a)P and DNA were incubated in phosphate buffer-ethanol solution, a small portion of the 6-OH-B(a)P became covalently linked to DNA with a concomitant decay of most of the 6-OH-B(a)P to a mixture of B(a)P diones. The kinetics of covalent linkage were comparable to the lifetime of the 6-oxo-B(a)P radical in solution (Ts'o *et al.*, 1974). Single strand breaks were introduced into DNA during incubation with 6-OH-B(a)P. EDTA (10^{-5} M) completely inhibited the production of single-strand breaks but it also inhibited adduct formation by at least 50% (Ts'o *et al.*, 1976). Synthetic 6-OH-B(a)P is more toxic than B(a)P to Syrian hamster embryo (SHE) fibroblasts in culture and is capable of inducing morphological transformation of these cells. Compared to B(a)P treatment with 6-OH-B(a)P requires a much shorter time to reach a plateau of maximal transformation frequency (Schechtman, 1975).

B(A)P DIONE/B(A)P DIOL REDOX CYCLES: GENERATION OF REDUCED OXYGEN SPECIES

In spite of their relative ease of isolation from metabolising systems, the BP diones are not unreactive compounds. They readily participate in reactions involving free radicals under physiological conditions which apparently lead to DNA damage and cellular injury and death (Lorentzen and Ts'o, 1977; Lorentzen *et al.*, 1979). Like other quinones, the three BP biones are electron deficient and particularly prone to participating in one-electron transfer reactions. Their oxidation potentials at neutral pH are very low (Lorentzen and Ts'o, 1977; Moriconi *et al.*, 1962), and they readily accept electrons even from mild biological reducing agents such as NAD(P)H and glutathione in the absence of oxygen. The B(a)P diols (hydroquinones) formed by reduction are extremely sensitive to oxygen. When exposed to the atmosphere these B(a)P diols are immediately and quantitatively reoxidised to the quinone, producing an equivalent of hydrogen peroxide.

$$\text{B(a)P diol} + O_2 \rightarrow [\text{B(a)P semiquinone radical}] \rightarrow \text{B(a)P dione} + H_2O_2$$

Reduction (B(a)P dione → B(a)P diol)

These autoxidations of B(a)P occur by one-electron steps. This is indicated by experiments which demonstrate that EPR spectra of the three semiquinone radical anions can be obtained by careful exposure of the synthetic diols in alkaline solution to small amounts of air. Thus, one-electron transfer from B(a)P diol to molecular oxygen takes place, producing the transient superoxide and semiquinone radicals; the superoxide radical rapidly dismutates to molecular oxygen and hydrogen peroxide, the latter being a detectable product of the autoxidations. This one-electron transfer mechanism is further supported by the fact that solutions of BP diols exposed to air readily reduce nitro blue tetrazolium, a common reagent used for the detection of superoxide radical.

The extreme lability of the B(a)P diols make their metabolic detection, as such, unlikely. However, Falk *et al.* (1962) identified glucuronide conjugates of the B(a)P diols in the bile of rats treated with B(a)P, and this indicates that reduction of B(a)P dione metabolites had taken place *in vivo*. Other more general evidence exists indicating that a wide variety of quinone compounds are substrates for reductases in cells (Bachur *et al.*, 1977, 1978, 1979; Iyanagi and Yamazaki, 1969).

Small amounts of BP dione induce the oxidation of a much larger amount of NADH to NAD^+ in the presence of a reductase, NADH dehydrogenase from *Clostridium Kluyveri* (EC 1.6.99.-). This ability has also been observed using purified rat liver microsomes in place of the reductase. A nearly equivalent amount of H_2O_2 is produced in this B(a)P dione-induced oxidation of NADH, indicating that oxygen is the ultimate electron acceptor.

Single-stranded breaks are introduced into T7 DNA by B(a)P diones as measured by alkaline sedimentation (Lorentzen and Ts'o, 1977). This capacity to cause DNA degradation was greatest for the 1,6 isomer, followed by the 3,6 and 6,12 isomers. DNA damage induced by B(a)P diones is substantially enhanced by the presence of Cu^{2+} or NADPH and suppressed by the presence of EDTA or by the removal of oxygen by N_2 flushing. These data suggest a free radical mechanism of DNA strand breakage involving the B(a)P dione and oxygen.

The three B(a)P diones are highly toxic to cultured mammalian cells. This is indicated by the inhibition of uptake of [^{3}H]thymidine into the DNA of Syrian hamster embryonic fibroblasts in the presence of B(a)P diones. The 1,6 and 3,6 isomers are more cytotoxic than the 6,12 isomer, but all three are much more cytotoxic than B(a)P. Furthermore, experiments in this laboraotry have shown that the cytotoxicity of B(a)P diones to cultured cells is dependent on molecular oxygen. The replacement of oxygen by nitrogen in both the culture medium and the atmosphere around the cells substantially reduces the capacity of the B(a)P diones to inhibit cellular DNA synthesis and to cause cell death. The products of oxygen reduction, viz. $O_2^{\cdot -}$, H_2O_2, $OH^{\cdot}$ and B(a)P semiquinone radicals (products of B(a)P diol oxidation) are candidates for the specific reactive species directly responsible for cellular injury.

ROLE OF SUPEROXIDE IN DNA STRAND SCISSION

Superoxide ($O_2^{\cdot -}$) is the initial reduced oxygen species produced upon univalent reduction in oxygen. It dismutates readily according to the following reaction:

$$HO_2^{\cdot} + O_2^{\cdot -} + H^+ \rightarrow H_2O_2 + O_2$$

The rate constant at physiological pH is $1 \times 10^5\ M^{-1}s^{-1}$. DNA strand scission was determined after incubating T7 DNA with KO_2, preincubated KO_2 (dismutated products) and reagent grade H_2O_2 using band sedimentation through alkaline NaCl (Studier, 1965). After 15 min of incubation, the number of strand scissions introduced into each intact T7 DNA strand by equivalent amounts of KO_2 or dismutated products ($O_2^{\cdot -}$/DNA base=10) was calculated to be 2.7 and 1.3, respectively. The products of KO_2 dismutation (H_2O_2 + O_2) and reagent grade H_2O_2 produced the same number of DNA strand scissions when incubations were carried out under identical conditions. Inhibition of strand scission by very small amounts of the chelator, diethylenetriaminepenta-acetic acid (0.1 μM) indicate that $O_2^{\cdot -}$ and H_2O_2 alone are not effective agents in breaking DNA. The complete protection observed with catalase and metal chelators strongly suggest that H_2O_2 (produced by dismutation of $O_2^{\cdot -}$) and metal ions are directly involved in the strand scission observed with KO_2 and preincubated KO_2. The enhancement of H_2O_2-induced strand scission by the addition of exogenous $FeSO_4$ and $CuSO_4$ suggests that H_2O_2 manifests its activity by being converted to $OH^{\cdot}$ in a Fenton-type reaction.

$$H_2O_2 + Me^{n+} \rightarrow OH^{\cdot} + OH^- + Me^{(n+1)^+}$$

This is supported by data which demonstrates the inhibition of H_2O_2-induced DNA strand scission by $OH^{\cdot}$ scavengers such as ethanol, *tert*-butanol, DMSO, and NaN_3. Controls studied showed that these compounds do not react with H_2O_2. The $OH^{\cdot}$ is probably produced near the site of DNA cleavage by reaction of H_2O_2 with adventitious metal ions.

The rate of strand breakage is higher when DNA is treated with KO_2 compared to preincubated KO_2. This is probably the result of a metal-catalysed Haber-Weiss reaction in which adventitious metal ions are cycled by first being reduced by $O_2^{\bullet -}$ and then oxidised by H_2O_2 with concomitant production of $OH^{\bullet}$. Strand breakage induced by KO_2 is inhibited by superoxide dismutase because this enzyme removes the source of reducing power, i.e. the $O_2^{\bullet -}$, thereby inhibiting the reaction for production of reduced metal ions needed to continually generate $OH^{\bullet}$.

This system is not without complexities, since complications do arise in attempting to analyse some of the data. First, the addition of exogenous $FeSO_4$ or $FeCl_3$ (10 µM) to KO_2-DNA solutions did not result in any significant enhancement of DNA strand scission. This is in contrast to the data obtained with H_2O_2 where a 9-fold enhancement was observed with exogenous $FeSO_4$ 10 µM. The lack of enhancement may be due to complex formation between ligand (DNA?)-iron-$O_2^{\bullet -}$. Caspary *et al.* (1981) have electron paramagnetic resonance data to indicate that the $O_2^{\bullet -}$ signal is stabilised by Fe^{2+} or Fe^{3+} ions and suggested that an outer sphere ion pair complex is formed between ligand (maleate) bound iron and $O_2^{\bullet -}$. Secondly, the addition of exogenous $MnCl_2$ and $ZnCl_2$ does not result in an enhancement of DNA strand scission by H_2O_2 while there is a 1.5 to 2.5-fold enhancement with KO_2. This could occur if Mn^{++} and Zn^{++} do not produce $OH^{\bullet}$ efficiently in the presence of H_2O_2. This appears to be the case since incubation of thymine with H_2O_2 in the presence of $MnCl_2$ or $ZnCl_2$ (10 µM) results in a very small or no degradation of thymine as indicated by absorbance measurement while $CuSO_4$, $FeCl_3$ or $FeSO_4$ (10 µM) decrease the absorbance of thymine quite substantially. DNA strand scission induced by $O_2^{\bullet -}$ is enhanced by $MnCl_2$ or $ZnCl_2$ because this system is capable of cycling the metal ions between oxidised and reduced form. Thirdly, addition of sodium formate (0.1 M), an efficient $OH^{\bullet}$ scavenger, resulted in an increase in the rate and extent of strand scission. This increase rate probably results from further reaction of the formate radical anion formed as follows:

$$HCO_2 + OH^{\bullet} \rightarrow CO_2^{\bullet -} + H_2O$$

The lifetime of the $OH^{\bullet}$ is probably very short compared to the formate radical anion. Subsequent reaction of this more stable radical with DNA could result in the increase in strand scission observed.

The data demonstrate that DNA strand scission induced by $O_2^{\bullet -}$ involves an intermediate in common with ionising radiation, i.e., the $OH^{\bullet}$. It is well established that ionising radiation is carcinogenic and that $OH^{\bullet}$ formed is primarily responsible for DNA damage. Since there are many pathways for the formation of $O_2^{\bullet -}$ in mammalian cells, this radical may be the source of DNA damage that may eventually lead to somatic mutation, senescence or neoplastic transformation (Lesko *et al.*, 1980).

SUPEROXIDE DISMUTASE (SOD) ACTIVITY IN SYRIAN HAMSTER EMBRYO (SHE) FIBROBLASTS AND ITS ROLE IN OXYGEN TOXICITY

Evidence from prokaryotes indicates that $O_2^{\bullet -}$ is an important agent in oxygen toxicity and that SOD provides an essential defence (Fridovich, 1978). SOD activity has been measured in two types of SHE fibroblasts, viz. a highly tumourigenic line (BP6T) and a non-tumourigenic line (SHE 21f). SOD was assayed spectrophotometrically by measuring its ability to inhibit superoxide-mediated autoxidation of pyrogallol (Marklund and Marklund, 1974). The 10,000 g supernatant from sonicates of BP6T and SHE 21f cells contained 6.4 and 3.6 units of SOD activity per mg protein, respectively. Two types of activity (Cu:Zn SOD and Mn SOD) were shown to be present in BP6T sonicates by electrophoretic mobility in polyacrylamide gels and sensitivity to cyanide. Treatment of BP6T fibroblasts with 3 mM diethyldithiocarbamate (DDC), a copper chelator, for 1.5 h reduced the SOD activity to 1.3 units per mg protein (80% inhibition). The activity gradually returned to normal after removal of DDC and further growth in DDC-free medium (approx. 22 h). Gel electrophoresis revealed that only the slower band of activity (Mn-SOD remained after DDC treatment.

Figure 1 (left panel) shows that the relative cloning efficiency of BP6T cells is dependent upon the concentration of oxygen to which cells are exposed and the duration of exposure. In 1% oxygen the cloning efficiency is almost identical to that observed in air, although the growth rate in mass culture was slightly lower (population doubling time was about 12 h compared to 10 h in air).

BP6T cells were treated with 3 mM DDC for 1.5 h, washed several times, and then exposed to increasing oxygen tensions for various time intervals. As shown in Fig. 1 (right panel) the cloning efficiency was drastically reduced in 50 and 70% oxygen compared to control cells, while the cloning efficiency in 1% oxygen was slightly enhanced. Thus, the toxicity of 3 mM DDC is reduced when cells are grown in 1% oxygen where only low levels of reduced oxygen species are being produced. For a 48 h exposure the D_{37} was calculated to be 79% oxygen for control cells but only 39% oxygen for DDC-treated cells. It is suggested that the effects on cell survival produced by 3 mM

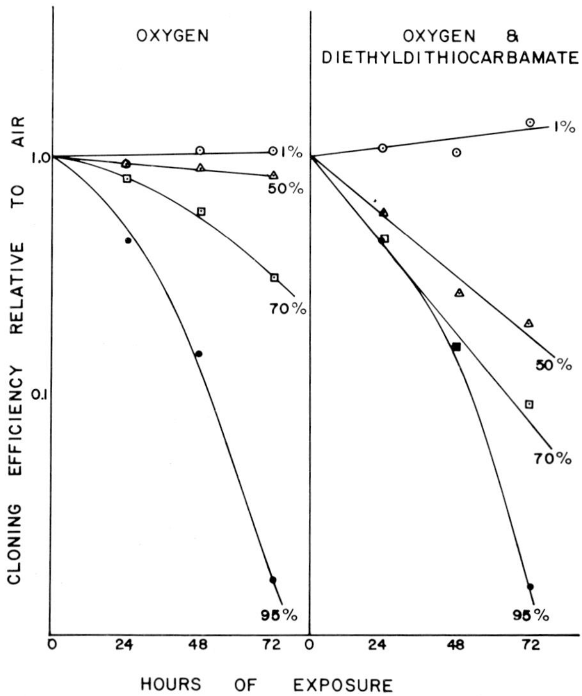

FIG. 1 Relative cloning efficiency of normal and diethyldithiocarbamate-treated BP6T cells after exposure to various oxygen tensions. Left panel: Values are relative to control exposed to air which exhibited a cloning efficiency of 70-80%. Right panel: Cells treated with 3 mM diethyldithiocarbamate in air, washed, seeded at clonal densities and then exposed to various oxygen tensions. Values are relative to a control treated with DDC and exposed to air. Cloning efficiency of the control was 40-50%.

DDC are due to inhibition of Cu:Zn SOD. In 95% oxygen DDC has very little effect on cloning efficiency. The cellular oxygen defence system is probably overwhelmed at this high oxygen tension and thus a large enhancement in toxicity would not be expected if the SOD level was diminished.

To examine the role of SOD in oxygen toxicity more closely we investigated the effect of DDC concentration on the incorporation of [^{3}H]thymidine into acid insoluble material after exposure of cells to air, 5% oxygen and 1% oxygen. Cells were treated for 1 h with 10^{-5}, 10^{-4}, 10^{-3} and 3×10^{-3} M DDC, washed and then examined for SOD activity and ability to incorporate [^{3}H]thymidine. There was no dimunition of SOD activity at 10^{-5} or 10^{-4} M DDC. Activity was reduced to 65-70% after treatment with 10^{-3} M DDC and to 40-45% with 3×10^{-3} M DDC. A biphasic response with respect to [^{3}H]thymidine incorporation was observed at all three oxygen tensions (Table 1). Toxicity was observed in all cases at 10^{-4} M DDC where there was no inhibition of SOD activity. Toxicity was dependent on oxygen tension at 3×10^{-3} M DDC where the SOD activity is inhibited; no toxicity was observed in 1% oxygen. This indicates that the effect seen in 3×10^{-3} M DDC is due to the production of high levels of reduced oxygen species in air, intermediate levels in 5% oxygen and low levels in 1% oxygen. Thus, SOD appears to provide an effective defence against oxygen radicals formed at normal oxygen tension and inhibition of this enzyme results in a toxic response.

The mechanism for the toxic response seen at 10^{-4} M DDC is unknown. A biphasic toxicity of DDC in human lymphocytes has been reported by Rigas *et al.* (1980). They postulate that the first toxic phase (10^{-4} M DDC) might be due to formation toxic chelates, of the type DDC...M^+, and that its reversal at higher DDC concentrations is due to formation of non-toxic chelates, DDC...M^+...DDC. It has been reported that chelates of oxidisable transition metals with equimolar amounts of strong chelator, X, can catalyse the production of $O_2^{\cdot -}$ (Michelson, 1974),

$$X...M^+ + O_2 \rightarrow X...M^+...O_2 \rightarrow X...M^{2+} + O_2^{\cdot -}$$

TABLE 1 Effect of diethyldithiocarbamate concentration on the incorporation of [^{3}H]thymidine into DNA of SHE fibroblast grown in various oxygen tensions*

Oxygen conc. in gaseous phase	DDC Molarity				
	0	10^{-5}	10^{-4}	10^{-3}	3×10^{-3}
Air	1.0	1.13	0.79	0.86	0.001
5%	1.0	1.19	0.78	1.06	0.56
1%	1.0	1.09	0.75	1.31	1.08

*Cells were treated with DDC at various oxygen tensions, washed, trypsinised and split into two fractions for measurement of SOD activity and incorporation of [^{3}H]thymidine into cellular DNA. Incorporation studies were carried out under the following conditions: 1×10^5 cells, 0.1 μCi of [^{3}H]thymidine/ml, 48 h, incubation in air, 5% oxygen or 1% oxygen. Values shown are ratios cpm control/cpm DDC-treated.

EFFECT OF EXOGENOUS SOD AND SELENITE ON THE CLONING EFFICIENCY OF DDC-TREATED BP6T CELLS

Cells were treated with 3 mM DDC and then exposed to air or 50% oxygen for about 48 h in medium supplemented with heat-inactivated serum containing up to 2100 units/ml of Cu:Zn SOD or 2×10^{-7} M selenious acid. Heat inactivation of the serum markedly reduced the cloning efficiency of control BP6T cells and DDC-treated cells compared to normal serum. Addition of exogenous Cu:Zn SOD had no effect on the cytotoxic effect of 50% oxygen, although the SOD activity of the DDC-treated cells was reduced to 20% of control. Addition of selenious acid, however, increased the cloning efficiency of DDC-treated cells 65% and 118% when these cells were exposed to air or 50% oxygen, respectively. Goldstein *et al.* (1979) reported that DDC inhibits glutathione peroxidase activity in mouse lung and liver *in vivo* and a selenium-dependent form of glutathione peroxidase which has activity towards H_2O_2 has been isolated from rat liver (Lawrence and Burke, 1976).

CONCLUDING REMARKS

One electron oxidations appear to be a very general phenomenon for the metabolism of carcinogens and in the metabolic reduction of oxygen to water. The subsequent generation of hydroxl radicals from superoxide produced in normal metabolic processes may be the source of DNA damage that leads to spontaneous mutation, aging and cancer. The relationship of the functional state of the cellular oxygen defence system to the above processes needs to be thoroughly investigated. Preliminary studies described in this report indicate that superoxide dismutase does provide an essential defence at normal oxygen tension. Leakage and malfunction of the oxygen defence system may be an important factor in the induction of a basal level of damage to the genetic apparatus. Quantitative data on the level of an unavoidable background risk that may result from oxygen radicals is essential before other avoidable risks present in the environment can be realistically evaluated.

REFERENCES

Bachur, N., Gordon, S. and Gee, M. (1977). *Mol. Pharmacol.* 13, 901-910.

Bachur, N., Gordon, S. and Gee, M. (1978). *Cancer Res.* 38, 1745-1750.

Bachur, N., Gordon, S., Gee, M. and Kon, H. (1979). *Proc. Nat. Acad. Sci. USA* 76, 954-957.

Caspary, W., Cohen, B., Lesko, S. and Ts'o, P. (1973). *Biochemistry* 12, 2649-2656.

Caspary, W., Lanzo, A. and Niziak, C. (1981). Manuscript in preparation.

Cavalieri, E. and Calvin, M. (1971). *Proc. Nat. Acad. Sci. USA* 68, 1251-1253.

Falk, H.L., Kotin, P., Lee, S. and Nathan, A. (1962). *J. Nat. Cancer Inst.* 28, 699-724.

Fridovich, I. (1978). *Science* 201, 875-880.

Goldstein, B., Rozen, M., Quintavalla, J. and Amoruso, M. (1979). *Biochem. Pharmacol.* 28, 27-30.

Hoffmann, H., Lesko, S. and Ts'o, P. (1969). *Rep. Div. Med. Chem.* 158th Nat. Meet. Am. Chem. Soc.

Hoffmann, H., Lesko, S. and Ts'o, P. (1970). *Biochemistry* 9, 2594-2604.

Ioki, Y., Kodama, M., Tagashira, Y. and Nagata, C. (1974). *Gann* 65, 379-380.

Iyanagi, T. and Yamazaki, T. (1969). *Biochim. Biophys. Acta* 172, 370-381.

Jeftic, L. and Adams, R. (1970). *J. Am. Chem. Soc.* 92, 1332-1337.

Kinoshita, N., Shears, B. and Gelboin, H. (1973). *Cancer Res.* 33, 1937-1944.

Lawrence, R. and Burk, R. (1976). *Biochem. Biophys. Res. Commun.* 21, 952-958.
Lesko, S., Ts'o, P. and Umans, R. (1969). *Biochemistry* 8, 2291-2298.
Lesko, S., Caspary, W., Lorentzen, R. and Ts'o, P. (1975). *Biochemistry* 14, 3978-3984.
Lesko, S., Lorentzen, R. and Ts'o, P. (1980). *Biochemistry* 19, 3023-3028.
Lorentzen, R., Caspary, W., Lesko, S. and Ts'o, P. (1975). *Biochemistry* 14, 3970-3977.
Lorentzen, R. and Ts'o, P. (1977). *Biochemistry* 16, 1467-1473.
Lorentzen, R., Lesko, S., McDonald, K. and Ts'o, P. (1979). *Cancer Res.* 39, 3194-3198.
Maher, V., Lesko, S., Straat, P. and Ts'o, P. (1971). *J. Bacteriol.* 108, 202-212.
Marklund, S. and Marklund, G. (1974). *Eur. J. Biochem.* 47, 469-474.
Massie, H., Samis, H. and Baird, M. (1972). *Biochim. Biophys. Acta* 272, 539-548.
Michelson, A. and Buckingham, M. (1974). *Biochem. Biophys. Res. Commun.* 58, 1079.
Moriconi, E., Rakoczy, B. and O'Connor, W. (1962). *J. Org. Chem.* 27, 2772.
Nagata, C., Inomata, M., Kodama, M. and Tagashira, Y. (1968). *Gann* 59, 289-298.
Nagata, C., Tagashira, Y. and Kodama, M. (1974). *In* "Chemical Carcinogenesis", Part A (Eds. P. Ts'o and J. DiPaolo) pp.87-111, Marcel Decker, New York.
Rhaese, H. and Freese, E. (1968). *Biochim. Biophys. Acta* 155, 476-490.
Rigas, D., Eginitas-Rigas, C., Bigely, R., Stankova, L. and Head, C. (1980). *Int. J. Radiat. Biol.* 38, 257-266.
Rochlitz, J. (1967). *Tetrahedron* 23, 3043-3048.
Schechtman, L. (1975). Ph.D. Thesis, Johns Hopkins Univ.
Studier, W. (1965). *J. Mol. Biol.* 11, 373.
Ts'o, P., Caspary, W., Cohen, B., Leavitt, J., Lesko, S., Lorentzen, R. and Schechtman, L. (1974). *In* "Chemical Carcinogenesis", Part A (Eds. P. Ts'o and J. DiPaolo) pp.113-147, Marcel Decker, New York.
Ts'o, P., Barrett, J., Caspary, W., Lesko, S., Lorentzen, R. and Schechtman, L. (1976). *In* "Aging, Carcinogenesis, and Radiation Biology" (Ed. K. Smith) pp.373-398, Plenum, New York.
Udenfriend, S., Clark, C., Axelrod, J. and Brodie, B. (1954). *J. Biol. Chem.* 208, 731.
Wilk, M. and Girke, W. (1969). *In* "The Jerusalem Symposia on Quantum Chemistry and Biochemistry. Physiochemical Mechanisms of Carcinogenesis", Vol. I (Eds. E. Bergman and B. Pullman) pp.91-105, Israel Academy of Sciences and Humanities, Jerusalem.
Wilk, M. and Girke, W. (1972). *J. Nat. Cancer Inst.* 49, 1585.

DISCUSSION

Willson: I am not familiar with the literature, Paul, but you did mention that you got the 6-hydroxy metabolite and subsequently you get the 3-6-quinone. Is there any evidence that you get the 3-hydroxy and then the 3-6-quinone?

Ts'o: A very good question. We have subsequently investigated the 3-hydroxy-benzo(a)pyrene and also the 1-hydroxybenzo(a)pyrene. They do form quinones but are much less reactive than the 6-hydroxybenzo(a)-pyrene. The 1-hydroxybenzo(a)pyrene manuscript (Caspary *et al.*, *Chem. Biol. Interact.*, *in press*) has just been accepted for publication last month. We talk less about these for one reason, namely, the 6-hydroxybenzo(a)pyrene is much more predominant vis a vis the 1 and 3, but the latter compounds do form.

Magee: I was very interested in your observation that the early hamster embryo cells are more readily transformed because in the transplacental carcinogenesis experiment of Druckrey, which many other people have subsequently confirmed, it is usually found that in the early stages of pregnancy cancers do not result when a directly acting carcinogen is given. Teratogenic effects are produced but there seems to be a certain discrepancy here which may be worth discussing. Secondly, and this is an entirely different question, I was very interested in the radical mechanism which you suggested for benzo(a)-pyrene. Where do you see the adducts coming in, which have been quite well characterised by Weinstein and Conney and others? The DNA adducts, what role do they have in carcinogenesis?

Ts'o: I don't know that I can give you a very complete answer to both your points. To the first one: if you cause too much damage to the embryo, it could hurt the foetus, and then it would not be born, or it could come out in odd shapes, etc. In order to have a "normal" foetus and then for the foetus to develop tumour cells, there must be a delicate balance. As you already know, Dr Joseph DiPaolo has used this kind of model in a different way in that you get the embryo out and you grind up the embryo to search for transformed cells, so you don't care if the foetus develops or not. Thus, I think you have an organisational problem against a cellular problem when you cause too much damage to the embryo. The second point I think is a very important question. We scientists like to extend our findings in a very broad way, so ordinarily when you find answer (a) you tend to think that answer (a) is *THE* answer. Other alternative answers (b), (c), (d), etc. are less significant. It remains to be shown which pathway of benzo(a)pyrene contributes what percentage to the induction of cancer in a given situation. For instance, there is no question that the formation of adducts of the diol epoxides are very effective in causing mutation. The effectiveness in causing transformation to carcinogenic cells is much more uncertain. Certainly, the forming of those DNA adducts by no way excludes other possibilities. For example, we already know that reduced oxygen species can be generated in benzo(a)pyrene metabolism and we know that $OH^{\bullet}$ can be generated in large quantity. I'd like to state that $OH^{\bullet}$ is the simplest carcinogen and the most well-known carcinogen to us after many years of radiation research. It is very clear that $OH^{\bullet}$ radical *can* be carcinogenic to man, but at what percentage, under what conditions and in which organs, and so on, comprise another set of questions. For example, we know that the generation of the $OH^{\bullet}$ radicals depends on the reducing power of the cell. So, smoking a cigarette simultaneously with drinking orange juice may cause the $OH^{\bullet}$ radical pathway to be more predominant than in another situation. It is not worth arguing about it at this time.

Slater: Can I follow that up with a speculation, basically trying to develop the question of Professor Magee. The work you've done on this 6-oxo-benzpyrene radical is very attractive to me and I wonder if perhaps what could happen is an intercalation of this radical species with DNA, followed by charge separation, if the intercalated benzpyrene has a donor base and an acceptor base on either side. Such a separation could be stabilised by the intercalation and by the entrapment of the intercalated substance, the formation of the negative charge on guanine would favour then the reaction with the diol epoxide so you would kinetically increase the rate of adduct formation from the epoxide by the intercalation of the radical. Do you think that might be an interesting line to develop?

Ts'o: Let me understand a little bit about the chemical reaction. The expoxide that you're talking about, do you mean the same epoxide on the molecule or a different epoxide?

Slater: A different epoxide - this is, of course, a rather different concept. Peter Magee was talking of adduct formation from the radical or adduct formation from the diol epoxide, and what I'm saying as a speculation of course, can the radical, as one molecular species, increase the adduct formation from another species, that is the diol epoxide, by actually causing charge separation after intercalation?

Ts'o: I'm just thinking about how to do the experiments.

Slater: I wasn't going as far as that! This is following up an idea which Patrick Riley and I had some time ago (Slater and Riley, 1978), if we intercate the benzpyrene, then form the radical *in situ*, and have an acceptor base above it and a donor base below then the radical can produce electronic redistribution leading to charge separation. The formation of the negative charge would be preferentially on the guanine because of its electronic properties. This would favour then the reaction with the incoming epoxide which is reacting as a carbonium species basically, because of this negative charge positive charge effect. Do you think this is worth considering, that is the radical favouring epoxide adduct formation?

Ts'o: I don't see anything wrong in terms of chemistry with it, the only argument one might consider is whether this activated intermediate is going to help itself attacking something on DNA or whether this reactive diol epoxide does need any help at all, none of which I know. It's all a question of chemical rate, however.

Slater: This would only be an increase on rate.

Willson: There is a simpler possibility. If the benzpyrene induces $OH^{\cdot}$ radical formation and this reacts with the DNA to give a DNA radical, then if a benzpyrene radical is also present, why can't the two just come together to give you an adduct? It's the nature of the adduct that one wants to know - what is its structure? Which adducts are important? Professor Magee said yesterday that with nitrosamines, methylation can take place in a whole range of tissues but only in some of these does cancer occur. What is the critical lesion - which are the most important? It may be those which are only present in very small yield. The apparent importance of some adducts may only be because they are the easiest ones to observe.

Magee: If I could comment on that, one of the suggested reasons is that the persistence of the methyl group varies greatly from one organ to another, and it does correlate rather well with organ specificity: it isn't just the methylation reaction, but how long the methyl groups may stay there. Different organs have different repair capacities and different capacities get rid of methyl groups. The brain can hardly do it, whereas the liver does it very quickly.

Ts'o: In one fundamental sense, one pathway leads to a 2-electron oxidation product, whereas the other pathway leads to a single electron oxidation product. In the general sense, which is more important in causing carcinogenesis? I don't think that we know the answer at this most fundamental level.

Mason: Iyanagi and Yamazaki (1970) investigated the reduction of benzoquinone and vitamin K_3 (menadione) by DT diaphorase, and they found that those quinones were reduced to the hydroquinone but not to the semiquinone. That may be of some interest in your work since I notice that you use the DT-diaphorase in your enzymatic reduction.

Ts'o: But you can also use rat liver microsomes with the NADP and the P_{450} reductase.

Mason: Yes, in the end it will not make any difference because the semiquinone is always in equilibrium with hydroquinone and quinone. In partial response to Professor Slater's earlier question, Iyanagi and Yamazaki (1969) investigated quinone reduction by the purified NADH-cytochrome b_5 reductase. They found a one electron reduction of both quinones to the semiquinone. In contrast to benzoquinone, menadione reduction is greatly increased by cytochrome b_5. As has been pointed out, benzosemiquinone has a very high redox potential and will not reduce oxygen or cytochrome b_5, whereas the menadione semiquinone has a lower redox couple and will reduce cytochrome b_5 as well as oxygen. The cytochrome b_5 may not necessarily be involved in the reduction of quinones in the way that it is in the reduction of cytochrome P_{450} by NADH.

Stier: Can I come back to Peter Magee's question on differentiation between the consequences of the two ultimate carcinogens, the epoxides and the 6-hydroxyquinones. In the one case you mentioned strand breaks are seen and in the other case one sees adducts to the DNA. What do you think about the usefulness of a diagnostic technique that was proposed by Regan and Setlow (1974) which uses the specificity of the repair enzymes which made a short patch repair in the case of the radical induced DNA damage and a long patch repair in the case of the adducts.

Ts'o: I think I would like to make a distinction at this time. The reactive species can form an adduct at some time, but can also cause formation of a DNA-DNA crosslink and DNA-protein crosslink, which are much more interesting to me presently, and we don't know very much about the ability of cells to reduce or to repair any crosslink. Thus, the agent causing DNA-DNA crosslink should give very different kinds of chemical reactions than those with epoxides, and this area has really been vastly under-investigated. And what we were talking about earlier, is that these agents (radicals, hydroquinones, quinone) can turn themselves into catalysts and produce enormous amounts of hydroxy radicals, practically *ad infinitum*, as long as there is reducing power, and as long as these agents are not being trapped. It seems to me this is a much more dangerous situation than this one-shot attack caused by the epoxide - that's what I'm referring to, though I have no knowledge what goes on inside the cell before transformation.

Slater: I'm very interested following up what you said about cross-links. What you have done in the last few years is to provide sound experimental evidence for some speculations in the literature. I can remember for example some years ago that Dr Riley and myself put forward an idea of crosslinking involving polycyclic hydrocarbon radicals and DNA, but we never did any actual experiments and the idea was met with quiet disbelief, so I am fascinated that you are now getting very strong evidence for some role of these polycyclic hydrocarbons as free radicals. I would certainly agree with you that they must have some role to play in the biological disturbances leading to cell damage although the diol epoxide work certainly is very strong with regard to adduct formation. Of course, cancer of the skin, caused by these substances, is increased by exposure to visible light, that would again favour some role for the free radical.

Ts'o: Yes. That was some of our very early work, our first paper on this was published about 1963 - it involved benzopyrene, DNA and shining light, and you got the formation of covalent bond.

Slater: Yes, it's also been shown in whole animals as well. Rats were painted on certain areas of skin with polycyclic hydrocarbons and then either kept in the dark or exposed to light. There was an increase in the incidence of skin tumours in animals exposed to light suggesting an important role for photo-excited intermediates.

REFERENCES to Discussion

Iyanagi, T. and Yamazaki, I. (1969). *Biochim. Biophys. Acta* 172, 370-381.

Iyanagi, T. and Yamazaki, I. (1970). *Biochim. Biophys. Acta* 216, 282-294.

Regan, J.D. and Setlow, B.B. (1974). *Cancer Res.* 34, 3318-3325.

Slater, T.F. and Riley, P. (1978). *Int. J. Quant. Chem.* Quantum Biology Symposium No.5, pp.143-148.

Treatment of Malignant Melanoma with 4-Hydroxyanisole

P.A. RILEY, B.D.G. MORGAN, T. O'NEILL, D.L. DEWEY and A.R. GALPINE

INTRODUCTION

The most important contribution to the pigmentation of the mammalian integment is that due to an indolic polymer of uncertain structure known as melanin. Melanin is synthesised by a population of specialised dendritic cells (melanocytes) which contain the enzyme tyrosinase. This enzyme catalyses the oxidation of the amino acid tyrosine in a series of reactions identified and described by Raper (1928). The first step in the reaction pathway is the incorporation of oxygen into the phenolic ring of tyrosine converting the monophenolic substrate into the diphenol, dihydroyxyphenylalanine (dopa). Subsequent stages of the oxidation consist of dehydrogenations of dopa and its derivatives.

It has been recognised for some time that, because of the relative reactivity of *ortho*-quinones, their production during melanogenesis could render the production of melanin hazardous to the melanocyte (Hochstein and Cohen, 1963). Under normal circumstances, however, melanocytes are protected from the possible cytotoxic action of intermediate oxidation products of melanogenesis. However, the discovery that the melanocytotoxic action of certain phenolic depigmenting agents is associated with intermediate products of their oxidation by tyrosinase (Riley, 1969a, b, 1970) suggested that, in addition to their depigmenting action, these agents might have therapeutic potential in the clinical management of malignant melanoma. One of the most active depigmenting compounds was found to be the tyrosine analogue 4-hydroxyanisole (4-OHA). This agent was shown to be selectively taken up by melanogenic cells and to be cytotoxic to

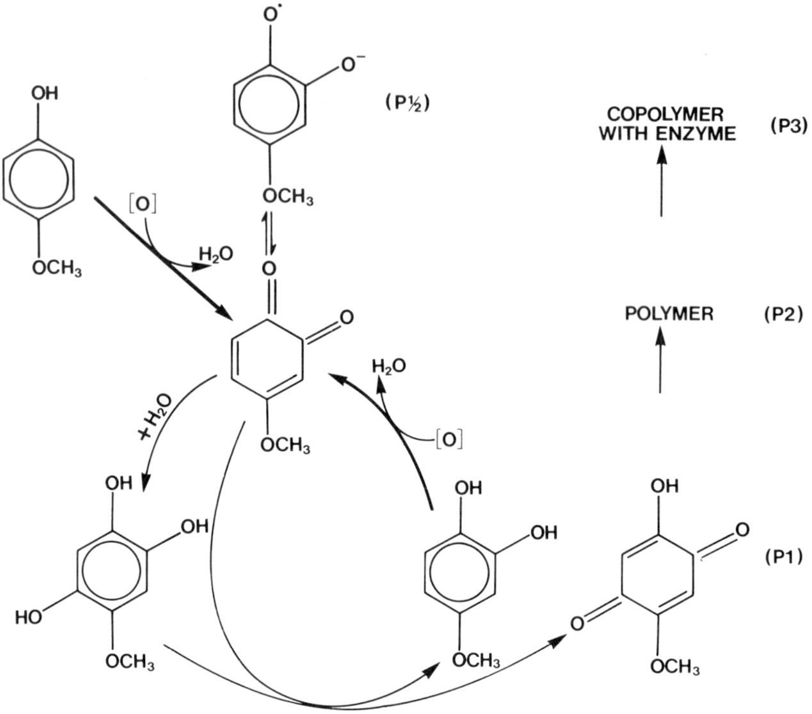

FIG. 1 Proposed schematic outline of the oxidation of 4-OHA. The initial reaction is a tyrosinase-catalysed formation of anisyl orthoquinone which, in the presence of sufficiently high concentrations of 4-OHA undergoes a single-electron reduction to give the transient initial product ($P\frac{1}{2}$) shown as the anisyl semiquinone radical anion. The formation of the product (P1) is by a condensation step with water followed by vicarious oxidation by the orthoquinone to give the hydroxy paraquinone derivative, which on further condensation gives the polymeric products (P2) and (P3).

primary cultures of melanocytes in micromolar concentrations when added to the culture medium. Examination of the relative toxicity to non-melanogenic cells of the spectroscopically identifiable tyrosinase oxidation products of 4-OHA indicated that there is a cell cycle-specific toxic action of the first product (P1) which is probably attributable to thiol binding by a paraquinone (Fig. 1). The time-course of the generation of a cytotoxic effect showed, however, that the most toxic material was generated very early in the incubation of 4-OHA with tyrosinase (Galpine, 1980), suggesting the transient

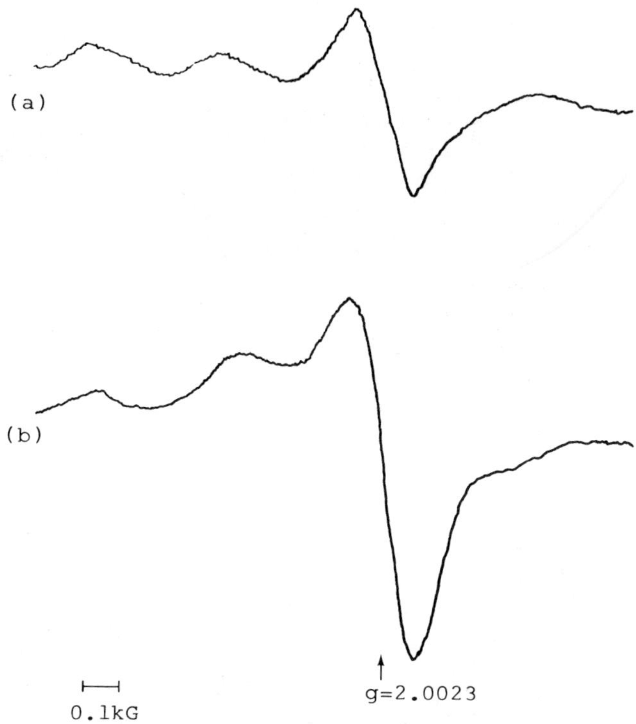

FIG. 2 Electron spin resonance signals from biopsy samples of black guinea-pig skin placed in quartz tubes and examined at -160°C. Trace (a) shows the signal due to the melanin content of the epidermis of a control animal treated topically with a cream base only. Trace (b) shows the signal from the partially depigmented skin of an animal treated locally for 8 d with a cream containing 20% 4-OHA. The increased intensity of the signal and the shift in the spectrum indicates the existence of a new radical species, possibly an anisyl semiquinone.

formation of a highly reactive oxidation product ($P\frac{1}{2}$) such as a semiquinone radical (see Fig. 1) which could initiate damaging reactions in the cells such as lipid peroxidation (Riley, 1970) or the indirect generation of $OH^{\cdot}$ radicals through superoxide anion formation (Riley, 1981). This latter mechanism might be favoured by evidence that addition of superoxide dismutase does not protect cells from the toxic action of $P\frac{1}{2}$ (Galpine, 1980). The putative identification of the early transient product ($P\frac{1}{2}$) as a semiquinone radical rests at present on the generation of a strong ESR signal (Fig. 2) in the partially depigmented skin of black guinea-pigs treated topically with 4-OHA (Riley, 1970).

4-Hydroxyanisole exhibits little generalised toxicity when given parenterally; large single doses (2 g/kg) produced methaemoglobinaemia and transient convulsions in "*to*" strain mice. Animal studies in mice bearing transpantable Harding-Passey melanomas showed that tumour regression occurred in animals receiving 4-OHA in doses (500 mg/kg total) well below those producing detectable systemic toxicity (Dewey *et al.*, 1977). A preliminary assessment of the possible clinical usefulness of 4-OHA in the treatment of malignant melanoma has been made (Morgan *et al.*, 1981) and a summary of the results of this clinical pilot study are presented below.

MATERIALS AND METHODS

Patients

The patients selected for the trial had histologically proven primary or secondary malignant melanomas which were unsuitable for treatment by conventional means. Eleven patients were included in the initial series of clinical tests. The cases are summarised in Table 1. Nine patients were female and 2 male. The average age was 52 years with a range of 3 - 83. The 3 year old child treated in this series had an unusual hypopigmented melanoma of the scalp with widespread secondary deposits. One patient was treated for a calcaneal metastasis diagnosed radiologically. The other cases exhibited well-defined lesions: 2 on the arm, 4 on the leg and 3 on the face and neck. In these cases the lesions to be treated were photographed and their size estimated by measurement of orthogonal diameters before, during and after treatment. Regression of tumour was taken to have occurred if a sustained decrease in size was recorded.

4-Hydroxyanisole

4-OHA was obtained from Koch-Light Ltd., Colnbrook, Bucks, UK, and checked for purity by gas chromatography after recrystallisation. The solution for infusion was freshly prepared on each occasion and consisted of a 2% solution in physiological (0.9%) saline sterilised by filtration (pore size = 0.22 μ). This solution could be stored for short periods at room temperature in containers covered with aluminium

TABLE 1 Summary of cases treated with 4-OHA

Case No.	Age (yrs)	Sex	Treated site	Route of administration	Dosage schedule (n x g/d)	Total dose (g)	Evidence of tumour regression
1	42	F	Arm	Intravenous	1 x 2	2	No
2	46	M	Arm	Intravenous	5 x 1	5	No
3	3	F	Scalp	Intravenous	21 x 4	84	No
4	31	F	Neck	Intravenous	3 x 1	6	No
				Subclavian artery	3 x 2	6	No
5	76	F	Leg	Intravenous	1 x 1 1 x 2 2 x 4	11	No
				Femoral artery	1 x 1 4 x 2	9	No
6	40	F	Leg	Intravenous	5 x 1 1 x 1 1 x 2 2 x 4	16	No
				Femoral artery	21 x 1	21	Yes
7	75	F	Leg	Femoral artery	80 mg/d increasing to 280 mg/d over 57 d	11	Yes
8	83	F	Face	Ext. carotid artery	10 x 2	20	Yes
9	53	F	Heel	Femoral artery	1 x 1 9 x 2 6 x 4 5 x 5	68	Yes
10	50	M	Mouth	Ext. carotid artery	1 x 2 8 x 4 5 x 8*	98	No
11	76	F	Leg	Femoral artery	1 x 2 19 x 8*	154	Yes

* in two separate infusions of 200 ml.

foil to protect it from light. Storage at 4°C resulted in gradual crystallisation of the 4-OHA from solution.

Routes of Infusion

Two routes of infusion were employed: intravenous and intra-arterial. Intravenous administration was by a continuous drip. Intra-arterial infusion was either by repeated injection (as in cases 7 and 9) or by bolus infusions into a cannulated artery (in cases 4, 5, 6, 8, 10 and 11).

RESULTS

Intravenous 4-Hydroxyanisole

The first patients to be treated had the drug administered by intravenous infusion. Patient 1 was given a total dose of 2 g 4-OHA infused in a sline drip into the left antecubital vein during 24 h, patient 2 received 5 g in a series of daily infusions of 1 g for 5 d by the same route. There were no adverse reactions. Case 3 was given a total of 84 g of 4-OHA intravenously over a 3-week period at a rate of 4 g/d. In this case significant methaemoglobinaemia resulted necessitating a transfusion of 1 pint of blood but no other side effects were observed. None of these cases showed any clinical improvement.

Combined Intravenous and Intra-arterial Administration

Cases 4 - 6 were treated initially with intravenous 4-OHA and subsequently by arterial injection with the intention of making a comparison of the effects of treatment by these different routes. Patient 4, with a melanoma on the neck received a total of 12 g 4-OHA; 6 g intravenously and 6 g infused into the subclavian artery. Patient 5 received 20 g total dose; 11 g intravenously and 9 g into the femoral artery. Neither of these cases showed any clinical improvement of their melanoma. A temporary "tingling" or "glowing" sensation in the area infused was reported during arterial perfusion. No adverse symptoms were reported. Case 6 received a total of 37 g 4-OHA of which 21 g was given by daily intra-arterial injections into the femoral artery. A significant clinical improvement was noted following intra-arterial therapy. The tumour became partially depigmented and decreased in size.

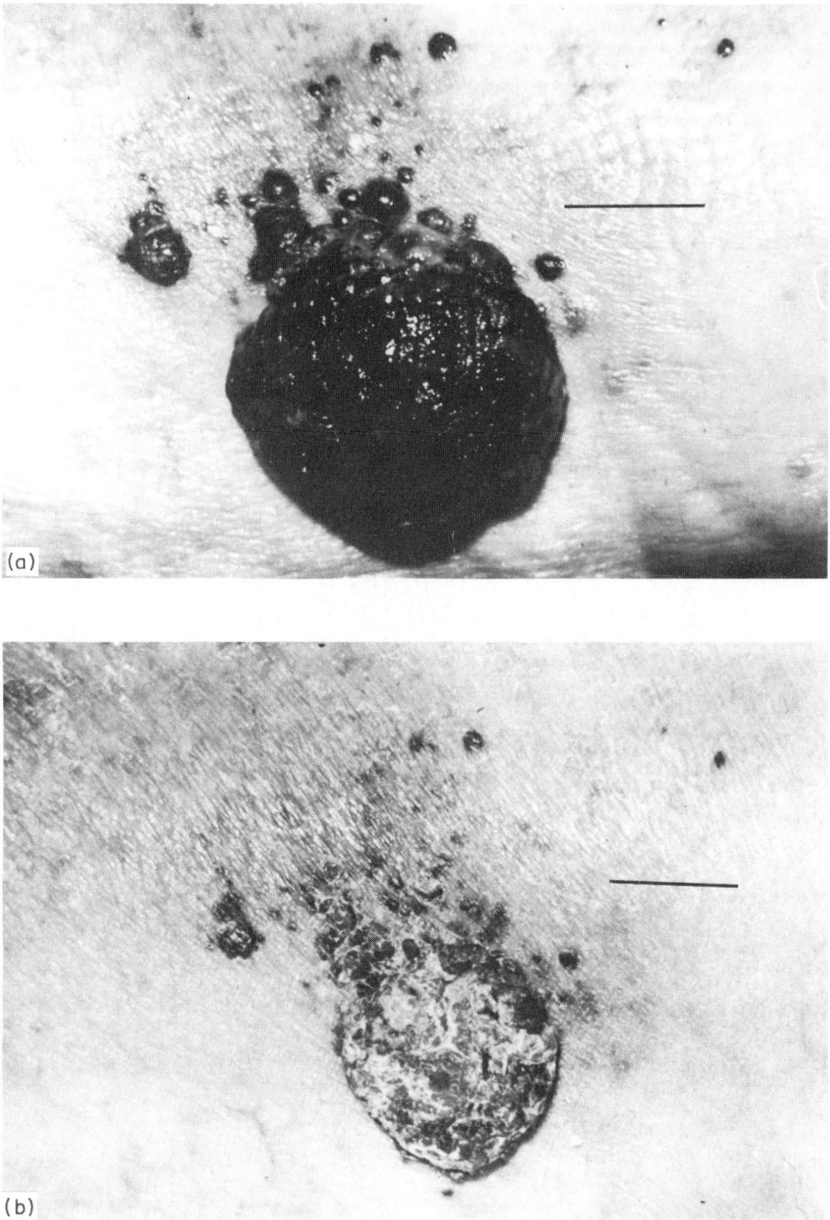

FIG. 3 (a) Nodular melanoma on the leg (case 7) before treatment. The scale bar represents 2 cm and the area of the main tumour was 17.3 cm^2. (b) After intra-arterial infusion with 4-OHA (see text for details). The area of the tumour mass at this stage was 9.9 cm^2. (Scale bar = 2 cm).

Intra-arterial Administration

The remaining 5 patients were all treated by the arterial route receiving progressively increasing doses. Case 11 received a total of 154 g of 4-OHA. The dosage schedules are summarised in Table 1. The external carotid artery was perfused in 2 cases (8 and 10). In one of these cases, where the melanoma was in the mouth, there was no clinical improvement despite the infusion of a large total dose (98 g) over a period of 2 weeks when therapy was discontinued. In the other case a marked improvement in a recurrent melanoma on the left cheek was observed. The 3 patients treated by arterial infusions of 4-OHA into the femoral artery (cases 7, 9, 11) showed a good response to therapy). Figure 3 shows the result of 4-OHA infusion in a 75 year old female in mild congestive cardiac failure and on steroids for asthma. She presented with a nodular melanoma and satellites on her right leg which had increased in size rapidly over the preceding 6 months (Fig. 3a). She was treated by daily injections of 4-OHA given into the femoral artery over a period of 6 weeks to a total dose of 10.7 g. The primary tumour became depigmented and reduced in size (Fig. 3b). It reamined as a fibrous scarred area for $3\frac{1}{2}$ years when the patient died in congestive cardiac failure. In case 11 multiple cutaneous metastases of malignant melanoma on the leg regressed following arterial perfusion with 4-OHA (Figs. 4a and b). Evidence that skeletal metastases are also susceptible to treatment with 4-OHA was shown in case 9. This 53 year old female had a primary nodular malignant melanoma of her right temple treated by wide excision and skin graft. There was local recurrence and lymph node metastases and these were treated surgically. Two years after the initial treatment, she developed a metastasis in the calcaneum (Fig. 5a). The pain prevented her walking. 4-Hydroxyanisole was administered via the femoral artery over 20 d giving a bolus dose daily in 200 ml of saline over 4 h to a total dose of 62 g. The inflammation, pain and swelling of the heel settled and she was able to walk again, initially in a plaster of Paris splint, but later without any support. There was radiological evidence of recalcification (Fig. 5b). Unfortunately, she was found to have hepatic metastases and died about a year later. At autopsy the calcaneum showed a series of ringed bands of residual tumour cells

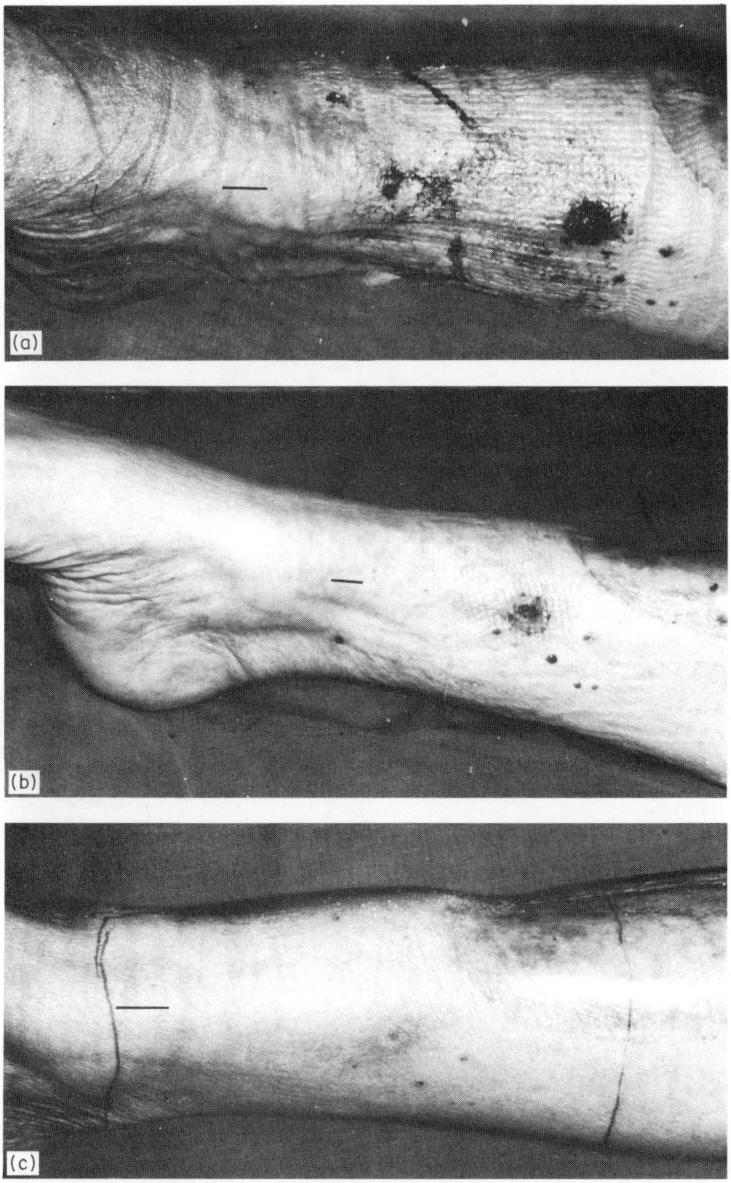

FIG. 4 (a) Melanoma with several satellite lesions on the right leg (case 11) before treatment. The main tumour area was 4.3 cm^2 (scale bar = 2 cm). (b) Appearance of the lesions after intra-arterial infusion with 4-OHA. (Scale bar = 2 cm). (c) Appearance of the right leg 72 d after cessation of treatment. A scarred area marks the site of the main tumour. The satellite lesions also exhibit a cicatrising regression. (Scale bar = 2 cm).

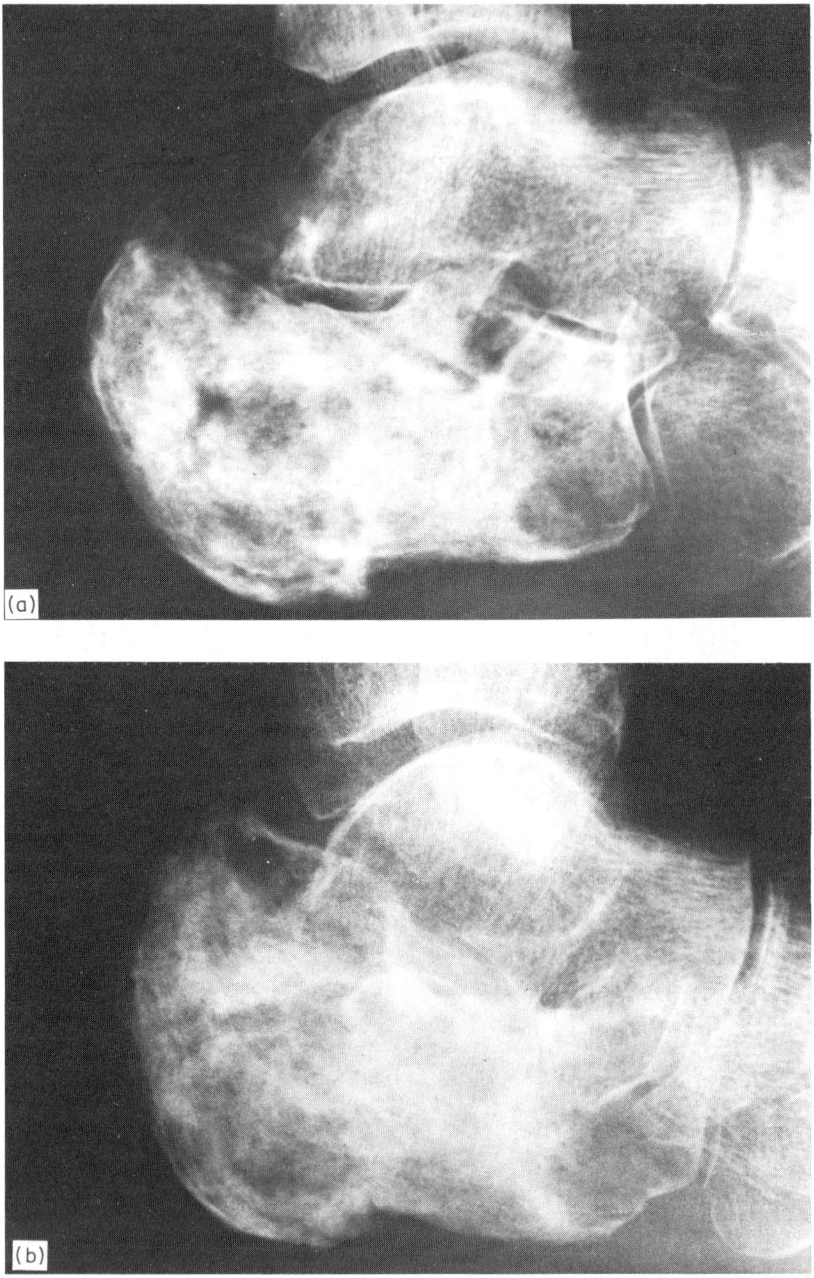

FIG. 5 (a) Radiograph showing calcaneal metastases before treatment (case 9). (b) Radiological evidence of recalcification after treatment with 4-OHA by infusion into the femoral artery.

with fibrosed and recalcified central zones consistent with the radiological findings.

DISCUSSION

The results of intra-arterial administration of 4-hydroxyanisole indicate that, by this route, the drug has a localised and therapeutically useful cytotoxic action on melanoma cells. Intravenous administration was without effect, suggesting that the rate of degradation of the agent is rapid. This is in agreement with the work of Frenk and Ott (1971) and Paslin (1973) who observed that subcutaneous or intraperitoneal administration of phenolic depigmenting agents (including 4-OHA) to transplantable-tumour-bearing animals did not arrest the growth of melanomas or extend the life-span of the animals carrying these tumours, whereas injection of 4-OHA into lesions was effective. Reports of the clinical effectiveness of intra-lesional 4-OHA (Webster *et al.*, 1981) is also in agreement with this interpretation. At present little is known about the pathways of degradation of 4-OHA. It is likely that, in common with other phenolic substrates, it is conjugated in the liver and excreted in the urine. The quinone derivatives may also be metabolised in the liver by the microsomal system (Bachur *et al.*, 1978). Certainly the half-life in the blood of 4-OHA in human subjects is very short; estimates of the rate of loss from the circulation have shown that 4-OHA is scarcely detectable in venous blood samples taken directly after intra-arterial injection of 1 g. Future studies may indicate how the circulating levels of hydroxyanisole may be maintained. Initial hopes that 4-OHA would inhibit the growth of disseminated metastases of malignant melanoma have not been realised but it may be possible to use analogues which will extend the biological half-life of the drug and enable the active component to reach distant sites.

The absence of toxic side effects may be, in part, attributed to the rapid elimination of 4-OHA. Methaemoglobinaemia was the only complication resulting from 4-OHA administration. Other potential hazards of treatment are those connected with arterial injections, e.g. thromboembolic phenomena, haematomas, infection and fluid overload, but none of these complications was encountered in our pilot study.

SUMMARY

In vitro studies on the depigmenting agent 4-hydroxyanisole (4-OHA) have shown that this substance has a selective toxic effect on melanocytes. The mechanism is dependent on the formation of a cytotoxic intermediate product of tyrosinase oxidation, probably a semiquinone free radical, and the possibility of using 4-OHA as a therapeutic agent in malignant melanoma was investigated. A preliminary clinical trial, undertaken on selected patients employing intravascular administration of 4-OHA to treat specific lesions indicates that the agent is selectively toxic to melanoma cells when locally administered by intra-arterial infusion.

ACKNOWLEDGEMENTS

This work was supported by the Cancer Research Campaign and the National Foundation for Cancer Research. We are also indebted to the Thomas Rowatt Memorial Fund for financial assistance.

We thank Mr S. Harrison, Mr D. McNeil and Mr R. Sanders for referring patients for treatment.

REFERENCES

Bachur, N.R., Gordon, S.L. and Gee, M.V. (1978). *Cancer Res.* 38, 1745-1750.

Dewey, D.L., Butcher, F.W. and Galpine, A.R. (1977). *J. Pathol.* 122, 117-127.

Frenk, E. and Ott, F. (1971). *J. Invest. Dermatol.* 56, 287-293.

Galpine, A.R. (1980). *Ph.D. Thesis*, University of London.

Hochstein, P. and Cohen, G. (1963). *Ann. N.Y. Acad. Sci.* 100, 876-886.

Morgan, B.D.G., O'Neill, T., Dewey, D.L., Galpine, A.R. and Riley, P.A. (1981). *Clin. Oncol.* (in press).

Paslin, D.A. (1973). *Acta Derm. Venereol.* 53, 119-122.

Raper, H.S. (1928). *Physiol. Rev.* 8, 245-282.

Riley, P.A. (1969a). *J. Pathol.* 97, 193-206.

Riley, P.A. (1969b). *J. Pathol.* 97, 185-191.

Riley, P.A. (1970). *J. Pathol.* 101, 163-169.

Riley, P.A. (1981). *In* "Proc. XI Int. Pigment Cell Conference". University of Tokyo Press (in press).

Webster, T.J.T., Whitehead, R.H. and Hughes, L.E. (1981). *Br. J. Cancer* 43, 729 (Abst.).

DISCUSSION

Swartz: That is very interesting work and very much of interest to ongoing studies in our laboratory. I have a suggestion on the mechanism of action that is a little bit different from what you suggested. What comes to mind (although perhaps with a little more thought will go away as quickly as it came) is that where you see the lack of effect of the drug, it seems to be in the well oxygenated areas. By analogy with the hypoxic sensitisers one might think of a mechanism of action where a toxic intermediate, maybe the semiquinone, is the active agent and, in the presence of oxygen, an electron is transferred from the semiquinone, inactivating it. That of course also would be analogous with the kind of systems which Ron Mason has been talking about.

Riley: Yes, that is a very interesting explanation. Of course, we do need an explanation for why the smaller lesions are unaffected and also why it is that we don't get generalised depigmentation in the areas which we are perfusing.

Adams: In relation to that, hypoxia seems to develop in tumours of small diameter (about 2 mm) although the proportion of hypoxic cells is small. In your talk you mentioned amelanotic cells. If they are present as a sub-population, aren't they more sensitive to other chemotherapies?

Riley: Yes, I think that is a very valid point because it is true that amelanotic cells are more sensitive to other chemotherapeutic agents.

Adams: And they are present aren't they in most melanomas?

Riley: Yes.

Connors: Patrick, intravenous injection doesn't work because it's a pharmacokinetic problem, isn't it?

Riley: Yes, it is - the drug is broken down very quickly, in fact we have tried to estimate the amount of 4OHA which is in the venous blood directly after intra-arterial infusion and it's scarcely detectable by the methods that we are using.

Connors: What you want is a prodrug that slowly releases the active drug.

Riley: Yes - something that would prevent it from being degraded.

We are doing studies at the moment to try to determine what the extra-tumoural routes of degradation are.

Connors: I have just been to a meeting on drug targeting where they had this problem and they get round it very simply by binding the drug to a dextran chain of appropriate molecular weight which is very slowly broken down. This can be done with your drug using one of those OH groups.

Riley: Thank you very much. We'll take that suggestion up.

Lohmann: Can you explain why the transient intermediate P_1 interacts with G_1 cells only?

Riley: The answer is "No", but cells in late G_1 are supposed to be quite sensitive to quinones aren't they? It may be because the quinone interferes with the electron transport processes, but I really do not know the answer.

Lohmann: May I ask another question please? In quite a few hospitals cisplatin is being used in preliminary trials upon melanomas. Do you have any experience with that compound and if so, how do the results compare with the ones you have reported here?

Riley: I have no experience of the use of cisplatin in the treatment of melanoma.

Connors: Cisplatin has been claimed to be effective in combination in melanoma but I do not know of any large clinical trial. May I just ask, in G_1 is there more tyrosinase than there is in S or in G_2?

Riley: I suppose it is likely to be more active in G_1, and it may be that melanoma cells would be more sensitive in G_1, but in our toxicity testing system we were using non-melanogenic cells. We were actually doing the incubation beforehand and then adding what we thought was the product, so I suppose that to explain the G_1 sensitivity to P_1 what we should be looking for is some kind of receptor for quinones. We are fairly confident that P_1 is a *p*-quinone of some kind, so presumably we would be looking for some process sensitive to quinones that would render the cells intoxicated.

Lohmann: If the concentration of tyrosinase has not been changed in the cases that you have observed, does this mean the occurrence of a so-called facilitated interaction between the substrate and the enzyme? Or does the reaction depend upon the concentration of the enzyme?

Riley: We have been measuring tyrosinase activities in biopsy material but unfortunately not in those which have been treated with 4OHA so I cannot properly answer you, but I would hope that if we can change the protocol so that we can use 4OHA perfusion in relation to some other procedure in cases where we are not so restricted, then it would obviously be very interesting to see what the correlation is between tyrosinase activity and 4OHA efficacy.

Willson: In your Table at the beginning you showed a number of compounds that produced depigmentation. A number of these were metal chelating agents and tyrosinase is a copper dependent enzyme. Is there any possibility that the radicals produced under these conditions complex with copper and inactivate the enzyme in this way?

Riley: I am sure that that is quite likely to happen. My feeling is though that from the point of view of cytotoxicity, inactivating the enzyme would be of relatively little importance. What we are observing is some effect that is more general than simply inactivating the enzyme. This is true both for tyrosine analogues and the cisteamine compounds. These agents produce specific melanocyte toxicity (Riley, 1981). The 8-hydroxy quinoline effect is a little bit more difficult to interpret because melanocytes are still present in the tissue after treatment with it (Searle and Riley, 1979).

Willson: The number of patients in your study is very small. What is the incidence of spontaneous remissions with this kind of tumour?

Riley: One of the reasons why we cannot draw any broad conclusions from this work is because it is known that malignant melanoma is a "funny" tumour and sometimes you do get spontaneous remissions. Against this of course is the fact that our intravenously treated patients did not respond and I think the time scale is also against this simply being spontaneous remission.

Willson: A small number of patients actually favours you in this respect. The chances that the remission you observe are not connected with the treatment will be small.

Swartz: Where these "funny" things seem to happen with melanomas, they appear to be related to an immune response. The sort of pattern that you are getting, for example the response not occurring in the small, actively perfused samples, is against this being an immune response and it is probably a chemical response.

Riley: Yes, thank you. Of course, it is possible that we could get a subsequent immune response as a result of the toxic effect on the cells, releasing some internal antigen or something of that sort.

Lohmann: Is copper involved in the overall reaction mechanism despite the fact that it doesn't show up in either the absorption or the EPR spectrum of tyrosinase?

Riley: I don't know that what I'm going to say is very illuminating but H.S. Mason's laboratory has shown that there is some form of copper-related radical produced during the catalysis, so I think it is clear that copper is involved in some form of catalytic radical formation.

Slater: Would you like to comment on the report in "Nature" last year (Bram *et al.*, 1980) about ascorbate and copper in relation to melanoma?

Riley: Well, I am told that although the mechanism reported for it is very plausible (Bram *et al.*, 1980) it is probably not significant in biological terms since the ascorbyl radical is stable. Ascorbate addition to primary cultures of melanocytes failed to show any cytotoxic effect, in fact if anything, it slightly protects against damage by other agents (Riley *et al.*, 1975).

Dianzani: My first question concerns your hypothesis that hydroxy anisole promotes lipid peroxidation. Have you any experimental evidence about this? Have you measured lipid peroxidation before and after hydroxy anisole?

Riley: Yes. I looked at this some years ago with Barbara Sawyer and Michael Wolff. What we were looking for was malonaldehyde production in an *in vitro* system, using mushroom tyrosinase to ensure that we got production of our intermediates, and we showed a very, very slight increase in malonaldehyde production under these conditions (Riley *et al.*, 1975), but I must admit I was not very confident that this could account for the toxic effect which we had observed on the cells. Perhaps, however, malonaldehyde production is not the best marker of lipid peroxidation initiated by a semiquinone.

Dianzani: My second question refers to the experiment which showed that the big tumours were influenced more than the little ones. I saw in your slides that the centre parts were more affected than the peripheral areas. Can this be explained on the basis of a difference in nutritional state of the large and small tumours? It is possible that central cells are not fed as well as those cells located at the periphery.

Riley: Yes, I think this is relevant to the point that Professor Adams was making that the degree of oxygenation may be a significant factor.

Adams: It seems such a good system experimentally. There are, however, a lot of better experimental tumours available. There are human tumours that can be grown as xenografts. Some of the old murine tumours are highly immunogenic, and the use of human tumours in immune-suppressed mice seems to me to be a very good idea.

Riley: We would be very interested to try that.

Adams: Well there are a number at the Royal Marsden which are at your service.

Magee: There is a chemically induced melanoma in the hamster (Shubik *et al.*, 1956) which might be useful if you are interested in a primary tumour.

Riley: Thank you, we would be interested in other animal models; the Harding-Passey tumour has its limitations. There is also some similar work on the B-16 melanoma and there are very great difficulties of interpretation with these particularly as in many B-16s there is hardly any measurable tyrosinase activity.

Adams: It is also antigenic as well.

Mason: How did you decide which chemical to use in the clinical trials? I am just curious as to how you go about making that decision from your original list.

Riley: Well, by the time we came to put anything into clinical trial 4OHA was the only one I knew enough about. I think by that time the decision had been made to use tyrosine analogues since they were relatively non-toxic.

REFERENCES to Discussion

Bram, S., Froussard, P., Guichard, M., Jasmin, C., Augery, Y., Suiossir-Barre, F. and Wray, W. (1980). *Nature (London)* 284, 629-631.

Riley, P.A. (1981). Proc. XI Int. Pigment Cell Conf., pp.439-445, University of Tokyo Press.

Riley, P.A., Sawyer, B. and Wolff, M.A. (1975). *J. Invest. Dermatol.* 64, 86-89.

Searle, C.E. and Riley, P.A. (1979). *In* "Hair and Hair Diseases" (Ed. C.A. Oxfanos), pp.911-929, Fischer, Stuttgart.

Shubik, P., Della Porta, G., Rappaport, H. and Spencer, K. (1956). *Cancer Res.* 16, 1031-1032.

INDEX